Bil

# VAGINAL SURGERY

## THIRD EDITION

**ILLUSTRATED BY**

**Allison Boisselle**
Illustrator
Department of Obstetrics and Gynecology
Brown University Program in Medicine
Providence, Rhode Island

**Melford D. Diedrick**
Former Director of Medical Illustration
School of Health Sciences
State University of New York at Buffalo
Buffalo, New York

# VAGINAL SURGERY

## THIRD EDITION

## David H. Nichols, M.D.

Fellow, American College of Obstetricians and Gynecologists; Fellow, American College of
  Surgeons; Fellow, International College of Surgeons
Professor and Chairman, Department of Obstetrics and Gynecology, Division of Biology and
  Medicine, Brown University, Providence, Rhode Island
Lecturer, Obstetrics and Gynecology, Tufts University School of Medicine, Boston
Obstetrician and Gynecologist-in-Chief, Women & Infants Hospital of Rhode Island
Surgeon-in-Chief, Department of Gynecology and Obstetrics, Rhode Island Hospital,
  Providence, Rhode Island

## Clyde L. Randall, M.D.

Fellow, American College of Obstetricians and Gynecologists; Fellow, American College of
  Surgeons; Fellow, Royal College of Obstetricians and Gynecologists; Fellow, American
  Gynecological and Obstetrical Society
Emeritus Professor, Gynecology and Obstetrics, State University of New York at Buffalo
Former Chief, Gynecology and Obstetrics, SUNY Affiliated Hospitals, Buffalo, New York
Johns Hopkins Program of International Education, Gynecology and Obstetrics, 1975-1980

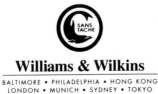

**Williams & Wilkins**

BALTIMORE • PHILADELPHIA • HONG KONG
LONDON • MUNICH • SYDNEY • TOKYO

A WAVERLY COMPANY

*Editor:* Carol-Lynn Brown
*Associate Editor:* Victoria M. Vaughn
*Copy Editors:* Susan Vaupel and Shelley Potler
*Design:* Saturn Graphics
*Illustration Planning:* Wayne Hubbel
*Production:* Raymond E. Reter

Copyright © 1989
Williams & Wilkins
428 East Preston Street
Baltimore, Maryland 21202, USA

Accurate indications, adverse reactions, and dosage schedules for drugs are provided in this book, but it is possible that they may change. The reader is urged to review the package information data of the manufacturers of the medications mentioned.

*Printed in the United States of America*

First Edition 1976
Second Edition 1983

**Library of Congress Cataloging-in-Publication Data**

Nichols, David H., 1925-
  Vaginal surgery.

  Includes bibliographical references and index.
  1. Vagina--Surgery.  I. Randall, Clyde L.  II. Title.
[DNLM: 1. Vagina--surgery. WP 250 N617v]
RG104.N52 1989   618.1'5059   88-27977
ISBN 0-683-06494-0

94

12 13 14 15

To Lorraine and Vernie
who have been with us all the way.

"And this is the reason why the cure of many diseases
is unknown to the physicians of Hellas,
because they are ignorant of the whole,
which ought to be studied also;
for the part can never be well
unless the whole is well."

SOCRATES IN THE CHARMIDES OF PLATO
*Translated by B. Jowett, vol. i, p. 11.*
From Kelly HA: *Operative Gynecology.*
New York, D. Appleton & Co, 1898

# Preface to the Third Edition

This is a book for the gynecologic surgeon, cognizant of an increasingly large number of women, many of them older, to whom restoration of quality of life has become more important than ever. At the same time, health care is becoming more expensive. In order to be affordable, when surgery is to be performed, it must be done correctly the first time.

Doing this safely requires appropriate surgical judgment, effective preoperative preparation and risk evaluation, and practiced precision in surgical technique. Good surgical judgment implies the ability to detect the important elements of a clinical situation, rank them in order of importance, and to develop an appropriate and cost-effective solution that will be correct the majority of the time.

Transvaginal surgery embraces, in general, less operating time, less depth of anesthesia, and reduced risk of pulmonary or gastrointestinal complication than does the abdominal counterpart. Although it does not necessarily prolong life, properly done it enhances the quality of life immeasurably.

Development and rediscovery of gynecologic surgical techniques that are responsive to newly recognized needs are clear evidence of surgical evolution. This new edition is written for those surgeons who want to develop or improve these skills in their own practices.

We have drawn extensively from the experiences and data of Henry and Swash's *Colpoproctology and the Pelvic Floor,* which has opened a new dimension in research-documented progress in reconstructive pelvic surgery. The operative experiences and recommendations detailed in the recent second English edition of Käser, Iklé, and Hirsch's *Atlas of Gynecological Surgery,* and a rereading of Halban's *Gynäkologische Operationslehre,* Mattingly and Thompson's sixth edition of *TeLinde's Operative Gynecology,* Howkins and Stallworthy's *Bonney's Gynaecological Surgery,* Peham and Amreich's *Operative Gynecology,* McCall and Bolton's translation of Martius' *Gynecological Operations,* Malpas' *Genital Prolapse and Allied Conditions,* and Krige's *Vaginal Hysterectomy and Genital Prolapse Repair* to name but a few, have been of great help. Hadra's *Lesions of the Vagina and Pelvic Floor* as well as Paramore's *The Statics of the Female Pelvic Viscera* and Werner and Sederl's *Abdominal Operations by the Vaginal Route* constantly serve as sources of surgical inspiration.

Particular gratitude is expressed to our publisher, Williams & Wilkins, and to our editors, Carol-Lynn Brown, Laurel Craven, and Vicky Vaughn for their patience and help, and to our secretaries, Donna Coppola, Susan Lowe, and Kathy Hawes for their typing skills and infinite understanding.

David H. Nichols, M.D.
Clyde L. Randall, M.D.

# Preface to the First Edition

For untold generations women have known that vaginal relaxation may develop soon or perhaps years after childbearing. An initial sense of relaxation was known to precede a more noticeable and uncomfortable degree of prolapse. Discomforts and dysfunctions of varying degree became annoying and at times distressing, for some to a point of virtually disabling women already overburdened with the work and responsibilities of a household and family.

Without reparative vaginal surgery, the problems of those women who develop genital prolapse would have remained unchanged to this day. In many communities skillful management of vaginal delivery now usually includes prompt and adequate repair of vaginal floor and perineal damage. Although such care will minimize later need for a posterior colporrhaphy and perineorrhaphy, the most skilled management of labor and delivery is not as likely to avoid the damage which predisposes the parous woman to the later development of a cystocele, or a degree of prolapse that eventually indicates repair.

Now that the risks of elective vaginal surgery should be minimal, physicians should be mindful of the possibility that women are often annoyed or distressed by a degree of prolapse that can almost always be corrected by restorative surgery. In fact, the recognition and evaluation of indications and the performance of remedial surgery for the problems associated with genital prolapse have become a primary responsibility and major activity of the gynecologic surgeon.

We believe that successful reconstruction and relief of the discomforts of genital prolapse depend upon an accurate knowledge of the probable etiologic factors plus an appreciation of the specific principles involved in an effective repair. Success is not assured by rote repetition of a gynecologist's routine method of repair, even when the technical steps as described might be expected to result in a satisfactory repair. It is our conviction that optimal results can be assured only when the procedure selected and the technique employed is tailored to the problem recognized and the tissues available for accomplishment of the repair.

Somewhat difficult to learn, and equally difficult to teach, much of vaginal surgery seems to have been rediscovered from generation to generation. A heritage all too readily lost, the techniques of vaginal surgery must be sought for, recorded carefully, and practiced, if competence and skills are to be maintained.

Each bibliographic footnote consulted will provide valued references and is likely to enable the interested reader to develop new and improved techniques.

Simply making the vagina smaller is neither the goal, nor the purpose of vaginal reconstructive surgery. While the goal is actually a restoration to the normal of symptomatic alterations in anatomy to an anatomically correct and asymptomatic status, this implies, of course, not only restoration of anatomic relationships but also the important physiologic restoration with which the former is indelibly entwined.

This concept is not difficult to accept, but there may be differences of opinion when one seeks to establish an understanding of what the normal really is, and thus to express the definitive goals of vaginal reconstructive surgery. It was to this broad point that the concept for this book developed. The anatomic relationships, particularly of the supporting tissues of the woman's reproductive organs, so carefully detailed and examined in the anatomic texts, seem to describe an entirely different set of interorgan relationships than we have observed in the living body, and the significance of these differences will be discussed in detail in the chapters which follow.

Our investigations into the clinical significance of pelvic anatomy have disclosed some unexpected and meaningful differences in tissue interrelationships which seem responsible for the support and function of the pelvic organs in the living, as compared to the relationships previously assumed as a result of observations noted by others in the embalmed cadaver. The differences observed might well be likened to a comparison of grapes and raisins. The objectives of surgical reconstruction obviously must be designed to restore the characteristics of the living, and should, therefore, not be based upon the somewhat bizarre, somewhat unnatural and certainly nonfunctioning relationships that are apparent in the nonliving cadaver.

We believe the development of operations utilizing concepts based upon cadaver studies have led to unphysiologic and unnatural objectives of reconstruction. The modifications and new techniques suggested are attempts to emphasize physiologic reconstructions and restore the more usual and normal relationships which are characteristic of functioning gynecologic anatomy. Conclusions based upon studies of fresh gross anatomy have encouraged the evolution of certain of the technical details and the surgical procedures which we believe likely to aid in the realization of improved results. At least in our hands their use has resulted in patients realizing greater degrees of comfort than had previously been achieved by the employment of some of the older but still commonly used techniques.

There seems need to repeatedly emphasize that a protruding uterus is the result of genital prolapse and not the primary cause of the symptomatology. For this reason hysterectomy, although usually a desirable part of the surgery employed to assure a satisfactory reconstruction, is not the essential feature and does not of itself assure the success of the repair or relieve the patient of the discomforts of a prolapse. On the other hand the currently widespread use of postmenopausal estrogen replacement therapy seems certain to account for an increasing incidence of iatrogenic endometrial hyperplasia and postmenopausal dysfunctional uterine bleeding. This probability alone, we believe, provides a reasonably valid indication for coincident hysterectomy, whenever repair is indicated; and hysterectomy can be accomplished with little increased risk to the patient.

In the presentation of this material, our primary objective is to encourage others to carry on similar studies and thus help to preserve and improve a heritage of surgery for the satisfactions of succeeding generations of surgeons and their patients. We acknowledge with sincere gratitude our dependence upon the works of many others. We have drawn heavily upon such classic texts and monographs as Paramore's "The Statics of the Female Pelvic Viscera," von Peham and Amreich's "Operative Gynecology," Kennedy and Campbell's "Vaginal Hysterectomy," Malpas' "Genital Prolapse and Allied Conditions," Martius' "Gynecological Operations," Gray's "Vaginal Hysterectomy," Bandler's "Vaginal Celiotomy," Smout, Jacoby, and Lillie's "Gynecological and Obstetrical Anatomy, Descriptive and Applied," Burch and Lavely's "Hysterectomy," and Krige's "Vaginal Hysterectomy and Genital Prolapse Repair." In our own studies the influence of many teachers will be recognizable though their basic contributions to our own concepts are not being individually recognized. Gratitude is also expressed to the editors and publishers of the journals, "Obstetrics and Gynecology," "The Amercian Journal of Obstetrics and Gynecology," "The Anatomical Record," "Postgraduate Medicine," and "Archiv für Gynaekologie" for permission to reprint portions of our studies which have appeared originally on their pages.

D.H.N.
C.L.R.
*1976*

# Contents

# CHAPTER 1

# Pelvic Anatomy of the Living

## GENERAL CONCEPTS

Vaginal surgery offers logical and effective methods for the restoration of distorted attachments and pathologic concentrations of pelvic connective tissues. Confusion and disagreements often arise, however, because concepts and definitions vary as to precisely what constitutes the normal state.

Effective vaginal surgery requires precise knowledge of the anatomy involved, an appreciation of the extent of individual variation, and an understanding of the effects of such physiologic processes as pregnancy, labor, delivery, menopause, and aging upon the tissues that are to be subjected to restorative surgery. Since the practitioner's knowledge of pelvic anatomy and his concept of normal anatomic relationships were first learned by study of the anatomy of the cadaver, many surgical reconstructions have been planned with the objective of recreating the anatomic relationships observed in the cadaver. Since these relationships are quite different from those of the living, many of the physiologic and symptomatic failures of gynecologic reconstructive surgery have been due to the intentional but erroneous development of cadaver-like relationships with unsatisfactory results that are both predictable and unfortunate.

Since the earliest days of medicine, dissections have been performed on, texts have been written about, and anatomy has been studied from elderly, often debilitated, and malnourished female cadavers. The anatomic interrelationships in such bodies are quite different from those found in the healthy, living, well-nourished, younger female. Furthermore, the standard anatomy textbook gives extensive description of only a small number of dissections and bases broad generalizations on this small number. There is no recognition of the large amount of variation that occurs quite normally and frequently between individuals and at different times of life.

The anatomic relationships of tissues and organs of an anesthetized patient are not quite the same as those of the patient who is wide awake; this is because of muscle paralysis from anesthesia, resting or baseline underdistention of the various organs, and the change in statics due to position. The horizontal position of the nonmoving surgical patient provides statics quite different from those of the vertical and active patient, whose pelvic organs are in varying stages of function and distention.

We shall, therefore, pursue in some detail the re-examination and redefinition of normal anatomy of the living. Moreover, every description of the procedures that follow will be similarly based on anatomic relationships observed in the living.

Vaginal reconstructive surgery is concerned with the return of abnormal organ relationships to a usual or normal state. There is no one site or degree of damage that must be repaired or restored; there are many, and they occur in

1

various combinations at various times of life, from different etiologic factors, in varying degrees, and with varying degrees of symptomatology and disability.

For years there has been heated discussion as to whether the more important factor concerned with vaginal position within the pelvis is that of suspension from above (cardinal ligament complex), a view championed by Fothergill (17), or of support from below (levator ani-pelvic diaphragm), as emphasized by Paramore (41) and Halban and Tandler (22). Mengert's (33) classic contribution in this area was to report an experiment whereby a tenaculum was applied to the cadaver cervix, a cord was attached to the tenaculum and run through a fixed pulley, and a 1-kg. weight was attached to the opposite end of the cord. One by one, starting at the top of the fundus, the lateral supports of the uterus and vagina were cut until prolapse of the uterus and vagina finally developed. It was only when the paravaginal tissues had been cut that prolapse occurred. "Marked descent of the uterus amounting to actual prolapse never occurred so long as any part of the upper two-thirds of the parametrial tissues were intact." This experiment convicingly emphasized the importance of the suspensory apparatus.

Bonney (3) strongly defended the position that both points of view were correct, i.e., the vagina is suspended from above and supported from below, and one or both systems could be damaged, causing genital prolapse of a type which reflected the site or sites of primary damage. It is important for the gynecologic surgeon to recognize the primary site of damage so that appropriate steps can be taken in surgical reconstruction to minimize the chance of postoperative recurrence of the genital prolapse. Damage to the suspensory system can give rise to eversion of the upper vagina, often with elongation of the cervix and cul-de-sac hernia; damage to the lower supporting system is more likely to be associated with eversion of the lower vagina, including cystocele and rectocele.

Anatomy texts have described vaginal position in terms of the relationships evident in the cadaver (15, 20, 61) and usually refer to the vagina as an almost straight and hollow tube extending posterosuperiorly toward the sacral promontory (Fig. 1.1). This concept developed because this relationship is usually demonstrable on sagittal sectioning of the cadaver (Fig. 1.2). When such a concept becomes the objective of reconstructive surgery for the relief of genital prolapse, however, the result may be an unusual deviation of the vagina. In some instances, the vaginal vault has been sewn to the sacral promontory or even to the anterior abdominal wall, the latter causing the vaginal axis to ascend in an almost vertical or anterior direction (16, 40).

Studies of usual depth and axis of the nulliparous vagina in the living (Figs. 1.3 and 1.4) provide impressively different information (9, 18, 36, 51, 52), especially when considering the unanesthetized patient.

The organs of the female pelvis are readily distensible within certain maximal limits. Bladder, vagina, or rectum distend quite independently in the course of their normal functions. Each is able rather quickly to resume its usual or resting shape, dimension, and relationship after such individual and functional distention has been relieved. Functioning in concert, they reinforce one another; the histologic components which permit such a range of activity include combinations of varying amounts of smooth muscle, striated muscle, elastic tissue and collagen.

### Smooth Muscle Fibers

Smooth muscle fibers are in a constant state of activity, helping to maintain tone, but permitting cellular elongation whenever necessary with no significant increase in tone. Smooth muscle cells will lengthen readily until a limit of

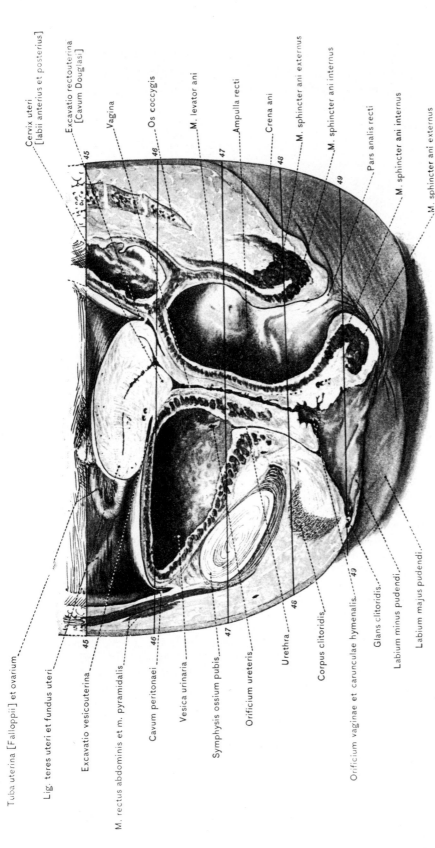

Tuba uterina [Falloppii] et ovarium

Lig. teres uteri et fundus uteri

Cervix uteri
[labii anterius et posterius]

Excavatio rectouterina
[Cavum Douglasi]

Excavatio vesicouterina

Vagina

Os coccygis

M. rectus abdominis et m. pyramidalis

M. levator ani

Cavum peritonaei

Ampulla recti

Vesica urinaria

Crena ani

Symphysis ossium pubis

M. sphincter ani externus

Orificium ureteris

M. sphincter ani internus

Urethra

Pars analis recti

Corpus clitoridis

M. sphincter ani internus

Orificium vaginae et carunculae hymenalis

M. sphincter ani externus

Glans clitoridis

Labium minus pudendi

Labium majus pudendi

**Figure 1.1.** Drawing of a sagittal section through the embalmed cadaver shows the axis of the vagina to be in an almost vertical position. It is displaced anteriorly by the dilated rectum, a relationship often found in the living. (From Carter et al: *Cross-Sectional Anatomy: Computed Tomography and Ultrasound Correlation.* New York, Appleton-Century-Crofts, 1977.)

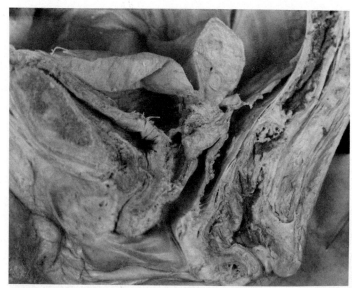

**Figure 1.2.** Photograph of a sagittal section of cadaver pelvis and almost vertical vaginal axis is shown, maintained by postmortem changes and chemical tissue fixation. (From Nichols DH, Milley PS, Randall CL: Significance of restoration of normal vaginal depth and axis. *Obstet Gynecol* 36:251–256, 1970.)

elasticity is reached. Once this elastic limit is attained, the cells will behave like an inactive fascial tissue. The response to mechanical or chemical stimuli is mediated involuntarily through the autonomic nervous system and spinal reflex arcs. Although smooth muscle will maintain tone, it is of limited value for support because cellular length will increase with increased stress up to a point of maximum distention. The syncytium of smooth muscle also evidences rhythmic contractions. The number of smooth muscle cells present within given tissues appears likely to be constant throughout the mature lifetime of the individual and does not significantly decline with age.

*Clinical Applications.* Review of the literature describing reconstructive surgery for the repair of genital prolapse suggests that smooth muscle bands within the subperitoneal tissues have been consciously, although perhaps not deliberately, utilized in the most successful repair operations. That these tissues are mainly composed of smooth muscle was suggested by Fothergill (17) in 1907, who first suggested operating within the avascular lines of cleavage between the vagina and bladder, followed by fascial overlapping of the vesicovaginal and rectovaginal septa. An amputation of the usually elongated cervix in the repair of prolapse was later added. Apparently under the impression that he was working with layers of fascia, Fothergill was, in fact, overlapping layers that were predominantly smooth muscle fibers. He was effectively shortening and reinforcing musculofibrous groups capable of considerable support. We must now realize that the essential accomplishment in a successful repair operation is the restoration of the normal functioning and supportive abilities of the smooth muscle content of this "fascial layer" and is not the result of a duplication and strengthening of a nonelastic connective tissue.

### Striated Muscle

Striated muscle also responds rapidly to stress and maintains tone and equilibrium. Striated muscle lacks inherent rhythmic contractions. The cells

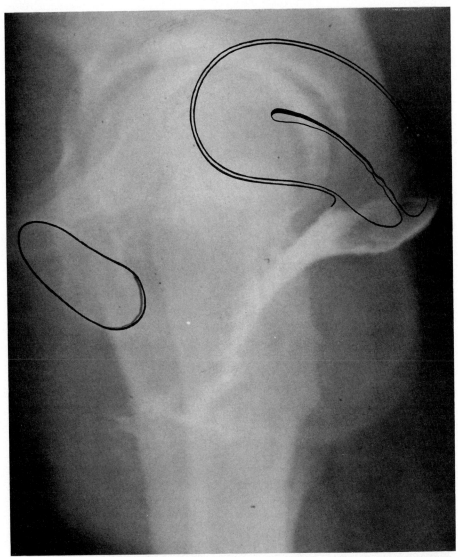

**Figure 1.3.** A normal vaginal depth and axis is shown. Colpogram of a healthy 25-year-old nulligravida standing at rest. The vaginal walls have been painted with barium paste. The perineal curve of the lower vagina is shown along with the more horizontal axis of the upper vagina. The position of the symphysis is outlined to the left, and the position of the uterus outlined to the right. St. Francis Hospital, X-ray 69-3159, courtesty of Dr. Paul J. deMarsovsky, Radiologist. (From Nichols DH, Milley PS, Randall CL: Significance of restoration of normal vaginal depth and axis. *Obstet Gynecol* 36:251–256, 1970. Reproduced with permission of the The American College of Obstetricians and Gynecologists.)

tend to maintain a constant length by contracting in response to strain. This favors maintenance of equilibrium as well as tone of supporting tissue. Smooth muscle helps to maintain tone but, since it more readily permits elongation, does not effectively tend to restore or maintain equilibrium. Striated and smooth muscle have complementary activities that permit and contribute to functional changes within the limitations of the pelvic supporting tissues.

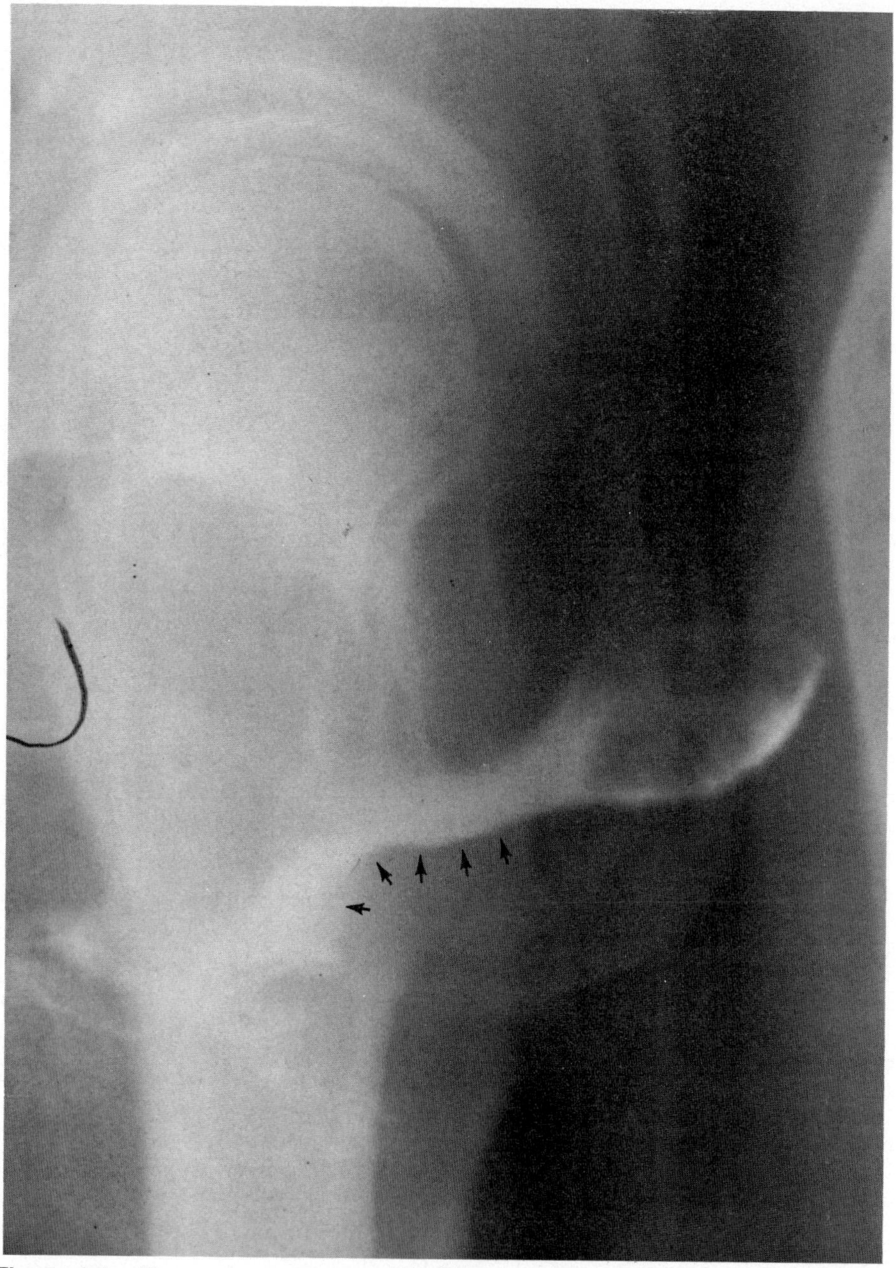

**Figure 1.4.** The same patient is straining, as by a Valsalva maneuver, which accentuates the horizontal axis of the upper vagina. The effect of the anterior margin of an intact levator plate is shown by the arrows. (St. Francis Hospital, X-ray 69-3159, courtesy of Dr. Paul J. deMarovsky, Radiologist; from Nichols DH, Milley PS, Randall CL: Significance of restoration of normal vaginal depth and axis. *Obstet Gynecol* 36:251–256, 1970. Reproduced with permission of the American College of Obstetricians and Gynecologists.)

### Elastic Tissue Fibers

Elastic tissue is made up of fibers constructed in irregular networks that are especially well-developed in tissues usually subject to stress. These fibers respond to stress with stretching, but they resist such stretching by a natural tendency to return to their original state, much in the same manner of a rubber band. The quantity of elastic tissue decreases with age, but the extent to which this is hormone-related and reversible is not known. The histogenesis of these fibers is unknown, although they are apparently produced by fibroblastic cells or histocytes. They do not seem to have an innervation, and the decrease in their number with aging probably partially accounts for the differences in composition and recurrence rate of cystoceles and other manifestations of genital prolapse in women long past menopause in contrast to those still in the reproductive years.

Collagen fibers are also arranged in an interlacing meshwork; but, unlike elastic tissue fibers, they do not stretch. With age they swell, fuse, and become hyalinized. Because they are flexible, they permit movement without stretching, much like a piece of string or rope.

Bone and cartilage are inflexible, firm and strong, and resist sudden strain and stress but respond to prolonged stress and strain by gradual changes in architecture. This response appears to be both age- and hormone-related.

## ANATOMY

### Relationships of Ureter to Vaginal Hysterectomy Ligatures

Hofmeister and Wolfgram (25) studied the reasons why the ureter is less often injured during vaginal procedures than during abdominal procedures even though it is more difficult to palpate or see. They performed vaginal hysterectomy in an x-ray department with multiple consecutive x-ray visualizations, radiopaque ureteral catheters, and wire sutures on the uterine pedicles.

It was possible to demonstrate that anterior retraction through the anterior peritoneal opening lifted the ureter as much as an additional 1 cm. away from the zone of danger.

The distance demonstrated during the vaginal hysterectomy procedures varied from over 2.1 cm. at the level of the parametrial areas during the hysterectomy to 1 cm. when the tube and ovary were removed by clamping the infundibulopelvic ligament. During the repair of the bladder, the needle was measured as 0.9 cm. distant from the ureter (25).

These studies suggest that the traction applied to the cervix during vaginal hysterectomy in combination with adequate retraction involving the anterior vesicouterine peritoneal fold provides protection against ureteral trauma not equaled during abdominal hysterectomy. They further demonstrated in these studies that the closest distances between the operator's clamps and the ureter were at the level of the infundibulopelvic ligament during salpingo-oophorectomy and during subsequent cystocele repair when the operator's needle was 0.9 cm. distant from the ureter.

### Anatomic Systems Responsible for Pelvic Support

It is evident that there are at least six different anatomic systems responsible for varying degrees of support of the birth canal. These can be injured or damaged separately or in various combinations, but they must be individually recognized and identified if restorative surgery is to achieve its stated goal. The following significant anatomic support systems are evident and will be considered separately in greater detail: (a) the bony pelvis, to which the pelvic soft tissues ultimately attach; (*b*) the subperitoneal connective tissue retinaculum and the broad ligaments, including the smooth muscle components and round ligaments; (*c*) the cardinal and uterosacral ligament complex; (*d*) the urogenital diaphragm, including the pubourethral ligaments; (*e*) the pelvic diaphragm, and particularly the pubococcygeus component and the levator plate; (*f*) the perineum, including the perineal body.

Although each of the above is a separate anatomic unit, they are often interrelated, and additional components may exert synergistic, supportive, or even sphincter-like action, e.g., the intact bulbocavernosi contracting in concert with the pubococcygei exert an almost sphincter-like effect on the vaginal outlet (Fig. 1.5). It is uncommon for any of these anatomic units to be individually defective, other than by congenital anomaly. With this exception, damage to these individual units may be either primary or secondary, generally in combination. Successful reconstructive surgery depends upon recognizing the combination of different types of damage. Equally important is the

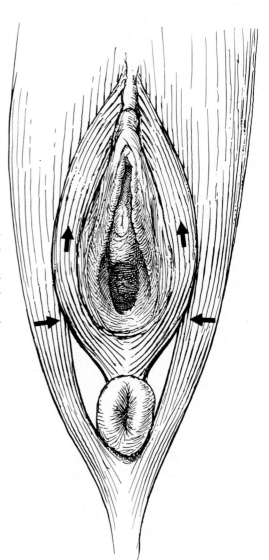

**Figure 1.5.** Contraction of the levatores ani exerts some side-to-side compression of the lower vagina. This may reinforce voluntary contraction of the intact bulbocavernosi at a somewhat lower level, steadying the perineum and constituting a sphincter-like effect.

recognition of active etiologic agents to which corrective attention can be drawn.

## Bony Pelvis

The bones of the pelvis are the ultimate fixed attachment of the pelvic soft tissues, and can be defective and, thus, deficient in support as a result of either congenital anomaly (e.g., exstrophy of bladder) or trauma (fracture, avulsion, or surgery). Significant deficiency should be taken into consideration when a plan of repair is being formulated.

## Broad Ligaments

The broad ligaments provide routes for entrance and egress of blood vessels and lymphatics supplying the organs they sheathe. They supply the genital system except when they are pathologically strengthened, for example, when severe fibrosis and scarring develop as a result of endometriosis, previous infection, cancer, previous surgery, or radiation therapy.

Severe fibrosis may prevent the descent of the uterus. Prolapse of the lower birth canal and cervix may then develop, often with pronounced and sometimes with extreme elongation of the cervix. Some relative independence of these various levels of support may explain, in the reverse situation, why independent surgical supension or fixation of the uterus may not arrest the development and progression of cystocele, rectocele, and descent of the cervix. The round ligaments provide only accessory support to maintain anteversion of the uterus, permitting the stability of a uterine axis under normal circumstances with a narrow angle relative to the upper vagina.

## Cardinal and Uterosacral Ligament Complex

These ligaments include a fine meshwork of muscle fibers and are part of the suspensory apparatus that serves to hold the cervix and upper vagina over the levator plate.

The blood vessels and lymphatics from the hypogastric plexus enter and leave the uterus and vagina along their lateral margins, as the vessels connect with their origin from the main internal iliac (hypogastric) vessels. These vessels are surrounded by strong perivascular fibroareolar sheaths closely attached to their adventitia. The histology of these so-called ligaments has been studied by many observers, perhaps most accurately by Range and Woodburne (47). They found that these ligaments consist principally of blood vessels (largely veins), nerves, lymphatic channels, and areolar connective tissue; the connective tissue is more dense lateral to the cervix and vagina. Collagen bundles parallel the veins, and the connective tissue contains many smooth muscle fibers associated with the adventitia of the blood vessels. They found that the loosely arranged connective tissue mesh strands become stretched or elongated longitudinally in the direction of a force applied to them. (Fig. 1.6).

Von Peham and Amreich (44), Richter and Frick (53) and Luisi (30) realized that this rich network of blood vessels lateral to each side of the upper vagina and cervix is strengthened by the connective tissue and muscle sheaths surrounding the valveless blood vessels. They named this the horizontal connective tissue ground bundle. At the cervix of an anteverted uterus this lateral paravaginal condensation of tissues makes a rather abrupt turn anteriorly, following, as it turns, the axis of the lateral side of the cervix (Fig. 1.7); thus, the cardinal ligament is in reality the same as the horizontal connective tissue ground bundle and serves to supply and to hold both cervix and upper vagina in place over the levator plate.

Campbell (4) studied the anatomy and histology of the uterosacral ligaments. He found that they were attached to the posterolateral aspect of the cervix at

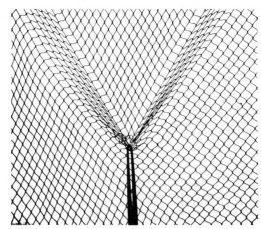

**Figure 1.6.** The effect of traction on the connective tissue fibers of the cardinal and uterosacral ligaments is demonstrated. A forceps has been applied to the center of a piece of plastic net, and traction has been applied, demonstrating the distortion of the pelvic tissues resulting from traction on the cervix. Condensation and obliteration of intra-areolar spaces account for "ligaments" apparent at operation, reinforced by blood vessels, lymphatics, and nerves and their sheaths, both of which enter and exit along the lateral margin of the upper vagina. (From Nichols DH, Milley PS: Clinical anatomy of the vulva, vagina, lower pelvis and perienum. In Sciarra J(ed): *Gynecology and Obstetrics*, 1977, reproduced with permission of Harper & Row.)

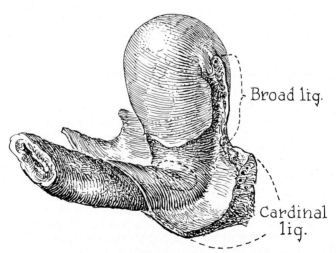

**Figure 1.7.** The cardinal ligament is shown as it attaches to the lateral portions of both cervix and upper third of the vagina. Notice that it follows the angulation of the intersecting axis of these two organs. (From Nichols DH, Milley PS: Clinical anatomy of the vulva, vagina, lower pelvis, and perineum. In Sciarra J(ed): *Gynecology and Obstetrics,* 1977, reproduced with permission of Harper & Row.)

the level of the internal os and to the lateral vaginal fornices. Although nearest the cervix, these ligaments are definite bands of tissue covered by peritoneum; they become thinned out as they course posteriorly, forming the superior boundary of the cul-de-sac of Douglas. The posterior third of each uterosacral ligament is fan-shaped and consists of more delicate strands of tissue that attach to presacral fascia opposite the lower portion of the sacroiliac articulation. There is much individual variation in the thickness and strength of these ligaments, and they do increase in prominence when tension or traction is applied to them. Histologically, the anterior or cervical third of these ligaments contains, in order of prominence: smooth muscle, fibroelastic connective tissue, blood vessels, sympathetic and parasympathetic nerves, and lymphatics. The intermediate third is made up of a connective tissue network with prominent sympathetic nerve ganglia and a few scattered strands of smooth muscle and some lymphatics. The posterior or sacral third is composed almost entirely of loose strands of connective tissue with a few blood vessels, nerves, and lymphatics. For these histologic reasons, it seems unlikely that under physiologic conditions the ligaments that primarily convey the pelvic parasympathetic nerve fibers from the sacral plexis to the lateral aspects of the uterus have any significant supportive function. They may assist in maintaining the position of the uterus and upper vagina over the levator plate. As a general principle, nerves in the body are usually arranged in positions protecting them from trauma, so it is unlikely that the primary purpose of these ligaments is to provide for the suspension of the uterus. The connective tissue elements of these ligaments are to a large measure enmeshed with those of the lower portion of the cardinal or transverse cervical ligaments and are, from a practical point of view, not only inseparable but constitute a surgically useful complex. The proliferation of connective tissue in this complex observed during surgery in patients with genital prolapse is probably a secondary pathologic hypertrophy. This hypertrophy is most likely a secondary line of defense in the body's attempt to compensate for the loss of homeostasis caused by increased intraperitoneal pressure or as a result of deficient support from a weakened levator plate.

### Urogenital Diaphragm and the Pubourethral Ligaments

Milley and Nichols (35) studied the connective tissue supports of the urethra and confirmed the observations of Zacharin (64), that the urethra is suspended from the pubic bone (Figs. 1.8 and 19) for most of its length by arched, bilaterally symmetrical anterior, posterior, and intermediate pubourethral ligaments. These studies further showed, as was suggested by Curtis et al. (9), that the anterior and posterior ligaments were formed by reflections of the inferior and superior fascial layers of the urogenital diaphragm (Figs. 1.10 and 1.11). The intermediate ligament represents a fusion of these fascial layers.

The posterior pubourethral ligament blends with the arcus tendineus of the levator ani. When the arcus tendineus was cut, however, the pubourethral ligament retained an attachment to the connective tissue inferior to the pelvic diaphragm. The posterior pubourethral ligament was a reflection of the superior surface of the urogenital diaphragm.

The pubourethral ligament is attached mostly to the lateral sides of the urethra, although some fibers are almost in apposition. Smooth muscle bundles are present that run parallel to the long axis of the ligaments.

Histologic section showed the pubourethral ligaments to consist of dense collagen, both smooth and striated muscle, and elastic fibers. The striated muscle might represent a pubourethral continuation of some fibers of the pubococcygeus.

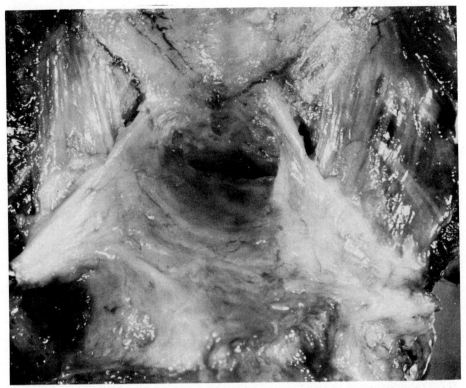

**Figure 1.8.** View of the cadaver pelvis is shown from above. The symphysis pubis is at the top of the picture, and traction to the pubourethral ligament has been applied by the hemostat shown on the *left,* accentuating the independent origin of this ligament from the posterior surface of the pubis but showing confluence posteriorly with the fascia of the pelvic diaphragm enclosing the pubococcygeus. (From Zacharin RF: The suspensory mechanism of the female urethra. *J Anat* 97:423–427, 1963.)

Study by light and electron microscopy and neurohistochemistry (63) showed that the tissue contained smooth muscle bundles associated with numerous nerve fibers. The enzyme content and fine structure of these were similar to those believed to represent cholinergic autonomic nerve tissue (acetylcholinesterase positive). Therefore, the term "ligament" is a misnomer, as these structures contain contractile elements under neural control.

The remainder of the urogenital diaphragm is sandwich-like, composed of superior and inferior fascial layers separated from one another by a layer of striated muscle, the deep transverse perineal. There is minimal striated muscle extending in this area to the wall of the urethra. In general, sphincters of the body under voluntary control are formed by concentric layers of striated muscle. This is not true for the urethra, although some external sphincter action is provided in the midportion of the urethra by pressure from the nearby pubococcygeus muscle and in the distal urethra by pressure from the bulbocavernosi.

The urogenital diaphragm runs between the inner surfaces of the ischiopubic rami and is pierced in the midline by urethra and vagina; by attachment to these structures, it assists in holding them in place. The posterior fibers of the

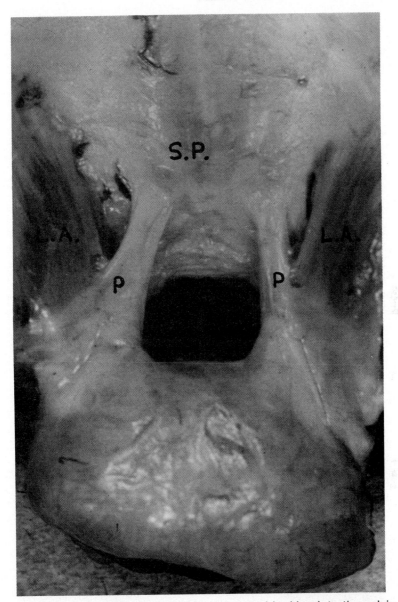

**Figure 1.9.** A fresh cadaver dissection is illustrated looking into the pelvis from above. The pubic symphysis *(S.P.)* is seen at the upper portion of the photograph. The bladder has been displaced posteriorly showing the posterior pubourethral ligament *(P)*. The darker colored levator ani *(L.A.)* arising from the arcus tendineus is seen lateral but distinct from the pubourethral ligaments. (From Zacharin RF, Gleadell LS: Abdominoperineal urethral suspension. *Am J Obstet Gynecol* 86:981– 994, 1963.)

urogenital diaphragm are fixed to the perineal body. When one is in the standing position, the urogenital diaphragm is almost horizontal in sagittal section; for this reason its fixation to the perineal body contributes to the support of the urethra and vesicourethral unction, lessening the tendency of these structures to rotate around the attachment of the pubourethral ligament to the pubis. The superficial perineal muscles and ischio- and bulbocavernosus

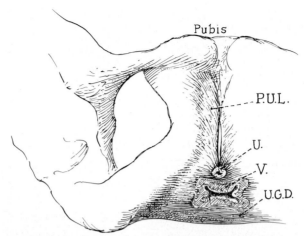

**Figure 1.10.** Frontal view of the urogenital diphragm *(U.G.D.)* shows its continuity with the anterior pubourethral ligament. The fascia of the urogenital diaphragm is reflected onto both anterior and posterior aspects of the pubis at a level more superior and medial than usually described. The sides of the diaphragm do not appear to meet anteriorly to form a transverse perineal ligament, as in the male.

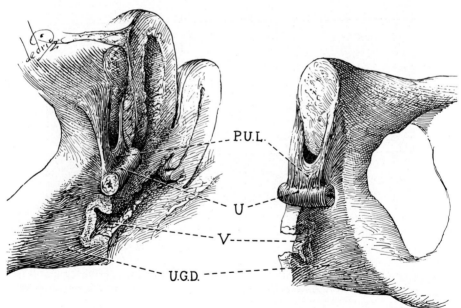

**Figure 1.11.** Sagittal view shows the relationship between the pubourethral ligament *(P.U.L.)* and urogenital diaphragm *(U.G.D.)* in the human female. The urethra *(U)* and vagina *(V)* are shown in their relationship to the urogenital diaphragm. Note the bladder sketched into the drawing at the left. (From Milley PS, Nichols DH: The relationship between pubourethral ligaments and urogenital diaphragm in the human female. *Anat Rec* 170:281–284, 1971; reproduced with permission of the Wistar Institute Press.)

muscles are superficial to the urogenital diaphragm, and appear to be considerably less important in urogenital support.

Ricci (50) mentioned that he did not doubt the existence of a urogenital diaphragm but had never seen one. Perhaps his failure to find one may have been because the attachments of the urogenital diaphragm to the urethra (pubourethral ligaments) are more on the superolateral aspect of the urethra than on the vagina.

*Anatomy.* The pubourethral ligaments are best demonstrated on a cadaver by sagittal section through the pelvis (Fig. 1.12) that permits their components to be visualized through its entire length; the anterior, intermediate, and posterior ligaments.

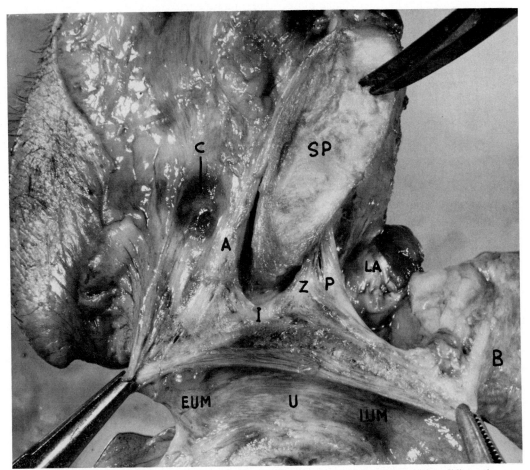

**Figure 1.12.** Sagittal section through the symphysis pubis *(SP)*, urethra *(U)*, and bladder *(B)*, shows the suspensory mechanism on tension. Traction to each end of the urethra results in some distortion that the length of the urethra has been exaggerated. Continuity between the anterior ligament *(A)*, intermediate ligament *(I)*, and posterior ligament *(P)* are shown along with expansion of the latter *(Z)* as it runs forward to become the intermediate ligament. The levator ani *(LA)*, clitoris *(C)*, and external urethral meatus *(EUM)*, are shown. (From Zacharin RF: The suspensory mechanism of the female urethra. *J Anat* 91:423–427, 1963.)

## Internal Urethral Sphincter

There has been a great deal of controversy concerning the nature of an internal urethral sphincter, but at no time have we found evidence of any significant amount of well-developed, physiologically useful, striated sphincter muscle under voluntary control. The urethral sphincter system consists primarily of smooth muscle and was described by Curtis et al. (9) as follows;

"The musculature of the bladder wall constitutes the internal sphincter, which is not a circular band at the neck of the bladder but a thickening of the muscle fibers beginning at the neck of the bladder and extending throughout the urethra, reinforced by fibers from the urogenital diaphragm, which constitute the external sphincter."

An analysis of anatomy and theory concerning the physiology of the bladder, trigone, and urethra was detailed in 1972 by the late John A. Hutch (27), emphasizing a bladder "base plate." He concluded:

"These studies force me to conclude that the bulk of the urethra is continuous with the deep trigone and, like the deep trigone, is derived from the Wolffian duct. It is this connective tissue that gives the urethra it tubular shape, the tough texture of the trigone, and limits its expansibility. Fortunately, imbedded in the collagen are many rings of circularly oriented smooth muscle. It is the tonus of this smooth muscle that keeps the lumen of the urethra constantly closed. In the female, this collagenous tube runs from the urethral meatus to the bladder neck. Its posterior wall continues upward into the base of the bladder, where it widens to form the deep trigone. It terminates by forming a tube-like structure at each cranial lateral border (Waldeyer's sheath). This is an oversimplification, because in most humans the tube fails to reach the bladder neck by about 0.5 to 0.10 cm. on the anterior wall. The defect that results is filled in by the detrusor loop. . . . It is this trigonal tissue that lends strength to the safety mechanism, giving form and shape and toughness to the urethra and to the bladder base. The rings of smooth muscle incorporated into the urethral portion constitute the basic primitive urethral sphincter that allows urine to accumulate in the bladder. The superficial portion (of the trigone), on the other hand, plays no role in the dynamics of the bladder neck, but it is primarily concerned with the competency of the urethral orifice." (Pages 78–79).

"There is a difference between the distribution of the periurethral striated muscle in male and female subjects. In both sexes there is more striated muscle along the anterior wall than along the posterior wall of the urethra, and in both sexes the striated muscle occupies the inferior one-half of the anterior urethral wall. Striated muscle on the anterior wall of the urethra does not reach the bladder neck in either male or female subjects. The junction between the smooth and striated fibers on the anterior wall is not a sharp horizontal line, but rather an oblique line formed by the tapering, outer smooth muscle layer downward and inward, while the striated muscle moves upward and outward. Striated muscle is less prominent and less consistent along the posterior wall of the urethra. In female subjects, striated muscle is sparse along the inferior half of the posterior wall of the urethra, probably because the vagina fuses so tightly to the urethra in that area." (Page 91).

"The internal sphincter is a double loop system formed by the base plate from the middle circular layer and the detrusor loop from the outer longitudinal layer. The base plate, which forms the top loop is located in the base of the bladder, and its tonus is constantly forcing the apex of the trigone forward. The detrusor loop, which forms the bottom loop, is located in the very top of the urethra forming most of the anterior and lateral walls of the urethra at the bladder neck. The loop is so positioned that the apex of the trigone fits snugly into its concave surface. Since the detrusor loop continues into the posterior surface of bladder as the right and left lateral posterior outer longitudinal layer, its force is constantly directed backward in direct opposition to the base plate, which is pushing the apex of the trigone forward. This is the heart of the closing mechanism of the bladder neck when the bladder is at rest and passively filling with urine.'' (Pages 106–107).

''For the internal sphincter to work properly, the base plate must be flat so that the fundus ring holds the apex of the trigone tightly into the concavity of the detrusor loop. At birth, all parts of the internal sphincter are present, but it does not function properly because the base plate is rounded. The same is true in stress incontinence. Here, the young girl is born enuretic and gains perfect control when her base plate flattens. Later in life when her anterior vaginal wall sags, the bladder descends, the bladder base becomes funneled, and she develops stress incontinence. A surgical procedure that elevates the bladder neck to a point where the base plate can flatten out restores her control.'' (Pages 116 and 117).

''Any operation that opens into the urinary tract or that plicates the urinary tract in the region of the trigone, bladder neck, or urethra in an effort to narrow the caliber of these structures is harmful. In cases of stress incontinence these delicate structures are all present and will work again if they are placed in their proper position. Cutting into them or suturing them only diminishes their chance in recovery. To operate successfully for stress incontinence we must attempt to re-establish a normal relationship between the urethra, the base plate, and the symphysis (as demonstrated by a lateral cystogram) through proper positioning of the anterior vaginal wall.'' (Page 145).

### Arcus Tendinei

There are two arcus tendinei on each side of the pelvis. The arcus tendineus of the levator ani runs from the back of the pubis to the ischial spine. Somewhat medial to this is the arcus tendineus of the endopelvic connective tissue. There is individual variation of the distance between these two arci at their origin and lateral extent, although they come together at the ischial spine. It is the arcus tendineus of the levator ani that provides a soft tissue attachment for the connective tissue bundle of fibers that is attached to the anterior vaginal sulcus (Figs. 1.13–1.15).

The urethra is both suspended (urogenital diaphragm) and supported (vagina) (Fig. 1.16). When hypermobile, this may be surgically remedied either by suspension or by support, *or by both!*

### Pelvic Diaphragm

The levator ani, with its superior and inferior fascial covering, constitutes the pelvic diaphragm and functions primarily as a tail wagger in pronograde four-legged animals. The assumption of an upright posture by man was accompanied by loss of the tail as a functioning appendage. The levator ani served an entirely different purpose as a result of the postural rotation of the pelvis. The comparative anatomy of this evolution has functional significance and relevance to the physiology of pelvic statics and is well worth the reader's study of the information available in the works of Thompson (58), Power (45), and Smout et al. (54).

Thompson wrote in his classic but not well-known treatise;

''As the pubococcygeus has lost its influence as a tail wagger over the caudal vertebrae, its influence over the rectum has increased and a large number of fibers losing their connection with coccyx pass round the rectum to form a sling; change of the commencement of which is seen in certain marsupials and carnivores.''

It is these detached fibers which form a loop around the rectum that Holl has called the puborectoralis or sphincter recti.

Some fibers, however, do retain their attachment to the coccyx, and this is occasionally torn during labor and delivery. This gives rise to the unusual pain

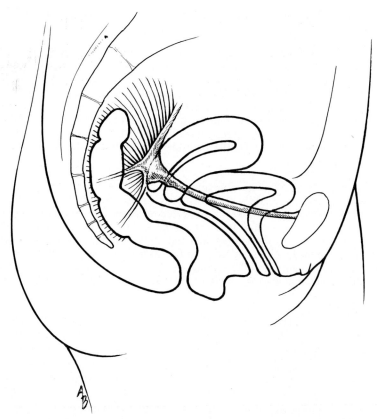

**Figure 1.13.** Schematic drawing showing the normal relationship between the vagina and the arcus tendinei. The arcus tendinei run between the back of the symphysis pubis to the ischial spine on each side of the pelvis.

of coccydynia which, as Malpas has pointed out, is elicited in certain patients by any activity that raises intra-abdominal pressure even momentarily. The pain is due to the detachment of the muscle from the bone rather than any affection of the bone itself, explaining why excision of the coccyx (coccygectomy) is generally both irrational and unrewarding. Most patients with chronic coccydynia need a preineal repair, not an excision of the coccyx. Power (45) noted the clinically significant embryology;

"The recti group of thoracoabdominal muscles arise through the ventral extension of the thoracic myotomes into the body wall. As the body wall develops, extensions of the myotomes migrate ventrally into these walls and the ventral ends of these extensions fuse together to form a ventral longitudinal muscle column from which the rectus abdominis and other elements are ultimately developed. The levator ani muscle, as shown by its nerve supply, is undoubtedly derived from the fourth sacral myotome. In the view of C.P. Martin, as the cloacal membrane migrates from the umbilical cord to the extension of the linea alba, an extension of the tendency of the myotomes to form a longitudinal muscle column on each side of the linea also occurs. Accordingly, we might expect that in cases where the os pubis is absent or imperfectly developed, the lower end of the rectus abdominis and the ventral end of the puborectalis ought to be structurally continuous."

This was observed by Power in the dissection of a stillborn fetus in which the pubis was totally absent on the right side and showed the rectus abdmoninis

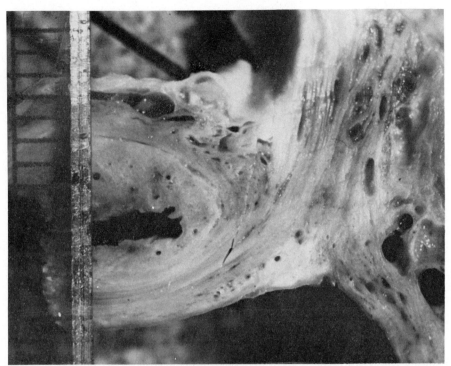

**Figure 1.14.** A fortuitous section through the urethra *(left)* and vagina *(below)* shows some of the distinct fibromuscular support of the former. The ventral support of the anterior fornix by its attachments to the arcus tendineus and cardinal ligament are shown on the *right.*

passing without interruption into the puborectalis. Finally, Power noted that the width of the true pelvis is only about one-third that of the abdomen. Consequently, the viscera in the pelvis fill up most of the pelvic floor and separate the peritoneum from the pelvic diaphragm. The viscera really are lying embedded in a mass of connective tissue that forms the layers of the endopelvic fascia. It is, therefore, easy to see why hernias through the pelvic floor are rare. The pelvic diaphragm is not a thin muscular layer in contact on its deep aspect with the peritoneum like the anterior abdominal wall. The vagina, in fact, forms the one weak spot on the pelvic floor, and it is here alone that we find hernias, such as cystocele, rectocele, and prolapse.

The levator ani, acting reciprocally with the striated muscle of the anterior abdominal wall, has assumed much responsibility not only for support of both pevic and abdominal contents, but for the maintenance and the equilibrium of intra-abdominal pressure (41, 42, 59). This reciprocal contraction has both an embryologic (45) and neurologic basis (59), and permits increase in intra-abdominal pressure, as with coughing and sneezing, to be applied equally to all sides of the intrapelvic organs and, thus, preserve their equilibrium of position. Whenever one of the other components is pathologically weakened or temporarily inactivated (the splinting effect of a tight corset), the other component will no longer contract reciprocally, and pressure upon one side of the pelvic organ may become greater than upon another side, permitting the organ to descend (geintal prolapse). If this movement carries the organ outside the physiologically effective pelvic cavity, the result will permit the transition of pressure to the content of such a displaced organ to be directed unequally. If

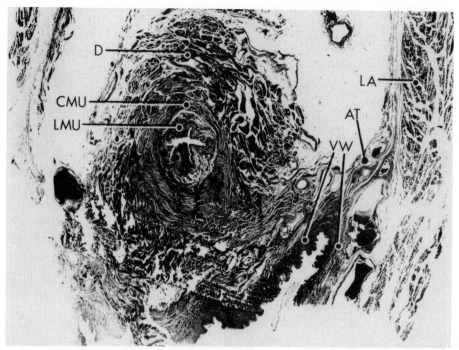

**Figure 1.15.** Photomicrograph of cross-section of pelvis of a 33-year-old cadaver is perpendicular to the intramural urethra. Coarse detrusor fibers of the bladder *(D)* surround the urethra, and the outer circular smooth muscle of the urethra *(CMU)* is seen surrounding the internal longitudinal smooth muscle layer *(LMU)*; note the attachment of the anterior sulcus of the vaginal wall *(VW)* to the arcus tendineus *(AT)* which overlies the levator ani *(LA)*. (From DeLancey JOL: Correlative study of paraurethral anatomy. *Obstet Gynecol* 68:91–97, 1986. Histologic sections provided by Dr. Thomas M. Oelrich, with permission of the American College of Obstetricians and Gynecologists.)

the vesicourethral junction has been displaced outside the pelvic cavity, increase in intra-abdominal pressure, which would normally be borne by both the intraperitoneal or intra-abdominal portion of the urethra and the bladder together and equally, will be borne by the bladder alone, increasing intravesical pressure more than intraurethral pressure, with resultant urinary incontinence (14).

Long ago, Dickinson (12) wrote:

"I venture to affirm that there is no considerable muscle in the body the form and function of which are more difficult to understand than those of the levator ani, and about which such nebulous impression prevail. The muscle sling, attached to the pubis in front, encircles like a collar the rectum and vagina. Its action in women is to drag the lower end of the vagina and rectum forward, level to the symphysis."

Sturmdorf (56) summarized its function as follows;

"The levator ani diminishes the force of intra-abdominal pressure upon the pelvic contents by deflecting the direction of that pressure, augments the resistance to pressure by closing the uterovaginal angle, and obstructs the pelvic outlet against the pressure by compressing the vaginal canal. It is the tensor of the pelvic fascia, the antagonist of the diaphragm and the abdominal muscle, contracting when these opposing muscles

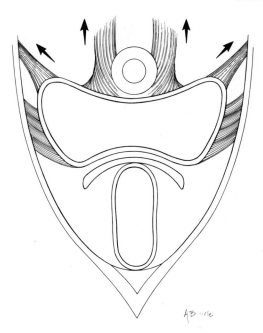

**Figure 1.16.** The urethra is both suspended (*central arrows* show the attachments and pull of the pubourethral ligament portions of the urogenital diaphragm) and supported (*lateral arrows* indicate the attachments of the vagina by intermediate connective tissue to the arcus tendineus).

contract and relaxing when they relax. When intact, it maintains the equilibrium of the pelvic organs; when its integrity is impaired, equilibrium is disturbed.''

Critchley, Dixon, and Gosling's study (8) of the periurethral and perianal parts of the levator ani using histochemical and electron microscopic techniques provides a quantitative comparison of the striated muscle fiber populations in these areas. Both regions consist predominantly of type I (slow twitch) fibers together with a small number of type II (fast twitch) fibers. However, marked differences have been demonstrated between the two regions with regard to proportions of the two fiber types, diameters of the constituent fibers and the distribution of muscle spindles. (Type I fibers maintain tone over long periods of time. Type II fibers contract suddenly over short periods of time.)

"Collectively, the results of the present study have shown that the levator ani muscle cannot be considered to comprise a single morphological or functional unit since its constituent parts perform different functions according to their anatomical location. Clearly the present results are of considerable importance when interpreting EMG recordings obtained from a single site in the levator ani. It is evident that the recordings obtained from one region alone do not provide an accurate indication of the functional status, either of other parts of the levator ani, or of the muscle in its entirety.''

The levator ani is composed of the three general portions named according to the origin of insertion of each. The medial and anterior division is the pubococcygeus, which, from the gynecologist's clinical point of view, is the most significant component of the levator ani.

Taking origin from the face of the pubis, about 1.5 cm on each side from the center, substantial portions sweep downward and posteriorly along the sides of the urethra, vagina, perineal body, and rectum, providing what appear to be clinically significant attachments of these muscles to the connective tissue along the sides of the urethra, the vagina, the rectum, and the upper portions of the perineal body. Since there appears to be considerable variation in the strength and integrity of these attachments, there is a corresponding variation in the degree to which these muscles offer support and help to resist damage of both internal and external genitalia.

There appear to be specific bundles of pubococcygeus fibers extending medially that contribute to the posterolateral investment of the urethra (pubourethralis) and provide a sling-like posterior support to the rectum (puborectalis).

The puborectalis may be a distinct development of the most medial portion of the pubococcygeus. It passes alongside the vagina and rectum to meet at the anterior extremity of the levator plate and forms a strong muscular sling behind the rectum. It is continuous with the deep external anal sphincter.

Bacon (1) believed the puborectalis to be a distinct muscle intimately associated anteriorly but distinctly separated posteriorly from the pubococcygeus; the two muscles appear to have a common origin except that the pubococcygeus arises on a higher plan. The puborectalis arises from the lowest portion of the symphysis pubis and from the deep layers of the triangular ligament. It passes downward and backward on either side of the vagina and lateral aspect of the rectum and fuses posteriorly in the midline, providing muscular support for the anorectal junction. Thus, the puborectalis, which serves an inportant role in rectal continence, relates only to the lower rectum and upper anal canal along both the posterior and lateral aspects.

There is much individual variation in the nature and strength of such muscular slips, however, which perhaps explains the discrepancies in anatomic literature. The views differ so widely that some authors deny altogether the existence of these muscle bundles, while others have contributed quite detailed descriptions with drawings and photographs of their relationships and distribution.

According to the careful dissections of Joachimovits (27), many individuals have a definite decussation of the puborectalis into clinically significant slips or prerectal bundles running from the belly of the muscles to the lateral margins of the perineal body. Superior to this area, at least in some individuals, there are muscle bundles running from the medial portion of the pubococcygeus to the posterolateral surface of the wall of the vagina and cranial toward the perineal body. These bundles have been designated as the pubovaginalis muscle, but the extent of this development is quite variable and probably accounts for the extremes of interpretation and opinion. As a result, the clinical significance of the components of the pubococcygeus must vary from one individual to another. These muscle fibers appear in significantly increased numbers in black women, which in combination with other inherited characteristics, particularly connective tissue strengths, may help to explain the lower incidence of certain types of genital prolapse among black women.

Frequently there are relatively strong connective tissue attachments between the pubococcygeus and the urethra along the junction between the lower and middle third of the vagina and cranialward to the lateral portions of the central perineal body. The clinical significance of these attachments appears chiefly in the recognition of the possibility that these fibers can be traumatically stretched or avulsed on either or both sides of the urethra.

Bacon and Ross (1) mentioned that the other levator components (pubococcygeus and iliococcygeus) sweep posteromedially to join each other behind the rectum and to insert into the coccyx;

"At the level of the anus, the levator ends in fibromuscular extensions which join with those of the longitudinal muscle of the rectum to insert into the anal canal at the intermuscular line. Some fibromuscular extensions of the conjoined tendon also pierce the subcutaneous portion of the external sphincter to insert into the skin about the anal verge as the corrugator cutis ani."

The right and left muscle bellies of the pubococcygei fuse in the midline posterior to the rectum (Fig. 1.17) and continue to the coccyx. This fusion constitutes the levator plate and upon it rest both the vagina and the rectum. It is the normal horizontal position of this supporting levator plate that accounts for the normally horizontal axis of the upper vagina. The levator plate is formed by the fused levator ani muscles extending posteriorly from a point of midline fusion just behind the levator hiatus to their coccygeal insertion. The rectum, vagina, and urethra pass through the hiatus. If the levator ani muscle is defective, the inclination of the plate will be downward and the hiatus will sag. Although Hadra (21) and later Halban and Tandler (22) recognized and defined the importance of the levator plate in providing pelvic support, the combination in the cadaver of rectal distension and absence of muscle tone made demonstration of the function of the plate difficult, and it remained for Berglas and Rubin (2) to demonstrate this plate in the living, and to relate pathologic displacement with various degrees of genital prolapse. This was accompanied by the direct injection of contrast material into the leavtor muscle and plate coincident with placement of the contrast material in the vagina, uterus, and rectum. Radiographs were taken of various patients at rest and while straining which clearly showed the integrity and horizontal position of the normal plate and tipping of the abnormal plate with bearing down coincident with genital prolapse.

Notice in Figure 16.7, redrawn from Berglas and Rubin (2), that the horizontal levator plate in a standing patient extends from the coccyx toward the midportion of the pubic symphysis but does not reach it. The anterior margin of the plate is separated from the posterior margin of the pubis by an opening called the genital or levator hiatus. When the supports of the plate are

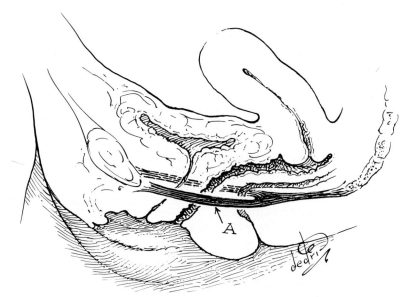

**Figure 1.17.** The vaginal axis of the erect or standing living female is shown. Notice the almost horizontal upper vagina and rectum lying on and parellel to the levator plate. The latter is formed by fusion of the pubococcygei muscles *(A)* posterior to the rectum. The anterior limit of the point of fusion is the margin of the genital hiatus, immediately posterior to the rectum. (From Nichols DH, Milley PS: Clinical anatomy of the vulva, vagina, lower pelvis, and perineum. In Sciarra (ed): *Gynecology and Obstetrics,* 1977; reproduced with permission of Harper & Row.)

damaged and it is permitted to tip, notice not only that the plate then permits the organs above it to "slide downhill" but also that the anteroposterior diameter of the hiatus is increased significantly, providing a larger portal for egress of prolapsing organs.

The function of the pubococcygeus muscle in the normal voiding mechanism is beautifully described by Muellner (37, 38). This concept emphasized the importance of voluntary skeletal muscle in the mechanism of continence. Muellner states;

"Before urination begins the diaphragm and the muscles of the abdominal wall contract, the intra-abdominal pressure rises, and the pubococcygei relax. As the pubococcygei relax, the neck of the bladder moves downward. This downward movement activates or initiates the contraction of the detrusor. At the same time, the contraction of the longitudinal fibers of the urethra, which are continuous with those of the detrusor, shorten the urethra and therby widen and open the internal urethral orifice. Urine is then expelled from the bladder.

At the conclusion of voiding, a contraction of the pubococcygei raises the neck of the bladder, the detrusor and urethral musculature relax, the urethra lengthens, the internal urethral orofice narrows and closes, and urination stops."

Gosling (19) describes the relationship between the levator ani muscles and the urethral wall and urethral junction as follows;

"The medial parts of the levator ani muscles (sphincter vaginae) are related to (but structurally separate from) the urethral wall. These periurethral fibers consist of an admixture of large-diameter fast- and slow-twitch fibers, together with muscle spindles. Therefore, unlike the rhabdosphincter, periurethral muscle possesses morphologic features that are similar to other "typical"voluntary muscles.

The levator ani plays an important part in urinary continence by providing an additional occlusive force on the urethral wall, particularly during events that are associated with an increase in intra-abdominal pressure, such as coughing and sneezing. This urethral occlusive force in the female is maximum at a level immediately distal to the maximum urethral pressure generated by the external urethral sphincter. Thus, in addition to providing support for the pelvic viscera, the periurethral parts of the levator ani also play an important active role in the urethral mechanisms that maintain continence of urine.

For micturition to occur, the pressure differential between the bladder and urethra muscle overcome the elastic resistance of the bladder neck. Immediately before the onset of micturition, the tonus of the rhabdosphincter is reduced by central inhibition of its motor neurones located in the second, third, and fourth sacral spinal segments. Such inhibition is mediated by descending spinal pathways originating in higher centers of the central nervous system. Concomitantly, other descending pathways activate (either directly or via sacral interneurones) the preganglionic parasympathetic motor outflow to the urinary bladder. This central integration of the nervous control of the bladder and urethra is essential for normal micturition. . . . . periurethral fibers are innervated by pudendal nerve and consist of an admixture of large-diameter fast- and slow-twitch fibers."

The intermediate portion of the levator ani, the iliococcygeus, is somewhat thinner and flatter than the pubococcygeus and measures between 0.5 and 1 cm. in thickness. Originating from the surface of the obturator internus fascia (from the so-called white line or tendinous arch of the levator ani, on a line running from the posterior pubis to the ischial spine), this muscle inserts along the lateral margin of the coccyx and lower sacrum.

The most posterior major division of the levtor ani is the coccygeus muscle, which takes its origin from the ischial spine and inserts along the fourth and fifth lateral margins of the coccyx and lower sacrum. Tandler (57) states "It lies intertwined with sinewy fibres on the front side of the sacrospinous ligament, and undergoes transformation into stronger more sinewy fibres at its points of insertion.'' The sacrospinous ligament is the ''tendon''or aponeurosis of the coccygeus muscle. Contrary to popular belief, though, the iliococcygeus is often convex in shape rather than concave (46). This is the result of pressure from fat within the ischiorectal fossa pushing on the soft belly of the muscle. This pressure, which is directed upward and medially, is developed when force is applied to the ischiorectal fat from below, when sitting or reclining (Fig. 1.18). When a loss of ischiorectal fat occurs as a result of massive weight reduction, the undersupport of the pelvic diaphragm is decreased, thus predisposing toward sagging of the levator muscle, tipping of the levator plate, and subsequent genital prolapse.

The normal contraction and tonus of an intact levator ani participate in maintaining adequate pelvic venous circulation. Thus, reconstitution of the levator by an appropriate colporrhaphy can be a factor in relieving perineal circulatory congestion and hemorrhoids, which will occasionally disappear several months after adequate perineal reconstruction.

### Rectal Continence

Contraction of the levator ani and puborectalis muscles exert pull upon the genital hiatus toward the pubis creating an angle in rectal inclination that functions effectively as a valve, according to the observations of Parks (43), and there is reflex reciprocity with the tone of the external anal sphincter. These muscles are innervated by the pudendal nerve and its accessory branches, and function in synergism.

Neuromuscular pressure receptors within the intrinsic striated muscular content of the levator ani are responsible for mediating this tone and they apparently communicate with the central nervous system by way of the pudendal nerve on each side of the body. The pudendal nerves generally arise

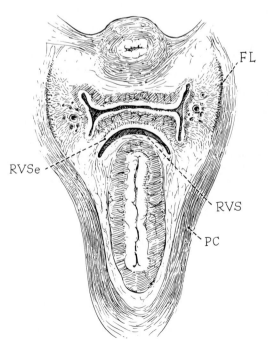

**Figure 1.18.** Cross-section of a female pelvis is shown through lower midportion of vagina. Note the convex configuration of the pubococcygeus *(PC)*. The rectovaginal space *(RVS)* is indicated between the rectum and vagina, as well as the position of the rectovaginal septum *(RVSe)*. The blood vessels in the connective tissue lateral to the vagina are shown. The fibers of Luschka *(FL)* are shown as they attach the paravaginal connective tissue to the sheaths of the pubococcygei. These connections tend to give the vagina an ''H''-shaped configuration. (From Nichols DH, Milley PS: Clinical anatomy of the vulva, vagina, lower pelvis, and perineum. In Sciarra J(ed): *Gynecology and Obstetrics*, 1977; reproduced with permission of Harper & Row.)

from spinal cord segments S3 and S4. Either congenital or acquired pathology of the pudendal nerve can alter the efficiency of its work and, thus, influence the ability and efficiency of these neuromuscular receptors to influence pressure and maintain this responsive muscular tone. Acquired damage may result from the trauma of stretching of the pelvic floor during childbirth and quite possibly from the chronic habit of excessive straining at stool (24).

The levator ani and the external anal sphincter differ from other striated muscles of the body in that they maintain a constant state of tone inversely proportional to the quantity of the rectal content. Because intestinal peristalsis continues around the clock, although at apparently various degrees of intensity, this aforementioned tone is responsible for our normal rectal continence both when we are awake and when asleep. Were it not for the effectiveness of this tone, we would be soiling ourselves regularly during sleep when the rest of our voluntary muscle system is relaxed.

Normal bowel function is to a large extent the product of habit. Defecation of sigmoid colon content is achieved by first voluntarily relaxing the pelvic diaphragm, unlocking the colic valve and relaxing the external anal sphincter. Modest increase in intra-abdominal pressure, as by bearing down, forces the stool content downward. The gastrocolic reflex pattern regularly assists by promoting intestinal peristalsis. A disorder of any of these steps predisposes to or causes constipation (29). Regular and excessive bearing down may stretch the anatomic integrity of the pudendal nerve and consequently weaken the muscles it innervates, occasionally resulting in a permanent loss of tone in the now denervated muscle of the pelvic diaphragm and external anal sphincter. The neuropathic loss of the tone of the anal sphincter permits it to relax at inopportune times producing rectal incontinence which may be most difficult to treat surgically. (The Parks group has suggested that this loss of voluntary muscle tone within the pelvic diaphragm may be associated with coincident urinary stress incontinence as well) (24).

### Perineal Body

The perineal body is a pyramidal fibromuscular elastic structure found in the midline between the rectum and the vagina on a line between the ischial tuberosities; it contains much elastic tissue. It is subject to individual variation in tone, thickness, and composition. It is somewhat like the hub of a wheel into which various muscles, i.e., the superficial and deep transverse muscles of the perineum, the bulbocavernosus muscle, the sphincter ani externus, and some fibers of the levator ani are inserted like spokes. It is bounded anteriorly by the vagina and posteriorly by the rectum. Studdiford (55) found that many smooth muscles in the perineal body serve as a distensible attachment to the levator ani and to the vagina. He believed this distensibility is important and, when lost through unrepaired perineal laceration, gives rise to rectocele and posterior vaginal eversion. Ranney (48) pointed out that the perineal body does not serve as a keystone, because its wide base points down, not up. If a keystone, it would by its very nature, fall down if pressure were applied.

The large number of nerve fibers and ganglia in the perineum distributed among the smooth muscle elements suggests a direct relationship with the smooth muscle, helping to emphasize its functional importance.

The large amount of smooth muscle within the perineal body provides it with physiologic distensibility, and when this characteristic has been lost, as occurs with unrepaired perineal body, the vaginal outlet becomes physiologically unstable.

Probably the most thorough recent study of the pelvic outlet in the female perineum has been reported by Joachimovits (22), who found a series of many anatomic dissections that the size, attachments, and strength of the perineal body are subject to wide individual variations. Because the living body is characterized by significant amounts of fibromuscular elastic tissues, the resulting tonus is capable of responding to physiologic requirements. The effects of tissue tone cannot be recognized in the cadaver, which accounts for the discrepancies in the anatomic descriptions of these structures.

When the perineal body appeared well-developed, Joachimovits found this pyramidal tissue readily divisible into two distinct parts; a distal fibrous portion practically covered by the superficial perineal muscles that penetrate the border of the urogenital diaphragm, and a cranial portion that attaches to the most caudal portion of the rectovaginal septum and contains considerably more smooth and striated muscle fibers. It is connected by smooth muscle bundles to the lowest portions of the anterior wall and contains some striated prerectal muscle fibers of the levator ani and fibers of the sphincter ani.

The two parts of the perineal body described by Joachimovits can be explained by the embryology of this structure. The structure develops from two vertical folds of the lateral wall of the cloaca that, early in development, grow as ventral and dorsal portions of the body. These folds fuse together in the midline to form a crescent-shaped fold of mesenchyme covered with epithelium (the urorectal septum), which serves to separate the rectum permanently from the urogenital sinus. The lower distal portion, arising from mesenchyme, more superficially located beneath the skin, has only secondarily combined with the larger dorsal part. Subepithelial masses of mesoderm adjacent to the distal cloaca contribute striated muscle bundles to each side of the perineal body as derivatives of these cloacal sphincters, which smooth muscle elements are contributed by the outer longitudinal muscles of the posterior vaginal wall and those of the anterior rectal wall. The caudal or superficial portion of the perineal body, by its attachment to the superficial perineal muscles, becomes fixed to the ischial tuberosities and is further fastened by its attachment to the bulbocavernosi. The external anal sphincter is anatomically weakened as a result of its divergence into laminae about the vagina. Bacon (1) has suggested that it is for this reason that severance of the subcutaneous external sphincter tends to result in retraction of the muscle ends, producing anal incontinence. If at any time the external sphincter has become detached from the perineal body, it should be reattached by the figure-of-8 suture technique of Campbell, as described in Chapter 12.

Our studies confirm that there is considerable individual variation in the strength and composition of the perineal body and the extent to which fibers of the pubococcygeus are attached to or interspersed with fibers of the perineum. With its double embryology, it is apparent that there can be genetically determined variations in strength of either the cranial or caudal division of the perineal body, or both, and these differences may help determine the noticeable ethnic dissimilarity in the severity as well as the types of genital prolapse. Most standard anatomy texts have described in much detail only one or two dissections of the perineum, with insufficient allowance for the phenomenon of individual variation in this area, which is quite widely distributed in nature.

Superficially, the pyramid of the perineal body is attached to Colles' fascia. The medial margins of the pubococcygeal muscles are in contact with the lateral surfaces of the perineal body at the border between its distal and proximal divisions. Although some prerectal fibers may insert on the lateral surface of the perineal body, the larger, more lateral bundles pass alongside the rectum and fuse into the levator plate as it extends to the coccyx.

Many smooth muscle cells extend as a ridge of variable thickness between the medial edges of the levator muscles in the midline. The attachment is greatest within the dorsal or deep division of the perineal body.

These prerectal bundles also received a secondary innervation along with the perineal muscles derived from the cloacal sphincter, and, as an aide to normal defecation, they can contract independently of the remainder of the levator complex. Their tonus increases (along with that of the pubovaginal bundles) while those of other levator fibers relax, thus pulling the perineal body forward and upward in a way that tends to neutralize variations in intra-abdominal pressure and helps prevent prolapse of the rectum during normal defecation. By way of contrast, the puborectalis bundles, that most medial portion of the pubococcygeus that comes together behind the rectum in the levator plate to form an alomst U-shaped sling for the rectum, contracts immediately after defecation, in unison with the remaining portion of the levator ani.

All of the attachments of the striated muscles to the perineal body are elastic to varying degrees. This elasticity probably varied within different phases of the individual's life cycle, along with the intrinsic elasticity of the connective tissues of the perineal body itself, becoming less evident with advancing years. Thus, the loss of an appreciable degree of the tissues' elasticity exposes the patient to increased risks of obstetric damage if parturition occurs during the latter years of the woman's reproductive life. Relative weakness of the individual's elastic tissue may, to some degree, be correlated with the development of subcutaneous abdominal striae during pregnancy, providing the so-called elastic index of Magdi (32 ), who noted the larger number of striae correlates with decreased elasticity of the perineum, suggesting, in such a situation, the desirability of earlier and larger episiotomy to prevent significant tissue damage.

Anteriorly, the attachment of the perineal body to the rectovaginal septum (see Fig. 1.27) at the site of this angle reinforces the anterior rectal wall; but disruption of this attachment between the rectovaginal septum and perineal body by tearing or attentuation contributes to the development of rectocele at this site. Generally, the perineal body is also lacerated, permitting low and midvaginal rectocele; but, if the perineal body remains intact, the rectocele may be seen higher within the vagina.

The length of the perineal body closely approximates the length of the urethra, as this is the normal level of lateral attachment of these organs to the connective tissue of the pelvic diaphragm (pubococcygeus). In the case of the urethra, this is aided considerably by the primary attachment of the pubourethral ligament, which, although primarily a portion of the urogenital diaphragm, is in a lateral relation to the fibers of the pelvic diaphragm.

### Superficial Perineal Muscles

The deep transverse perineii, arising from the inferior rami of the ischia, are enclosed within the layers of the urogenital diaphragm. The presence of the vagina interrupts the extent of the development, in contrast to the male, and only a few fibers cross the midline between rectum and vagina.

The superficial transverse perineii arise from the pubic rami and attach to both the perineal body and the deep portion of the external anal sphincter, but they are not of great clinical significance.

The internal anal sphincter is the lower border of inner circular smooth muscle of the rectum and is of secondary importance in control of anal continence.

The external anal sphincter is divided into three portions. The subcutaneous portion is continuous with fibers of the bulbocavernosus, both being derived from the cloacal sphincter and sharing common innervation and coordination of sphincter functions. Unrepaired laceration will usually result in anal incontinence, because the division, the superficial portion, is weakened in its attachment to the female perineal body by the mobility of the vagina. The muscle originates from the coccyx, encircles the anus, and inserts into the perineal body.

The deep external anal sphincter cannot be distinctly separated posteriorly from fibers of the pubococcygeus. In fact, Courtney (7) states that: "The deep external sphincter is a continuation of the puborectalis formed by decussation of its fibers through the central tendinous point of the perineum. The anterior part of the anorectal ring is completed by the deep part of the external sphincter, while laterally and posteriorly it is formed by the U-shaped muscle sling of the puborectalis." Thus, he considers the levator ani, particularly the puborectalis portion, and the deep external sphincter as anatomically and functionally one muscle, a view supported by Wendell-Smith (62).

## Blood Vessels of the Female Perineum

The vascular supply of the perineal structure is derived from the branches of the internal pudendal artery, which arises from the anterior trunk of the internal iliac. The internal pudendal leaves the pelvic cavity through the greater sacrosciatic foramen. As it ascends along the pubic ramus, it pierces the posterior layer of the urogenital diaphragm, travels for a short distance within the diaphragm, and perforates the anterior layer. The terminal branches include the artery to the bulbocavernosus muscle and the dorsal artery of the clitoris. The branches within the perineum include the external or inferior hemorrhoidal arteries and they originate as the pudendal artery rises anterior to the ischial tuberosity. The external hemorrhoidal arteries run across the ischiorectal fossa and are distributed to the anal sphincter and levator ani muscles. They are the chief sources of hemorrhage from all superficial wounds about the anus or ischiorectal fossa. These vessels have accompanying veins that empty into the pudendal veins.

The superficial perineal or vulvar artery is anterior to the external hemorrhoidal artery. It is distributed to the vulva, with branches to the muscles, and is a source of arterial hemorrhage in wounds of the vulva.

The transverse perineal artery is smaller, supplies the cutaneous surface of the perineum, and is a source of hemorrhage from laceration of the perineal body. The fourth branch is the artery of the bulb, a vessel of considerable diameter but of short length. It sends branches to the bulbocavernosus muscle.

The terminal branches of the internal pudendal artery, the artery of the corpus cavernosum, and the dorsal artery of the clitoris are the vessels that supply the erectile tissue of the clitoris. When the clitoris is amputated, the two dorsal arteries may require ligation. Bleeding from the vessels of the corpora cavernosa can usually be controlled by pressure, as the traveculae favor coagulation of blood.

The veins of the perineum are valveless and have free anastomosis with the large intrapelvic venous plexuses. Consequently, there can be alarming hemorrhage from wounds of the vulva and vagina, and massive hematomas are possible.

When the tone of the pelvic musculature is poor, venous return is impeded, and chronic congestion and varicosities, including hemorrhoids, may develop. These often improve after restoration of tone after reconstruction of the pelvic musculature.

Special properties of pelvic and perineal blood vessels include the following:

1. Although there are many large venous networks within the pelvis that are capable of considerable venous distention, these veins are almost entirely without valves.
2. Abundant smooth muscle fibers associated with adventitia of pelvic blood vessels probably account for at least part of the impressive quantity of smooth muscle found in the extra peritoneal connective tissue of the pelvis.
3. The warmth and heat of tissues undergoing erection (clitoris, bulbocavernosus muscle) demonstrate that most of the blood involved in the erectile process comes in fact from arteriolar direction and that the venous congestion is probably a secondary phenomenon.

## Vagina

Vaginal depth and axis are maintained as a result of multiple but varying anatomic supports along the length of the vaginal walls. The lower third is supported predominantly by attachment through intermediate fibers to the pelvic diaphragm and the arcus tendineus, urogenital diaphragm, and perineal body and indirectly by the same muscles and connective tissues to which the perineal body itself is attached. Support of the middle third is contributed by lateral fusion with fibers in the pelvic diaphragm. but even stronger lateral support is obtained by attachments to the inferior portions of the cardinal ligaments. The upper third of the vagina is adjacent to the rectum, which, in turn, rests on the levator plate but is not attached directly to the fibers of the pelvic diaphragm. The upper vagina and cervix are as a unit maintained in a position anterior to the levator plate by their lateral attachments to the cardinal and uterosacral ligaments.

The vagina is a fibromuscular tube, the walls of which are normally in apposition in the relaxed state; it is H-shaped in its central portion, the side walls being suspended by their attachment to the paravaginal lateral connective tissue from which they receive their blood supply and to the arcus tendineus. The vagina is lined by a stratified squamous epithelium with rugal folds, giving the epithelium accordian-like distensibility without laceration. The stratified squamous epithelium is rich in glycogen during reproductive years. A dense, thin layer of elastic fibers is found immediately beneath the epithelium. Beneath this is a well-developed fibromuscular layer. Smout et al. (54) have described a muscular meshwork of smooth muscle fibers predominantly oriented in a longitudinal direction in the innermost component but arranged circularly toward the periphery. The fibrous capsule external to this muscular coat is rich in elastic fibers and large venous plexuses. The vagina is attached to the lateral pelvic wall by condensations of connective tissue and smooth muscle intimately adherent to the adventitia of the vaginal blood vessels. This tends to fix the position from side to side, and the muscular elements supply a certain amount of tone, permitting it to adapt to changes in intravaginal and extravaginal pressure. There is a large amount of elastic tissue mingling with the fibromuscular connective tissue elements of the vaginal capsule. These permit distention and allow return to normal size. In the midline, the vagina can distend without interference from either the bladder or rectum. The relatively avascular vesicovaginal and rectovaginal spaces permit these organs to expand, contract, and slide somewhat independently of one another; thus, each causes minimal interference with the function of the other. The rectovaginal septum is fused with the posterior vaginal wall as the anterior lining of the rectovaginal space. Because the vagina is a distensible organ, its depth is best measured when it is in a relaxed or resting state. The posterior vaginal wall is approximately 10 cm long. Since the cervix is incorporated in the anterior vaginal wall, the length of the anterior vaginal wall plus cervix approximates the length of the posterior wall. The connective tissue adventitia of the vagina is continuous with that of the cervix.

The vagina is normally narrowest in its lower third where it tends to be constricted laterally by the adjacent portions of the levator ani. The vagina is largest in its middle and upper thirds. The connective tissue lateral to the lower third is attached to fibers of the pubococcygeal muscle (fibers of Luschka) and to fibers fixing it to the urogenital diaphragm. Luschka (31) discribed the connection as follows: "In the female the fibers originating from the upper pubic ramus pass alongside the vagina and are connected with it through strong connective tissue but do not end in the vagina."

### Vessels of the Vagina

In addition to the vaginal blood supply received from branches of the internal pudendal artery, diffuse anastomoses form between these and branches of the uterine, inferior vesical, middle rectal, and vaginal arteries. The confluence of these anastomotic branches forms longitudinal azygos vaginal arteries in the midline of the anterior or posterior vaginal walls, or both, according to Smout et al. (54) and Quinby (46).

A right and left vaginal artery, or occasionally two, arise (independently in most instances) from each internal iliac artery slightly cephalad and posterior to the origin of each uterine and inferior vesical artery. Occasionally, the vaginal artery arises as a division of a short common trunk with the uterine artery. This branching, however, occurs at the lateral extremity of each cardinal ligament and has great clinical significance. Alarming arterial hemorrhage, thus, may follow laceration or surgical trauma to the vagina, especially in the vault of the vagina, even though the uterine artery has been securely ligated. Occasional postoperative arterial vaginal hemorrhage coexistent with intact ligation of the uterine artery may thus require separate isolation and ligation of the vaginal artery or, failing this, hypogastric or internal iliac ligation.

Vaginal veins communicate with rich plexuses in the paravaginal tissues, perineum, rectum, and bladder.

### Normal Vaginal Depth and Axis

The vagina in the cadaver is usually depicted as an almost straight hollow tube extending vertically upward toward the sacral promontory (15, 20).

Early concepts describing a more horizontal upper vaginal axis of the living patient were discussed by Hadra (21) and objective evidence was based on the studies of impressions made on wax molds by Dickinson (12), and again in 1961 on similar studies by Morgan (36), who used molds of the vagina made from a rapidly solidifying dental impression paste. An expanded similar study was reported in greater detail by Richter (51) in 1966.

Radiographic colpography has demonstrated a distinct, superiorly convex, perineal curve in the lower vagina (18, 39) (Fig. 1.3). In the living, the upper vaginal axis lies in an almost horizontal plane when the patient is in a standing position. The upper vagina lies on the rectum, which, in turn, lies on and parallel to the levator plate. It is this almost horizontal position of the supporting levator plate that accounts for a similar axis to the upper vagina. The levator plate is formed by the fusion of the levator ani muscles posterior to the rectum, from just behind the levator hiatus to their coccygeal insertion (Fig. 1.7). The rectum, vagina, and urethra pass through the levator hiatus, and, if the levator ani muscle is defective, the inclination of the plate will be downward and the hiatus will sag. Although the cervix and upper vagina have considerable mobility, they are more or less anchored in position over the levator plate by the cardinal ligaments. The length and flexibility of these ligaments normally permit the cervix and upper vagina to be moved in any direction over the rectum on the levator plate but not anterior to the margin of the genital hiatus.

The vagina is maintained in depth and axis by different anatomic supports at different vaginal depths. The lower third is supported predominantly by connection between fibers received from the pelvic diaphragm and the urogenital diaphragm. The most posterior portion of the lower third is further attached to the perineal body and indirectly receives contributions from the various other muscles and connective tissue thickenings to which the perineal body itself is attached (Fig. 1.5). The middle third of the vagina receives some contribution from lateral fusion with a lesser number of fibers from the pelvic diaphragm, but even more lateral support is obtained from the lateral and most inferior portion of the cardinal ligaments that carry the main vaginal blood vessels both to and from their hypogastric origin. The upper third of the vagina receives almost no significant support from direct attachment to the fibers of the levator ani or pelvic diaphragm, but, in fact, rests on the rectum, which, in turn, rests on the fused pubococcygei of the levator plate. The upper vagina and the cervix together are maintained in position over this levator plate by their lateral attachments to the upper cardinal ligaments (44).

The vagina is "fixed" at two points, i.e., the urogenital diaphragm and at the "cardinal ligament" at the vault, and is flexibly suspended in between with connective tissue attachments to the arcus tendineus and pelvic diaphragm.

The sphincter-like effect of simultaneous contraction of the levator ani and the bulbocavernosi is illustrated in Figure 1.5. Huisman (26) believes "the real voluntary urethral sphincter is located in the pelvic floor musculature, e.g. the pubococcygeus muscle."

### Connective Tissue Planes and Spaces

Much of the beauty of soft tissue pelvic architecture derives from the abilities of the organs of the three primary systems in this area; urinary, reproductive, and rectal (gastrointestinal) to function independently of one another. Each is capable of the limits of its normal range of function without permanent alteration of the anatomy or function of its neighbors, i.e., the organs are capable of independent expansion and contraction.

There are connective tissue spaces (17, 44, 49) between these organs that permit this relatively independent function. The connective tissue spaces to be described, it must be emphasized, are potential spaces. They are filled for the most part with loose areolar tissue, are virtually devoid of blood vessels and nerves, and are readily converted to actual spaces by blunt dissection, often with the index finger. Before dissection, they are somewhat analogous to the space inside a folded, empty paper bag. These spaces are divided by connective tissue septa that not only afford mechanical support but also provide the physical routes of blood vessel, lymphatics, and nerve tissue to and from the pelvic organs. These structures are contained within the septa along reasonably constant routes and do not trespass on the connective tissue spaces. Although their location is quite regular within the septa, individual variations as to the site of the origin and their relative size are occasionally seen. The anatomic ligaments form natural barriers to the spread of infection, cancer, and hematomas. The septa, on the other hand, through their blood vessels and lymphatics, form natural routes for the transmission of infection and malignancy arising from the pelvic organs. A detailed knowledge of the anatomy of these spaces and partitioning septa is essential to the understanding of their actual and potential functional importance in both health and disease. From accurate knowledge and experience, the surgeon can know not only where to find major vessels and so avoid unnecessary surgical penetration of adjacent organs. To the gynecologic surgeon, this anatomic knowledge helps demarcate the likely limits and routes of direct spread of malignant disease and to determine the extent of necessary extirpation. To the surgeon concerned with pelvic reconstruction, the implications are obvious in the need to re-establish original relationships between the organs.

The connective tissue capsules or adventitia of the bladder, birth canal, and rectum are attached to the pelvis and at certain points to one another, by condensations of connective tissue that contain the principal blood vessels and lymphatics to and from these organs. Although these septa vary in strength and thickness from person to person, their relation and position are constant.

Potential spaces exist between these septa, and the spaces are filled with fat and loose areolar tissue but are essentially free of blood vessels and lymphatics (Figs. 1.19 and 1.20). These areas become actual spaces only by dissection, but this is easily accomplished bloodlessly and bluntly once access to the space has been gained by surgical penetration through a septum.

Safe extirpation or reconstructive surgery for benign pelvic disease requires identification, penetration, and invasion of the midline anterior and posterior spaces, but the oncologic surgeon requires penetration and dissection of the lateral spaces as well.

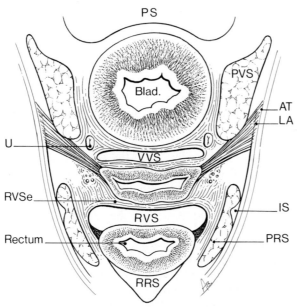

**Figure 1.19.** The connective tissue septae and spaces of the pelvis are shown. The paravesical spaces *(PVS)* are shown lateral to the bladder. The ischial spine *(IS)* is noted in the lateral wall of the pararectal spaced *(PRS)* on each side. The prevesical space *(PS)* vesicovaginal space *(VVS)*, rectovaginal space *(RVS)*, and retrorectal space *(RRS)* are shown in the midline. The rectovaginal septum *(RVSe)* is shown. Note to the attachment of the vaginal sulci to the arcus tendineus *(AT)* and ventral surface of the levator ani *(LA)*. The levator ani form the lateral wall of the pararectal spaces. The ureter *(U)* is shown. The rectal pillar separating the rectovaginal space from the pararectal space is of two layers (6) though these may be fused, as shown.

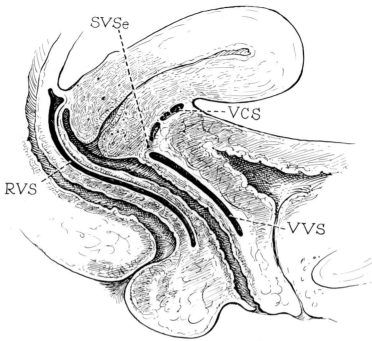

**Figure 1.20.** Median sagittal section through the female pelvis showing the midline connective tissue spaces between bladder, vagina, and rectum. The vesicocervical space *(VCS)* is separated from the vesicovaginal space *(VVS)* by fusion between the adventitia of the cervix and bladder called the supravaginal septum *(SVS)*. The rectovaginal space *(RVS)* is shown between the rectum and the vagina, extending from the perineal body to the bottom of the cul-de-sac of Douglas. The rectovaginal septum is a condensation of tissue attached to the posterior vaginal wall along the full length of the rectovaginal space.

In the operative procedures to be described later, it is essential that the operator become thoroughly familiar with the pelvic connective tissue planes and spaces, especially with their relationships to one another. A relatively simple diagram of the clinically significant anatomic relationships, as illustrated in Figures 1.21 and 1.22 should be kept in mind.

The bladder, vagina, and rectum have been indicated as in the coronal section. The cardinal ligament extends laterally from the central portion of the upper vagina and cervix. A vertical pillar extends along each side of these three essential pelvic conduits, from the pubis to the coccyx, intersecting the cardinal ligaments, and assures both attachment and continuity with the connective tissue capsules of each of the three essential organs. Fascial investments of striated muscle of the lateral pelvic wall form the lateral boundaries of these connective tissue spaces, now readily identifiable as the vesicovaginal, the rectovaginal and the retrorectal space, the space of Retzius, and laterally, the paired paravesical and pararectal spaces. In general, these connective tissue septa and spaces are relatively constant in their relationship to one another, and the gynecologic surgeon will do well to keep such a simple diagram in mind. It will be referred to in greater detail and in a less schematic fashion later in this chapter.

### Vesicovaginal Space

The vesicovaginal space lies in the midline and is bounded anteriorly by the bladder adventitia, laterally by the bladder septa or pillars, and posteriorly by

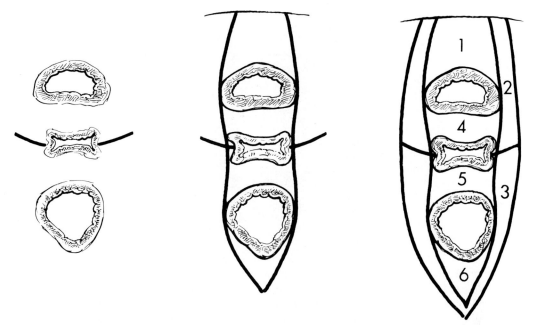

**Figure 1.21.** A schematic way of learning the names and relationships of the potential connective tissue spaces of the pelvis is shown. The drawing on the *left* shows, in the center, the vagina with cardinal ligament attached. A cross-section through the bladder is *above* and the rectum *below*. *Vertical lines* are drawn on either side of these three organs in the *center drawing*. They correspond to the bladder and rectal connective tissue septa and cross the cardinal ligament as shown. Two additional lines have been added to the drawing on the *right*, representing the obturator fascia and pelvic diaphragm. The potential connective tissue spaces of the pelvis, and their approximate relation to one another, are shown: *(1)* the prevesical space, *(2)* the paravesical space, *(3)* the pararectal space, *(4)* the vesicovaginal space, *(5)* the rectovaginal space, and *(6)* the retrorectal space.

the adventitia of the vagina. Superiorly, it ends at the point of fusion between the adventitia of the bladder and vagina. This point of fusion is called the supravaginal septum or vesicocervical ligament (44). From our dissections we have found that his point of fusion occasionally contains multiple fasciculi, oriented in the same general direction but occurring at slightly different levels (Fig. 1.20). Inferiorly, the vesicovaginal space is limited by the fusion of the urethral and vaginal adventitia.

**Supravaginal Septum**

There seems to be wide individual variation in both the strength and the extent of the supravaginal septum. At times, it seems, in fact, to be a nonentity, demonstrable only as the fascial capsule of the cervix through which the surgeon must dissect in the performance of vaginal hysterectomy in order to reach the anterior peritoneal plication. At surgical dissection, much of this tissue may be artifactual, but it represents the point of fusion between the connective tissue support of the bladder and that of the upper vagina and cervix. When a cystocele involves this area, adequate repair must involve identification and plication to assure restoration of the fascial capsule of the cervix. From our dissections we have found that this point of fusion occasionally contains multiple fasciculi, oreinted in the same general direction but occurring at slightly different levels. It is perhaps along the long fibers of this

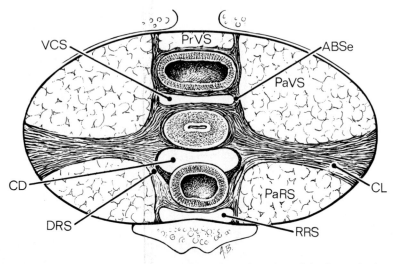

**Figure 1.22.** Diagrammatic cross-section of the female pelvis through the cervix is shown. The prevesical space *(PrVS)* is seen anterior to the bladder, and is separated from the paravesical spaces *(PaVS)* by the ascending bladder septa *(ABSe)*. The latter also separates the paravesical space from the vesicocervical space *(VCS)*. The cul-de-sac *(CD)* is separated from the pararectal spaces *(PaRS)* by the descending rectal septa *(DRS)*, the posterior sheath of which separates the retrorectal space *(RRS)* from the pararectal spaces. (After von Peham H, Amreich J: *Operative Gynecology.* Philadelphia, JB Lippincott, 1934.)

supravaginal septum that cervical cancer may directly invade the wall of the bladder. The connective tissues of this septum may be softened considerably in pregnancy with increase in elasticity to accomodate the necessary stretching as the uterus enlarges and for the contraction of the uterus in labor with minimal alteration in bladder function. This softening accounts for the ease with which the bladder may be bluntly separated from the lower uterine segment and cervix at the time of cesarean section, contrasting sharply with the need for sharper surgical division of these organs in the nonpregnant state.

Anterior entry between the vagina and the peritoneal cavity is often through anatomic areas somewhat different, depending on whether the approach is from the vaginal or from the abdominal side. This structural difference may help explain why the surgeon who customarily operates by the abdominal route may experience unexpected difficulty in separating bladder from cervix when he approaches hysterectomy vaginally; similarly, the surgeon who is more comfortable with performing hysterectomy through the vagina may wonder why unfamiliar difficulties may arise during the course of abdominal hysterectomy.

This anatomic difference is explained in Figure 1.23. A customary route of dissection is identified by the arrows. The vaginal operator may incise directly through the point of fusion between the bladder and the vagina, providing ready access to the anterior vesicouterine perineal fold. When this is not promptly evident, it is likely that the dissection has been carried beneath the connective tissue capsule of the uterus, well above the anterior peritoneal reflection. The peritoneum and the uterine connective tissue capsule will be peeled off from the anterior surface of the uterus. The abdominal operator, on the other hand, will first enter the anterior peritoneum, continuing the dissection beneath the connective tissue capsule of the uterus beneath or through the so-called

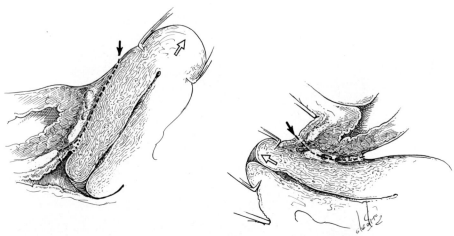

**Figure 1.23.**   The site and direction of anterior peritoneal incision often used in the so-called endofascial type of abdominal hysterectomy are shown by the *solid arrow* in the drawing on the *left.* This dissection, following the route of the *broken line,* is often beneath the connective tissue capsule of the uterus and must cut across the lower part of the supravaginal septum to reach the vagina, as shown by the *broken line,* or may enter the vagina behind most of the supravaginal septum, as shown by the *dotted line.* The *open arrow* shows direction of removal of the uterus. A desirable route of incision and dissection with vaginal hysterectomy is shown by the *solid arrow* in the drawing on the right. The supravaginal septum may be incised immediately after opening the vagina, and dissection may be carried superiorly between connective tissue capsules of uterus and bladder (the so-called vesicocervical space) until the anterior peritoneal plication is reached. Should the operator's dissection be beneath the connective tissue capsule of the uterus, he/she will find him-/herself tunneling interior to and failing to recognize peritoneum on the anterior surface of the uterus well above the anterior peritoneal fold. The *open arrow* shows direction of removal of the uterus. (From Nichols DH, Milley PS: Clinical anatomy of the vulva, vagina, lower pelvis, and perineum. In Sciarra J(ed): *Gynecology and Obstetrics,* 1977; reproduced with permission of Harper & Row.)

supravaginal septum to the vagina. The former is the essence of the so-called endofascial hysterectomy (5). Recognizing these differences and becoming comfortable with both techniques will provide valuable surgical experience and enable one to find the anterior vesicouterine peritoneal fold when operating through the vagina, as well as finding the longitudinal muscle layer of the vagina more safely when operating for benign disease through a transabdominal approach.

The continuity of the connective tissue capsule of the vagina and bladder is demonstrated in Figure 1.24, in which sagittal section had been obtained post-mortem through the vagina, cervix, and bladder of an aging patient with procidentia. Notice the continuity of this layer which must be transversed, as well as the looseness of the areolar tissues filling the potential vesicovaginal and vesicocervical spaces.

**Vesicocervical Space**

The vesicocervical space is the continuation of the vesicovaginal space superiorly above the supravaginal septum. The posterior border of this space is composed of the connective tissue adventitia of the cervix and vagina. These

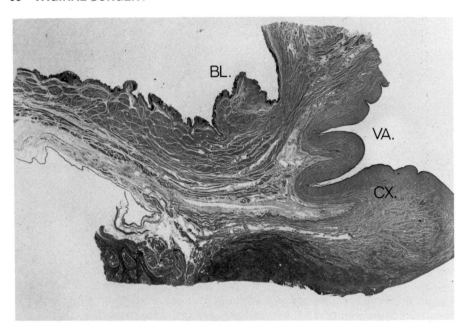

**Figure 1.24.** Photomicrograph is shown of sagittal section through bladder, *top left,* vagina, *top right,* and cervix, *lower right,* of autopsy specimen of elderly patient with untreated genital prolapse. Descent of the cervix *(CX)* had drawn it and vagina *(VA)* away from the bladder *(BL)*. An attachment (supravaginal septum) of the fibromuscular connective tissue capsule of the bladder to that of the vagina is shown. (From Nichols DH, Milley PS: Clinical anatomy of the vulva, vagina, lower pelvis, and perineum. In Sciarra J(ed): *Gynecology and Obstetrics,* 1977; reproduced with permission of Harper & Row.)

adventitia are continuous. The superior border is the peritoneum lining the vesicouterine peritoneal pouch. Cutting the supravaginal septum establishes communication by the vesicovaginal space and the vesicocervical space.

**Ascending Bladder Septa**

Although the ascending bladder septa are weak cephalad, they become the stronger bladder pillars (which contain efferent veins from the vesical plexus and ureter) by the addition of the lateral strong connective tissue portions of the cardinal ligament. Medially, they are loose in texture and contain fat and ureter. These septa attach to the lateral inferior extension of the bladder, connecting it to the upper surface of the cardinal ligaments, lateral to the cervix (Figs. 1.16 and 1.19). They contain some cervical branches of the uterine artery anteriorly into the sides of the bladder base.

**Prevesical Space of Tetzius**

The prevesical space is in the form of a triangle extending from the umbilicus laterally to the lateral umbilical ligament (obliterated hypogastric artery). Anteriorly, the transversalis fascia extends from the umbilicus to the pubis; it extends inferiorly to the cardinal ligament and the supravaginal septum. It is separated from the paravesical spaces by the ascending bladder septa. The prevesical space, thus, includes the area between the pubis and the anterior vesical wall roofed by the fascia between the medial umbilical ligaments.

The ascending bladder septum above the uterer contains many blood vessels, including the inferior vesical artery and large veins of the vesical plexus. Below the ureter, however, blood vessels are scant, and the tissues between bladder and vagina can be easily separated without hemorrhage.

### Paravesical Spaces

The paired paravesical spaces, right and left, are natural, fat-filled, pre-formed spaces that lie above the cardinal ligament and its prolongation (horizontal connective tissue ground bundle); they are bounded medially by the bladder pillars and laterally by the pelvic walls, the fascia of the internal obturator muscle, and the levator ani. The roof is formed by the lateral umbilical ligament (vesico fascia).

### Descending Rectal Septa

The descending rectal septa run alongside the vagina from the undersurface of the cardinal ligament and its vaginal prolongation to the lateral surface of the rectum and thence to the sacrum. Each septum contains two layers, which are often fused (6). They divide the rectovaginal space from the lateral pararectal spaces.

### Retrorectal Space

The retrorectal space lies in the midline between the sacrum and the adventitia of the rectum, between the posterior portion of the rectal pillars. This space communicates with the pararectal spaces above the uterosacral ligaments.

### Pararectal Spaces

The paired pararectal spaces are only potential and are not preformed. They lie below the cardinal ligaments and its vaginal prolongations. The medial border is formed by the rectal pillar, the lateral by the levator ani. The posterior portions extend backward above the ischial spine but under the cardinal ligament to the anterior surface of the lateral part of the sacrum. Behind the cardinal ligament the independent caudal portion of each side becomes continuous with the cranial portion of the opposite side.

The upper rectum is surrounded by a single circular pararectal space. The boundaries of this space, formed by communication of two pararectal spaces and the retrorectal space, are formed laterally and below by the cranial surface of the levator, above and medially by the rectum, descending rectal septa, and the cardinal ligament. It is made L-shaped by the horizontal part below the cardinal ligament and the cranial and ascending portion behind the cardinal ligament. The cranial portion of the space is bounded anteriorly by the cardinal ligament and posteriorly by the lateral part of the sacrum. The sheaths of the great vessels of the pelvic wall form the lateral border; the pararectal space is bordered medially by the rectal septa and ureteric sheath. The inferior or horizontal division is bounded below by the levator ani, above by the cardinal ligament, and medially by the rectal septum. The two pararectal spaces communicate with each other posterior to the rectum, where there is no limiting membrane.

### Rectovaginal Septum

The rectovaginal septum is a distinct fibromuscular elastic tissue layer fused to the undersurface of the muscularis of the posterior vaginal wall to form the anterior border of the rectovaginal space. It was described by Tobin and Benjamin (60) as the "anterior layer of Denonvilliers' fascia" and was the subject of a special investigation by Milley and Nichols (34) in 143 specimens ranging in age from 8 fetal weeks to 100 years. It is a peritoneal fusion fascia, subject to wide individual variation in size, strength, and consistency, and is normally well formed by the 14th fetal week. In its fresh state, it is translucent and in the coronal plane parallels the sacral curvature, also curving posterolaterally to become indistinctly fused with the parietal endopelvic fascia (Fig. 1.25). The septum, representing fusion of the walls of the fetal peritoneal pouch, extends from the caudal margin of the cul-de-sac of Douglas to the proximal edge of the perineal body. It is a fixation point for the upper or proximal border of the perineal body and is of considerable clinical significance, for if this attachment to the perineal body is avulsed, the anterior rectal wall may bulge with the straining of defecation, and the deflection of the fecal stream during normal defecation may be abolished, with resulting constipation. Midline laceration of the septum from excessive stretching during labor may cause obliteration of the rectovaginal space. Such pathologic fusion of anterior rectal wall to posterior vaginal wall decreases the effectiveness of defecation. Failure of this normal fusion to develop during early life may produce congenital enterocele with its inherent weaknesses. It is because of the strength contributed by the septum to the perineal body in the midline that spontaneous obstetric lacerations above the perineal body are more likely to occur in the posterolateral vaginal fornix than in the midline. Histologically, this septum consists of a fibromuscular elastic layer of dense collagen, abundant smooth muscle, and coarse elastic fibers, elements that are best demonstrated by specialized staining (Fig. 1.26). The surgical significance of reconstruction of this layer will be discussed in Chapter 12.

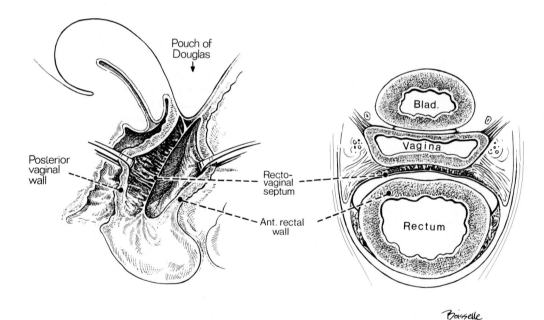

**Figure 1.25.** The rectovaginal septum is shown. Sections showing the partly dissected rectoseptum. It extends from the pouch of Douglas to the perineal body and forms the anterior surface of the rectovaginal space. Its adherence to the posterior vaginal wall is illustrated along with its posterolateral curve. (Adapted from Nichols DH, Milley PS: Surgical significance of the rectovaginal septum. *Am J Obstet Gynecol* 108:217, 1970; reproduced with permission of CV Mosby.)

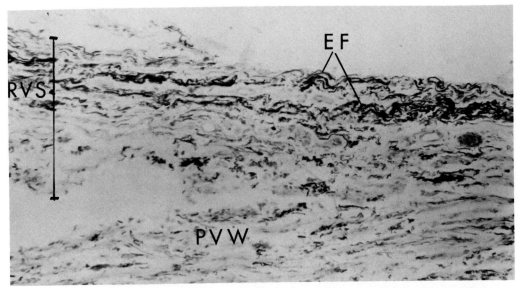

**Figure 1.26.** Sagittal histologic section through area of junction between the rectovaginal septum *(RVS)* and the posterior vaginal wall *(PVW)* is shown. The two have been separated at the *left* of the photograph by blunt dissection. Note the coarseness of the elastic fibers *(EF)* in the septum compared with those in the vagina. Orcein stain; X 106. (From Milley PS, Nichols DH: The human rectovaginal septum. *Anat Rec* 163:443–447, 1969; reproduced with permission of the Wistar Institute Press.)

### Rectovaginal Space

The functional independence of the posterior vaginal wall with respect to the anterior rectal wall depends upon maintenance of the relatively avascular midline rectovaginal space, which permits the two organ walls to slide with considerable independence over one another. The anterior wall of this space is formed by the rectovaginal septum, which is attached to the posterior vaginal wall and the fat-covered rectal adventitia. The lateral walls are separated from the pararectal spaces by a descending rectal septum (rectouterine) on each side. The roof is the peritoneum and rectouterine peritoneal pouch (cul-de-sac of Douglas), and the inferior margin of this space is the perineal body.

The rectovaginal space ends where the levator ani muscles are attached to the cranial portion of the perineal body (Fig. 1.27). This coincides with the caudal attachment of the fascia of Denonvilliers to the perineal body. The relative freedom with which the vaginal wall can move independently of both bladder and rectum undoubtedly facilitates the type of segmental damage discussed in regard to the etiology of prolapse. This is damage concentrated principally on the lateral supports of the vagina, which permits eversion of the vault of the vagina with the development of enterocele.

### Retrorectal Space

The retrorectal space lies in the midline between the sacrum and the adventitia of the rectum between the posterior portion of the rectal pillars. This space communicates with the pararectal spaces above the uterosacral ligaments. An extension of Richter and Frick's (53) third-dimensional concept of these connective tissue planes and spaces is presented in Figure 1.28.

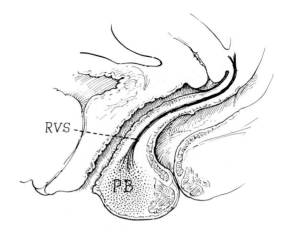

**Figure 1.27.** Sagittal section shows the relationship between the rectovaginal septum *(RVS)* as it blends with the superior border of the perineal body *(PB)*.

## Cleavage Planes

There are natural and potential cleavage planes (49) between organ systems in the female pelvis that, under certain stressful situations, permit segmental avulsion and pathologic sliding of one or more organ systems upon another. Although the existence of these specific segments of potential damage was well known to David B. Hart (23), their existence was demonstrated in the elegant and complex work of Halban and Tandler (22). It remained for Dickinson (11,

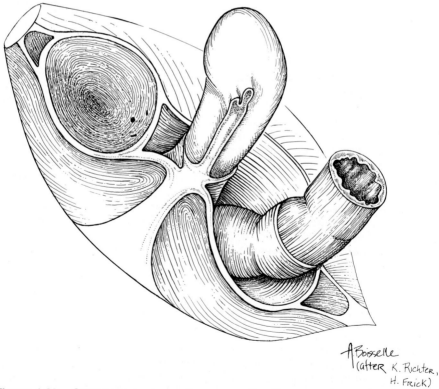

**Figure 1.28.** Stereograph shows the connective tissue septae and paravaginal spaces in relation to the bladder, uterus, and rectum. The spaces permit these three organs to function independently of one another (53).

13) to simplify and classify these characteristic segmental relationships and to draw meaningful conclusions concerning the importance of their role in cause, type, and selective treatment of genital prolapse.

We are in accord with Dickinson's concepts. Those which seem of practical significance may be summarized as follows:

1. There is a retropubic plane between the pubis and the urethra that is of clinical significance when the pubourethral ligament of the urogenital diaphragm becomes avulsed or stretched. This displacement permits the proximal urethra to rotate from its usual location, with consequent "wheeling"and rotational descent of the bladder neck (Fig. 1.29).

2. Another potential plane of cleavage exists between the posterior vaginal wall and the anterior wall of the rectum, i.e., in the rectovaginal space. The organ systems anterior to this space are, to a large extent, interconnected, especially in the upper two-thirds of the musculoelastic investments. There may be eversion of the upper vagina and cervix as a result of an over-stretchng of the cardinal and uterosacral ligaments. These structures together may first pull upon the anterior leaf of the cul-de-sac, causing a traction enterocele. As they slide over the anterior rectal wall, a sliding hernia is produced; if the hernia is progressive, it will pull upon the anterior rectal wall, aiding in the development of high rectocele. This development is further favored by the following mechanisms: high rectocele often coexists with enterocele because the peritoneal fusion fascia of Denonvilliers (rectovaginal septum) is missing above the lower point of the enterocele. This results in a loss of support to the anterior rectal wall and the posterior vaginal wall. Whenever a high rectocele is present, enterocele should be suspected. Its presence or absence should be determined with certainty; if

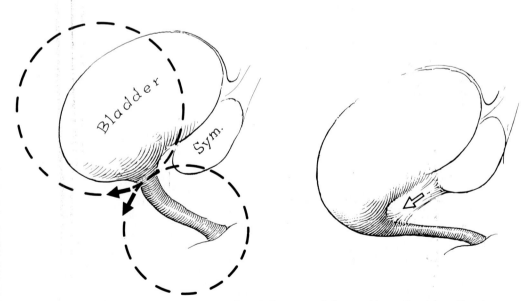

**Figure 1.29.** "Wheeling" or rotational descent of the vesicourethral junction is noted on the *left.* This may result at rest from pathologic elongation of the pubourethral ligaments, as shown on the *right,* with obliteration of the posterior vesicourethral angle forming one contributing factor for urinary stress incontinence.

found, repair should be accomplished as a separate step during high posterior colporrhaphy.

## References

1. Bacon HE, Ross ST: *Atlas of Operative Technic: Anus, Rectum and Colon.* St. Louis, CV Mosby, 1954.
2. Berglas B, Rubin IC: Study of the supportive structures of the uterus by levator myography. *Surg Gynecol Obstet* 97:677–692, 1953.
3. Bonney V: The sustentacular apparatus of the female genital canal, the displacements from the yielding of its several components and their appropriate treatment. *J Obstet Gynaecol Br Emp* 45:328, 1914.
4. Campbell RM: The anatomy and histology of the sacrouterine ligaments. *Am J Obstet Gynecol* 59:1–12, 1950.
5. Contamin R, Leger P: Anatomic principles of major gynecologic surgery: Abdominal hysterectomy. *Int J Gynaecol Obstet* 8:522–525, 1970.
6. Contamin R, Bernard F, Ferrieux J: L'Hysterectomie vaginale intrafasciale avec reconstitution de la paroi vaginale posterieure. *Gynecologie Pratique* 23:17–30, 1972.
7. Courtney H: Anatomy of the pelvic diaphragm and anal rectal musculature as related to sphincter preservation in anal rectal surgery. *Am J Surg* 79:155, 1950.
8. Critchley HOD, Dixon JS, Gosling JA: Comparative study of the periurethral and perianal parts of the human levator ani muscle. *Urol Int* 35:226–232, 1980.
9. Curtis AH, Anson BJ, McVay CB: The anatomy of the pelvic and urogenital diaphragms in relation to urethrocele and cystocele. *Surg Gynecol Obstet* 68:161–166, 1939.
10. DeLancey JO: Correlative study of paraurethral anatomy. *Obstet Gynecol* 68:91–97, 1986.
11. Dickinson RL: The vagina as a hernial canal. *Am J Obstet Dis Wom* 22:692–697, 1889.
12. Dickinson RL: Studies of the levator ani muscle. *Am J Obstet Dis Wom* 22:897–917, 1889.
13. Dickinson RL: Genital prolapse: Its operative correction based on a new study of cleavage lines and sliding segments. *Am J Obstet Dis Wom* 17:17–35, 1910.
14. Enhorning G: Simultaneous recording of intravesical and intrurethral pressure. *Acta Chir Scand* 276:4–12, 1961.
15. Eycleshymer AC, Schoemaker DM: *A Cross Section in Anatomy.* New York, Appleton-Century-Crofts, 1983, p 5.
16. Ferguson WH: New functional repair of post hysterectomy vaginal vault prolapse with Marlex mesh. *Am Surg* 30:227, 1964.
17. Fothergill WE: On the pathology and the operative treatment of displacements of the pelvic viscera. *J Obstet Gynaecol Br Emp* 13:410–419, 1907.
18. Funt MI, Thompson JD, Birch H: Normal vaginal axis. *South Med J* 71:1534–1536, 1978.
19. Gosling JA: The structure of the female lower urinary tract and pelvic floor. *Urol Clin North Am* 12:207–214, 1985.
20. Grant JCB: *An Atlas of Anatomy,* ed 2, Baltimore, Williams & Wilkins, 1943, p 123.
21. Hadra BE: *Lesions of the Vagina and Pelvic Floor.* Records, Philadelphia, McMullin & Co, 1888.
22. Halban J, Tandler J: *Anatomie und Atiologie der Genitalprolapse beim Weibe.* Vienna and Leipzig, Wilhelm Braumuller, 1907.
23. Hart DB: *The Structural Anatomy of the Female Pelvic Floor.* Edinburgh, Maclachlan and Stewart, 1880.
24. Henry MM, Swash M: *Coloproctology and the Pelvic floor.* London, Butterworths, 1985.
25. Hofmeister FJ, Wolfgram RC: Methods of demonstrating measurement relationships between vaginal hysterectomy ligatures and the ureters. *Am J Obstet Gynecol* 83:938–948, 1962.
26. Huisman AB: Aspects on the anatomy of the female urethra with special reference to urinary continence. In Ulmster U (ed): *Contributions to Gynecology and Obstetrics,* 10:1–31, Basel, Karger, 1983.
27. Hutch JA: *Anatomy and Physiology of the Bladder, Trigone and Urethra.* New York, Appleton-Century-Crofts, 1972.
28. Joachimovits R: *Das Beckenausgangsgebiet und Perineum des Weibes.* Vienna, Willhelm Maudrich, 1969.
29. Lennard-Jones JE: Constipation. In Henry MM, Swash M (eds): *Coloproctology and the pelvic floor.* London, Butterworths, 1985.
30. Luisi M: *Anatomica Clinica Ginecologica.* Milano, E Ambrosiana, 1978, p 64.
31. Luschka HV: *Die Anatomie des Menschen.* Tubingen, H. Lauppsche Buchhandlung, 1869, pp 143–149.
32. Magdi L: Obstetric injuries of the perineum. *J Obstet Gynaecol Br Commonw* 49:687–700, 1942.
33. Mengert WF: Mechanics of uterine support and position. *Am J Obstet Gynecol* 31:775, 1936.
34. Milley PS, Nichols DH: A correlative investigation of the human rectovaginal septum. *Anat Rec* 163:443, 1969.
35. Milley PS, Nichols DH: The relationship between the pubourethral ligaments and the urogenital diaphragm in the hu-

man female. *Anat Rec* 170:281–283, 1971.

36. Morgan KF Jr: Casts of the vagina as a means of evaluation of structural changes and treatment. *Calif Med* 94:30–32, 1961.
37. Muellner SR: The etiology of stress incontinence. *Surg Gynecol Obstet* 88:237–242, 1949.
38. Muellner SR: The anatomies of the female urethra. *Obstet Gynecol* 14:429, 1959.
39. Nichols DH, Milley PS, Randall CL: Significance of restoration of normal vaginal depth and axis. *Obstet Gynecol* 36:251–256, 1970.
40. O'Leary JA: Ventrofixation in the management of vaginal vault prolapse. *Surg Gynecol Obstet* 120:1296, 1965.
41. Paramore RH: The supports-in-chief of the female pelvic viscera. *J Obstet Gynecol Br Emp* 13:391–409, 1908.
42. Paramore RH: Some further considerations on the supports of the female pelvic viscera, in which the intra-abdominal pressure is still further defined. *J Obstet Gynecol Br Emp* 14:173–189, 1908.
43. Parks AG: Anorectal incontinence. *Proc Roy Soc Med* 68:21, 1975.
44. von Peham H, Amreich J: *Operative Gynecology*. Philadelphia, JB Lippincott, 1934.
45. Power RMH: Embryological development of the levator ani muscle. *Am J Obstet Gynecol* 55:367–381, 1948.
46. Quinby WC: The anatomy and blood vessels of the pelvis. In Meigs JV (ed): *Surgical Treatment of Cancer of the Cervix.* New York, Grune & Stratton, 1954, p 32.
47. Range RL, Woodburne RT: The gross and microscopic anatomy of the transverse cervical ligament. *Am J Obstet Gynecol* 90:460–467, 1964.
48. Ranney AL: *The Topographical Relations of the Female Pelvic Organs*. New York, Wood, 1883, pp 107–110.
49. Ricci JV, Thom CH, Kron WL: Cleavage planes in reconstructive vaginal plastic surgery. *Am J Surg* 76:354–363, 1948.
50. Ricci JV: *The Cystocele in America*. New York, Blakiston, 1950.
51. Richter K: Die physiologische topographic der weiblichen genitale in moderner sicht. *Zentralbl Gynackol* 89:1258, 1967.
52. Richter K: Lebendige anagomie der vagina. *Geburtshilfe Frauenheilkd* 26:1213, 1966.
53. Richter K, Frick H: Die anatomie der fascia pelvis visceralis aus didaktischer sicht. *Geburtshilfe Frauenheilkd* 45:282–287, 1985.
54. Smout CFV, Jacoby F, Lillie EW: *Gynecological and Obstetrical Anatomy*. Baltimore, Williams & Wilkins, 1969.
55. Studdiford WC: The involuntary muscle fibers of the pelvic floor. *Am J Obstet* 60:23, 1909.
56. Sturmdorf A: *Gynoplastic Technology*. Philadelphia, FA Davis, 1919, pp 109–114.
57. Tandler J: *Lehrbuch der Systematischen Anatomie,* vol 1. Leipzig, Vogel, 1926, p 370–371.
58. Thompson P: *The Myology of the Pelvic Floor.* London, McCorquodale, 1899.
59. Tilney F, Pike FH: Muscular coordination experimental studies in its relation to the cerebellum. *Arch Neurol Psychiatry* 13:289–334, 1925.
60. Tobin CE, Benjamin JA: Anatomical and surgical restudy of Denonvilliers' fascia. *Surg Gynecol Obstet* 80:373–388, 1945.
61. Uhlenhuth E: *Problems in the Anatomy of the Pelvis*. Philadelphia, JB Lippincott, 1953, p 161.
62. Wendell-Smith CP: The homologues of the puborectalis muscle. *J Anat Aust and NZ* 98:489, 1964.
63. Wilson PD, Dixon JS, Brown ADG, et al: Posterior pubourethral ligaments in normal and genuine stress incontinent women. *J Urol* 130:802–805, 1982.
64. Zacharin R: The suspensory mechanism of the female urethra. *J Anat* 97:423–427, 1963.

# CHAPTER 2

# Reduction of Maternal Injuries Associated with Childbirth

In the annals of medical and surgical literature, the reviewer expects to find record of cumulative knowledge which has been responsible for improving the effectiveness of treatment. In the practice of obstetrics and gynecology during the 20th century, however, preventative measures have proven to be most effective. Prophylactic measures now spare all but a very few American women from the life-threatening or disabling consequences of obstructed labor or obstetric hemorrhage and from the development of eclampsia or puerperal sepsis. In somewhat the same manner, it has been the measures employed to assure the earlier diagnosis of sexually transmitted disease and of carcinoma of the cervix, rather than more effective new treatments, which have been largely responsible for improving the gynecologic health of American women during this century.

A noteworthy omission, however, has been evident in the literature relating to the specialty of obstetrics and gynecology during the 20th century (8). Stated most simply, there seems to have been a lack of interest or documentation indicating study of the manner in which human parturition can be managed so as to minimize anatomic injuries in the maternal reproductive tract. Although the effectiveness of preventative measures has been generally recognized, obstetric practices seem to have neglected opportunities to initiate more effective efforts to lessen the maternal injury and subsequent disability possible and not infrequently attributable to the conduct of childbirth. It would seem as though there has been a rather general acceptance of the probability of injury and the need for subsequent repair of maternal tissues as unavoidable consequences of human parturition.

During the years while surgical repair of varying types and degrees of maternal injury has been thoroughly described, relatively little has been spoken or written to suggest techniques and procedures recommended to reduce the frequency and extent of maternal injuries. In the literature of the United Statese, there have been a few noteworthy exceptions. Gustafson (5), publishing a review from a clinician's point of view, entitled his 1940 report "The Prevention and Treatment of Cystocele in the Reproductive Age." He included several paragraphs in which variations in the management of labor and delivery were related to the maternal injuries that had been recognized postpartum. The well-documented study of Curtis and Anson (1) published in 1942, however, did not indicate major consideration of the factors seemingly accounting for the injuries of maternal soft tissues, which they described. Among the earlier studies, the report of Power (7) contributed importantly to the obstetrician's and gynecologist's knowledge of the anatomy often involved in the maternal injuries recognized after childbirth.

We believe the first significant objectively documented study comparing the management of labor and delivery with subsequent evidences of maternal soft tissue injuries was reported by Gainey (3) in 1943. No equally contributory study appeared in the American literature until Gainey's second report in 1955 (4), at which time documented evidences of specific injuries were compared in two series of 1,000 patients each. Each patient in both series had been delivered and the postpartum evidences of injury had been assessed personally by the author. There was, however, an essential difference in the management of labor in the two series. Episiotomy had been employed in the first group only when there was maternal or fetal indication—either to avoid "impending" perineal laceration or to hasten delivery because of "fetal distress." In the second series, in every instance, episiotomy had been done at the outlet station of the presenting part, after which all deliveries had been terminated by low or outlet forceps, except 27 instances that included forceps rotation and 40 breech presentations delivered as "breech assists," with forceps to the aftercoming head.

In Gainey's 1955 report (5), Table 2.1 provides evidence that there was significant protection of the vagina, urogenital diaphragm, and perineum when episiotomy was performed and delivery of the fetal head was controlled by "outlet" or "prophylactic" forceps. It is our conviction that Gainey's two reports should be studied carefully by every obstetrician-in-training, and not because of the suggested virtues of so-called "routine episiotomy and pro-

**Table 2.1**

**Comparison of Pelvic Soft Tissue Damage Between Primiparous Obstetric Patients Without Laceration and Those with Episiotomy**[a]

|                        | SERIES 1                                              | SERIES 2                                           |
| ---------------------- | ----------------------------------------------------- | -------------------------------------------------- |
|                        | Para I without Laceration (209 cases) (%)             | Para I with Laceration (590 cases) (%)             |
| Detached urethra       | 6                                                     | 5.6                                                |
| Relaxation             | 9                                                     | 1.9                                                |
| Left pubococcygeus     | 10                                                    | 1.9                                                |
| Right pubococcygeus    | 19                                                    | 6.4                                                |
| Left iliococcygeus     | 3                                                     | 0                                                  |
| Right iliococcygeus    | 2                                                     | 1.2                                                |
| Total levator atrophy  | 27                                                    | 11.2                                               |
| Detached urethra       | 6                                                     | 5.6                                                |
| Relaxation             | 28                                                    | 10.3                                               |
| Anovaginal damage      | 29                                                    | 1.2                                                |
| Cystocoele             | 15                                                    | 6.1                                                |
| Obliteration of fornix | 17                                                    | 3.6                                                |
| Rectocoele             | 7                                                     | <1                                                 |
| Detached R-V septum    | 8                                                     | <1                                                 |
| Anal sphincter damage  | 0                                                     | <1                                                 |

[a] From Gainey HL: Postpartum observation of pelvic tissue damage: Further studies. *Am J Obstet Gynecol* 70:800, 1955.

phylactic forceps.'' Rather, Gainey's studies illustrate the ability an obstetrician can develop to predict, assess, and record the damage that labor and delivery may do to maternal soft parts. It is evident that the concerned obstetrician may develop the ability to relate which preceded maternal injuries. The benefits of episiotomy presume a knowledgeable anatomically correct repair of the episiotomy.

Review of the obstetric literature as well as the annual reports of the teaching services suggests that most of the residency training programs in this country have not been teaching or encouraging the Gainey type of objective and systematic postdelivery appraisal of maternal injuries. Significant studies were made and reported, first by DeLee in 1920 (2) and by Gainey in 1943 and 1955. The literature indicates little effort, however, to prove or disprove the significance of the factors that those observers had recognized and reported. Their studies still await either confirmation or denial based on objective observations at least as well documented as the data DeLee and Gainey presented. Is the occurrence of the genital dysfunction due to maternal injury and the discomforts women experience because of pelvic relaxation of little or no concern to the obstetrician? Is the obstetrician-gynecologist justified in concluding "if it bothers her we can certainly do a satisfactory repair whenever she wants it done"? Such a willingness to disregard the possible effectiveness of prophylactic measures would not seem compatible with usual professional points of view. We believe there are indeed other factors that have accounted for the undeniable fact that the "teachers" of obstetric practice at the undergraduate, graduate, and continuing education levels have, for the most part, failed to emphasize how labor and delivery can best be managed in order to avoid or minimize maternal tissue damage.

For generations dedicated teachers of obstetrics have emphasized and personally practiced conservative obstetrics. A virtually universal willingness to perpetuate the conviction that "nature does it best" has made certain that each medical student and resident-in-training becomes sufficiently experienced in the observation of spontaenous delivery that they will recognize and remember the factors accounting for the abilities of the female to deliver normally, while at the same time appreciating the satisfactions of the "natural" delivery of a normal child (9).

We believe obstetricians and gynecologists might well consider Gainey's method as a reliable means of recording injuries and improving the results of the management of labor and delivery. It seems evident, however, that DeLee's teachings and the documentation in Gainey's studies were not published primarily as efforts to establish guidelines for the management of each stage of labor in order to minimize maternal injury. Both observers directed their attention, or at least seem to have directed their reports, to the obstetrician's management of the delivery itself, as related to the consequences of that management for mother and child. Although not intending to detract from the basic importance of DeLee's and Gainey's observations, we would suggest that the vaunted reliability of today's data collection systems might well be utilized in efforts to determine the relation of the conduct of both the first and second stages of labor with the eventual degrees and sites of maternal injury.

We believe it quite possible that too few questions have been raised in regard to the management of the first stage of labor. Operative interference seems no longer to be considered except in terms of delivery by cesarean section. Such procedures as Voorhees bags to tamponade intrapartum bleeding, Duhrssen's incisions to expedite completion of the first stage, or vaginal hysterotomy to effect delivery before completion of the first stage are, fortunately, no longer considered useful techniques to be learned by the obstetrician-in-training. On the other hand, much attention is now given to the quality of myometrial action during the first stage of labor, in terms of the effectiveness of uterine contractions. Factors accounting for a satisfactorily progressing first stage of labor are not within the consideration of this review except as those factors can be shown to relate to the degree of soft tissue injuries and the subsequent development of anything from a minor degree of relaxation to a disabling degree of procidentia. We would exclude, of course, from the gynecologist's concerns in regard to the effects of labor and delivery on maternal soft parts such immediately evident injuries as may account for immediate and often an alarming amount of bleeding. When laceration, evulsion, or inversion occurs, each requires the obstetrician's immediate attention. On the other hand, the types of obstetric injury not usually evident until months or years after trauma occurs are slow to develop. It is this type of maternal injury, the years afterward type of obstetric damage, with which the gynecologic surgeon usually gains an extensive experience.

## FACTORS ACCOUNTING FOR UTERINE PROLAPSE

One woman, often after a single pregnancy and the not obviously difficult labor and delivery of an average-sized child, may, within a very few years, develop a virtually complete prolapse of the uterus, with perhaps equally evident eversion and prolapse of the vagina. Another woman of the same age, in no better general health, after the delivery of one or several large babies, develops no demonstrable prolapse of the uterus and has surprisingly well-supported vaginal walls and a well-preserved perineum. Why do the forces of "normal labor" produce extensive injuries in one woman and no demonstrable damage to another woman whose bony pelvis and soft tissue also seemed adequate, comparable, and normal? We know there can be a neurogenic or a congenital factor, because an occasional woman, never pregnant and having no history of unusual trauma or weight bearing, will develop uterine and vaginal prolapse. Such a "predisposition" has, of course, been noted in victims of multiple sclerosis and in association with spina bifida occulta. In a majority of instances, however, only the trauma of labor and delivery seems to suggest an etiology, and so the question: Why prolapse later in some patients and not in so many others who were presumably exposed to the same forces of labor and delivery?

An obvious first suspicion suggests that not all labors involve the same stresses and strains on tissues supporting the uterus, cervix, and vagina. Factors accounting for the resistance offered may be as important as the factors that produce the strength and effectiveness of uterine contractions. As we better understand both we may gain increasingly reliable means of controlling or regulating the strength of contractions and the resolution of resistance.

Both the means of decreasing resistance by encouraging relaxation and the means of augmenting the forces of labor by the accurately regulated infusion of an oxytocic are now universally available. Both are controllable and may be helpful to mother and child when administered with the all-important vehicle of clinical judgment. Psychologic preparation for labor as well as sedation, analgesia, or regional blocking may all be effective aids to the progress of labor in addition to helping relieve the pains of childbirth. However, fatigue, impaired morale, and tissue depletion decrease tissue response and elasticity, and, when oversolicitous sedation is given, labor may be harmfully prolonged.

Well-meaning but ill-advised coaching by "supporting" personnel, whether an apprehensive but fatigued friend or the less personally concerned but "let's get it over with" type of labor room attendant, may result in increased maternal injury.

Fortunately, the majority of patients in labor do not seem to develop a desire to bear down with their uterine contractions until the presenting part begins to distend the pelvic floor. Most attendants at parturition have no difficulty visualizing the damage threatened when the woman in active labor, in ill-advised but understandably desperate efforts to "get it over with," bears down as forcefully as she can before her cervix is fully dilated and before the presenting part can readily descend in the vagina in response to the pressures being applied. When such premature bearing down does occur, certainly the tissues supporting both the fundus and the cervix in normal anatomic relationships with the bony pelvis and adjacent viscera must either succeed in resisting the woman's efforts to "deliver her uterus with the baby in it," or her efforts will result in considerably more stretching and detachment of uterine supporting tissues than would have occurred had there been no bearing down effort before the cervix was fully dilated. By the same mechanism, a disporportionately large fetus, and particularly a poorly flexed, unfavorably presenting vertex or breech (that must mold or adapt to the passageway before descent can occur), may account for the transmission of voluntary bearing down efforts on the patient's part to effectively increased stress and stretch on uterine support. Whenever descent of the fetus is not occurring, voluntary maternal efforts only result in increased stress on the tissues normally supporting the uterus and vagina within the maternal pelvis. It is not difficult to visualize and understand the mechanism by which the forces of labor, if not directed by knowledgeable advice in accord with intelligent management, can result in injuries predisposing the patient to the later development of uterine prolapse.

## INJURIES OF VAGINAL WALL SUPPORT

The mechanism of injury that results in the detachment of vaginal wall from its supporting tissue does not seem to be so generally understood. It is simple enough to recognize that overdistention of the vaginal walls during the birth of a large fetus may leave the vaginal walls stretched beyond the ability of tone-regaining involutionary processes to restore to a nonjredundant caliber. It is evident that a cystocele and/or rectocele would be a likely result.

The vagina can be damaged obstetrically by a single event or a combination of two events. Damage to the elasticity and integrity of the vaginal wall itself from overstretching by the presenting part of the fetus is one event. The other is stretching or avulsion of the lateral connective tissue segments that attach the vagina to the pelvic side walls (Fig. 2.1).

It is equally easy to visualize that laceration of the vaginal membrane could be expected when the forces making for distention are unevenly applied, as when a poorly flexed vertex or a compound presentation results in maximal distention of only one segment within the circumference of the vagina. The occurrence of so-called superior sulcus tears is perhaps the best example of a laceration of vaginal wall due to maximal need for or maximal resistance to distention in a segment of vaginal circumference.

Laceration or the effects of overdistention are readily visualized and understood. If they represented the extent of the vaginal injuries so frequently due to childbirth, repair of the damage would be no problem, and the results of vaginal repairs would be uniformly good. The more significant types of vaginal injury, however, and the ones not so readily and commonly visualized are the result of detachment of the vaginal wall from the supporting tissues accounting for the usual relation of the vagina to the bony pelvis and to the adjacent rectum, uterus, and bladder.

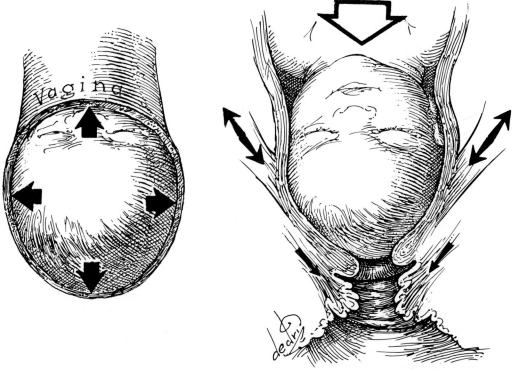

**Figure 2.1.** Types of cystocele are illustrated. A distention cystocele produced by overstretching of the walls of the vagina itself during childbirth is most often related to long labor or the development of some pressure necrosis, or occasionally to a short precipitous labor in which distention was so rapid that the vagina was not given time for elastic adaptation and distention. Defective connective tissue and elastic tissue in a wall of the vagina may also be a factor. Progression is usually slow until accentuated by the nutritional changes after the menopause, when estrogen withdrawal seems associated with more rapid progression. This type of cystocele, seen in the drawing to the left, can be recognized by the lack of rugal folds. A translocation or displacement cystocele is associated with the vaginal descent that occurs as a result of an overstretching or attentuation of the lateral connective tissue support to the vagina, illustrated in the drawing to the right. The lateral attachments of vagina and cervix are being stretched as they are pushed in front of the baby's head. In this traction type of cystocele the rugal folds of the anterior and posterior walls of the vagina are about the same size as those on the lateral vaginal walls.

To understand and anticipate the vaginal injuries commonly associated with parturition, the attendants should recognize that normally, and certainly in the labor of the primipara, at full dilation of the cervix the presenting part does not at that time emerge from the cervix and, for the first time, begin to descend into and through the vagina. Rather, the fully engaged presenting part, almost completely covered by thinned, beginning to dilate cervix, has in all probability occupied the upper third to half of the vagina for 2 or more weeks. As a result distention of the upper vagina, with accommodation of the engaging vertex or breech, has occurred very gradually, so gradually in fact that the patient may not be aware of the descent taking place until she notices a new awareness of heaviness, low backache, and at times rectal pressure, while at the same time breathing becomes somewhat easier, for ''lightening'' has occurred. Although such positioning or settling of the presenting part, and particularly the descent of the presenting part into the upper vagina, is not equally characteristic of relationships as the multigravida approaches term, such gradual descent of the presenting part and gradual dilation of the upper vagina does usually occur in the primigravida days or weeks before painful contractions (labor) begin. With the onset of effective labor, we should, therefore, visualize contractions as tending to draw the cervix up and over the presenting part, while the station of the vertex or breech may change relatively little during the process. It is important to recognize that the presenting part is not being pushed out of the cervix. More accurately, the cervix is being drawn up over the vertex or breech, during which time the presenting part will remain in the already dilated upper vagina.

It is desirable for the attendant to recognize why vaginal injury is more likely to occur in the multipara who experiences a hard but short labor, than in the primigravida who begins a labor of 8 or more hours' duration with the presenting part well engaged. After the initial labor of the primipara, when we might expect to find evidence that parturition had been most damaging to the vaginal walls and vaginal supporting tissues, examination several weeks postpartum often reveals the contour of the upper vaginal walls to be well preserved and the vaginal fornices well supported.

An equally surprising degree of preservation of vaginal caliber and fornices should not be expected, however, if the primigravida had gone into labor with the presenting part not engaged. With such a patient, should the cervix be approaching full dilation with the presenting part still not engaged, anticipating disproportion, abnormality, or malpresentation, delivery by cesarean section would probably be elected. Although there might prove to have been no disproportion or abnormality to have jeopardized the fetus, cesarean section under such circumstances would probably have preserved the integrity of the mother's pelvic supporting tissues and spared her from the development of a prolapse and eventually an extensive gynecologic repair.

When an unengaged presenting part begins to descend rapidly into the vagina as second stage pains begin, similar damage may occur whether the fascial planes are congenitally weak or unusually strong. Relatively weak or inadequate fascial attachments may be shredded by the forces of labor until there is so little remaining support that the vagina will eventually appear detached, redundant, and "prolapsing." In other instances, however, fascial support of the upper vagina is so strong as to actually resist dilation of the vagina by the presenting part. Under such circumstances the force of uterine contractions may tend to push an undilating, contraction ring-like segment of vagina ahead of the presenting part (Fig. 2.2). If this situation persists the forces of labor will be exerted, not so much on distending or dilating the vagina as upon the supporting fascia that is trying to hold that segment of vagina in its normal position within the maternal pelvis. In either case, after postpartum involution is complete, examination will show evidence that the tissues supporting the vagina are no longer able to maintain the concavity of the superior vagina fornices. Such redundant vaginal walls sooner or later give way to clinically evident vaginal eversion, often with associated uterine prolapse.

At the time of postpartum examination, as a rule, if there is evident descent and beginning prolapse of the uterus and cervix, the vaginal fornices may appear to be obliterated, with the vaginal walls bulging down along the cervix. When postpartum examination does reveal a lack of upper vaginal support, the examiner should realize that detachment of the upper vagina is likely to have occurred coincident with disruption (or at least a noninvoluting degree of lengthening) of uterine and cervical support. Under such circumstances,

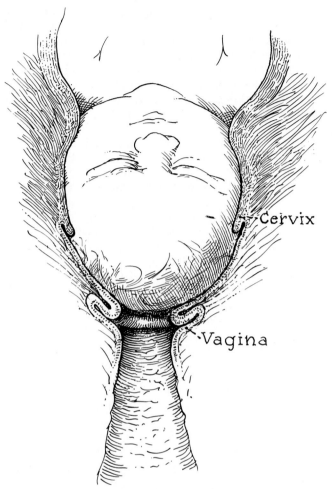

**Figure 2.2.** As the presenting part descends through the vagina in addition to the marked thinning out of the vaginal wall due to the very considerable increase in the diameter of the vagina, more potentially significant changes may be occurring in the connective tissue strands that normally maintain the position, relationships, and contour of the upper vagina. Effective uterine contractions serve to draw the lower uterine segment and cervix up over the presenting part. Such cervical dilation may occur without earlier or simultaneous descent of the presenting part into the upper vagina. When this occurs an abrupt or precipitous descent of the presenting part into an undilated vagina may result in a segment of undilated vaginal wall being pushed into an intusseception-like doubling of the thickness of the vaginal wall. A segment of vaginal wall so thickened results in still greater resistance to further descent of the presenting part.

prolapse to procidentia can be expected eventually to become evident although, fortunately, such an extreme degree of supporting tissue injury does not often occur.

## INJURIES OF UPPER VAGINAL SUPPORT

The obstetrician-gynecologist soon learns that prolapse may not develop and the upper vagina may appear well supported with well-preserved fornices, yet the patient may develop a marked cystocele or rectocele or both. As a matter of fact, at the time of postpartum examination, the obstetrician-gynecologist will, at times, not be surprised to find this type of injury in the para I whose obstetric history records the onset of labor after the vertex had been deeply engaged for 2 weeks and her completely effaced cervix was noted to be 2 cm. dilated at the onset of labor. Under such circumstances, the upper vagina had been slowly dilated and descent of the presenting part was not subjecting the vaginal supporting tissue to the stresses developed when a presenting vertex begins to descend rapidly through an undilated upper vagina. While it may be true that prolapse, cystocele, and rectocele are often noticeable in the same patient and there may be no history or earlier record to suggest that one type of relaxation occurred before the other, it is equally true that a rather marked cystocele or rectocele or both may develop without significant descensus or prolapse of the uterus.

It should be emphasized in the teaching of obstetric practice that voluntary effort (the traditional bearing down usually encouraged throughout the second stage of labor) can appreciably increase the type of vaginal injury that is most to be avoided: the overstretching and disruption of the connective tissue that normally account for the concavity of the upper vaginal fornices and the support of the upper vaginal walls in their normal relationship to the bony pelvis, bladder, and rectum. Admittedly, bearing-down effort usually seems beneficial to progress in the second stage of labor and is certainly of psychologic importance to both the parturient and those attending her. However, no one can predict in advance, and very few can determine during labor, whether such voluntary effort is actually supporting and abetting descent of the presenting part through dilating, relatively nonresisting vaginal walls. If there could be assurance that the vaginal walls were in fact offering little resistance to dilation, we would agree that voluntary bearing-down effort should be encouraged as soon as the cervix is fully dilated and descent begins. Under such circumstances the presenting part, with a contraction of the uterus, would tend to descend readily through the upper vaginal segment, especially if the upper vagina had previously been gradually dilated during engagement (preceding the onset of labor). Too often, however, the vaginal walls have not been so gradually dilated before the onset of the second stage, and then even with second stage contractions, the vagina does not distend adequately very readily and may, in effect, actually be resisting dilation and, therefore, be resisting descent of the vertex or breech. Vaginal resistance is likely to account for a noticeable lack of progress during the earlier part of the second stage, as illustrated.

Evidence of vaginal resistance to dilation and resistance to descent of the presenting part may at times be recognized by the formation of a ring-like segment of vaginal membrane, perhaps incompletely around the circumference of the vertex or breech. With each contraction and bearing-down effort, this resisting ring of vagina remains ahead of the presenting vertex or breech. Obviously, the force behind the descending fetus must be sufficient to cause the resisting segment of vagina to yield. Equally obvious, however, is hope that the force favoring descent will be just sufficient to result in dilation of the vaginal walls and not be so dominant as to push the undilated segment of vagina along ahead of the presenting part. When the resistance of the vagina does not permit dilation and progress with contractions, then adding appreciably (by voluntary bearing down) to the forces pushing the presenting vertex or breech against the ring of vagina that is resisting descent is likely to increase ischemia, lower tissue elasticity, and augment the development of the resisting, nondilating segment of vagina. As a result of this situation, the forces favoring descent of the presenting part, which normally account for vaginal dilation, begin to pull on the fascial fibers supporting the undilating segment of vaginal wall. Under such circumstances, descent can be accomplished only by pushing the undilated segment or ring of vaginal wall ahead of the presenting part.

In all probability, once a resisting contraction ring-like segment of vagina is pushed ahead of the presenting part, the damage to vaginal supporting tissue has been done. As the fascial attachments give way, the rim or roll of resisting, undilated vaginal wall irons out rapidly, and descent of the presenting part proceeds to the perineal stage. There is no evidence of the damage done until weeks later when postpartum examination reveals loss of vaginal rugae and a loss of the concavity of the superior vaginal fornices. The persistence of redundant vaginal wall and the development of eversion (with or without uterine prolapse) confirm that a satisfactory reattachment of vaginal wall support does not necessarily occur spontaneously during involutionary tightening of the pelvic fascial planes.

If those attending the parturient could determine the moment when disruption of the planes of connective tissue supporting the vaginal walls begins, there would seem to be a moment when one could do an episiotomy-like incision of the rolled-up, nondilating segment of vaginal wall. By letting the incised margins separate, the presenting part could descend without tearing or loosening the lateral attachment of the tissues supporting that portion of the vagina. Although such an incision should theoretically relieve the obstruction and solve the problem, for several reasons it would appear to be a procedure of no practical value.

Whether the parturient is a primagravida or a multipara, if she nears the second stage of labor with the presenting part not engaged, the segment of vagina likely to be torn from its attachments is the pericervical upper third, where fascial attachments are strongest but where an obstructing rim of undilating vagina would be difficult to visualize and incise. Of greater significance would be the probability that by the time development of a nondilating ridge of vagina became evident, the forces of labor would have begun shredding or loosening the connective tissue supporting that segment of vagina. To make matters worse, disruption of the fascial support of the vagina is the injury the obstetrician is most anxious to avoid. Detachment of the fascial support of the vagina in the posterior and lateral pericervical fornices is likely to result in a prolapsing vagina. This is a particularly undesirable result because repair will involve a technically difficult operation, with difficulty likely to be experienced in restoring vaginal support and depth while preserving a satisfactory vaginal caliber in an anatomically desirable axis (see Chapter 16).

Effective measures depend upon recognition of the possible consequences when the presenting part is not coming down into the vagina as full dilation of the cervix is near. At that time, the woman should be cautioned not to bear down until told to do so. Careful appraisal of the situation is particularly important. If uterine contractions at this stage are hard, long, and frequent, fetal oxygenation may be critical. Any type of regional blocking anesthesia is not likely to significantly alter the pattern of myometrial contractions. Precipitous second stage descent of the fetus and prompt delivery will give attendants opportunity to resuscitate the baby, but at a probable cost of considerable maternal "childbirth damage." Particularly if there is a tight perineal outlet, a partially asphyxiated baby will not tolerate prolonged compression of the head on the perineum. As previously emphasized, rapid descent of the presenting part through an undilated vagina is likely to damage vaginal supporting tissues to a degree resulting in eventual prolapse. If the problems have been anticipated and delivery by section can be done before vaginal supporting tissues are damaged, the baby will also benefit. There are very few situations where a cesarean is indicated (before an impending vaginal delivery can occur), but faced with an unengaged presenting part at full dilation with frequent and long uterine contractions, the risks to the baby and to the mother's pelvic supporting tissues warrant "interference." One cannot predict how much fetal damage may occur or how much maternal damage will eventually indicate repair, but we can recognize that under these circumstances an eventual prolapse can be prevented.

## PROPHYLAXIS

Perineal tissue vulnerability to permanent damage from stretching or tearing appears to correlate directly with the number and width of the striae gravidarum of the abdominal skin at term. When these are broad and coarse, laceration of the perineum is likely and early and adequate episiotomy is indicated; when few or absent the opposite may prevail (6).

When only cystocele and/or rectocele are evident, we believe it represents the easily visualized result of simple overdistention of the vaginal circumference to a degree that involuntary changes do not restore the original integrity of the vaginal wall. As a result, the thinned vaginal wall offers less than adequate resistance to any natural bulging tendency of the bladder and/or rectum to sacculate into the vaginal lumen. A precipitous type of rapid second stage labor can be readily visualized as likely to cause more damage to the musculofibrous layers responsible for the circumference of the vagina, and avoidance of a rapid tumultuous labor is desirable as a means of lessening injury of maternal soft tissues as well as a means of protecting the integrity of venous sinuses and the circulation of the fetal cranium. At the opposite end of the spectrum of myometrial behavior, when labor seems arrested in the second stage, or when disproportion impedes progress after full dilation of the cervix, relatively prolonged pressure of a large fetal vertex in the vagina may cause ischemia to a degree accounting for eventual focal necrosis within the musculoconnective tissue layer of the vaginal wall. A vaginal wall weakened by such effects of parturition may also eventually account for a cystocele and/or rectocele.

There are not many things the obstetrician may do during the perineal stage of labor to alter the relative stress of vaginal dilation on the anterior as compared to the posterior wall of the vagina. The most frequently indicated "interference" is the rotation of a peristently posterior vertex to an occiput anterior presentation. This rotation permits the normal mechanism of flexion and extension as the vertex emerges beneath the pubic arch to proceed with much less distention posteriorly than would have occurred during delivery of the head as an occiput posterior. No such alteration of presentation can be employed to protect the anterior vaginal wall and the tissue supporting the trigone and urethra. The performance of an adequate episiotomy has been shown to effectively lessen the degree of injuries to the supporting tissues in the anterior vaginal wall. In order for an episiotomy to be effective, however, it must be done before the perineum has held the extending vertex up against the infrapubic structures long enough to cause anterior wall damage.

It is possible to lessen the degree of vaginal wall injury that accounts for a cystocele or a rectocele by such management of labor as avoids tumultuous, precipitous labor or neglected arrest of progress in the second stage. Management will have a more evident effect on the site and degree of maternal injury, however, if our consideration is directed in efforts to minimize damage to uterine and vaginal wall supporting tissues, for it is here that significant damage could account for the eventual development of uterine prolapse and/or vaginal eversion.

We believe it should be a major objective of the obstetrician to recognize and minimize factors likely to cause stresses and possible damage to uterine and vaginal supporting tissues. It is evident that those attending the parturient should often encourage relaxation rather than voluntary effort, assuring the woman that her contractions will do the work, and avoid the old exhortation to "work with your pains and get it over with as quickly as possible." We believe it particularly important in the interests of preserving uterine supporting tissues and the integrity of vaginal support that the woman in labor be urged not to bear down and not to work with her pains at least until the cervix is known to be fully dilated and, almost equally important, not until the presenting part has traversed the upper vagina, descent is evident, and the presenting part is beginning to distend the perineum.

The shape of the bony pelvis significantly affects the probabilities of the types of maternal soft tissue injury that may occur (Fig. 2.3). Obstetricians have traditionally and consistently regarded the classical gynecoid type of bony pelvis as a desirable characteristic of the woman well suited to childbearing. It is also true, however, that the wide infrapubic arch characteristic of the

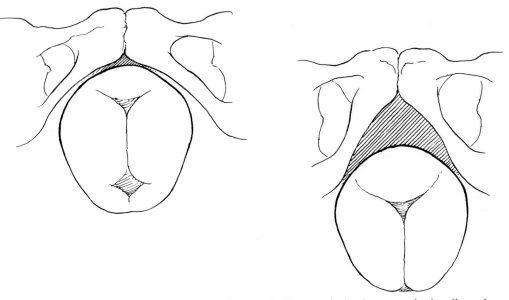

**Figure 2.3.**   The site and degree of obstetric damage in the lower vaginal walls and perineum may have been somewhat predetermined by the angle of the infrapubic arch. A widely arched gynecoid pelvis facilitates delivery of the baby's head but a wide bony arch provides little or no protection to the anterior vaginal wall and infrapubic tissues supporting the trigone and urethra, as shown in the drawing to the left. The relatively uncommon narrow angled arch of an android pelvis holds the descending and extending head away from the soft tissues supported above the anterior vaginal wall. A narrow bony arch forces the presenting part to require and cause greater distention posteriorly, as indicated in the drawing on the right. As a result when the bony pelvis is android the posterior vaginal wall, perineum, and rectum will be at greater risk, while relatively little damage should occur anteriorly.

gynecoid pelvis is frequently noted in the postpartum patient who shows extensive anterior wall damage, particularly a cystocele and urethrocele with, at times, little associated rectocele. At the time of postpartum examination of a patient with an android type of narrow infrapubic arch, however, one usually finds that the structures of the anterior vaginal wall have suffered relatively little damage, because the fetal head was obliged to distend the pelvic floor and perineum to a greater degree than the same sized vertex would have required to emerge through a gynecoid type of bony outlet. Consequently, lacerations of the pelvic floor and perineum are more frequent and urethroceles are less frequent when the patient has an android type of bony pelvis.

The obstetrician will know the dimensions and type of the bony pelvis and whether the management of labor and delivery is likely to involve consideration of disproportion. Some obstetricians will favor induction of labor before the fetal head becomes as large as it could become at full term. The majority, however, usually prefer to await the onset of labor, then appraise the situation and decide whether vaginal delivery or cesarean section is indicated.

Consideration of preventative measures suggests closely related questions. When is the optimal time to do an episiotomy? Does an episiotomy, done at an effective time in labor, actually help preserve the vaginal walls and particularly the integrity of the tissues supporting the uterus and vagina? Gainey's careful studies clearly demonstrate the effectiveness of episiotomy as a means of decreasing the extent of the soft tissue injuries that can be identified as the result of vaginal delivery. It is important to remember that the very considerable pressure that develops around the entire circumference of the vaginal wall as the presenting part dilates the vagina is increased when the integrity of the posterior vagina is reinforced by the musculature of the perineum. If the parturient has an android type of bony pelvis with a relatively narrow infrapubic arch, that bony structure holds the descending fetal vertex away from and lessens the distention of the anterior vaginal wall beneath the trigone and urethra. The usual gynecoid type of bony pelvis, however, with its wide infrapubic arch, does not protect the fascial support beneath the trigone and urethra from the distention that develops when the presenting part is forced anteriorly against the bony pelvis as the extending vertex comes against the musculature of the perineum.

Episiotomy is usually considered as a means of protecting the lower posterior vaginal wall and perineum from a laceration that could not be repaired as satisfactorily as an elected incision. It is important to remember also that resistance to lower vaginal dilation, which the perineal musculature places in the way of the presenting part, will be immediately lessened by an adequate episiotomy. It is evident, therefore, that when the parturient has an android type of pelvis, an episiotomy will be indicated to protect the pelvic floor and perineum from the laceration likely because of the greater distention necessary posteriorly before the vertex can emerge from beneath the infrapubic arch. It is equally important, if not equally evident, to remember, however, when the parturient has a wide gynecoid infrapubic arch, although there will be less distention posteriorly as the vertex comes under the pubic arch, that an adequate episiotomy will spare the tissues supporting the trigone and urethra from the damage likely to occur anteriorly if an episiotomy is not performed.

It is not equally clear, however, that episiotomy will of itself reduce the incidence of uterine prolapse and eventual procidentia. We believe it would be difficult to assemble data that would be convincing on this point, because the same intelligence in the conduct of labor that usually results in the election of an episiotomy would also be determining the management of the first and second stages of labor. It seems probable, therefore, that during labor the factors that increase the probability of eventual prolapse would have been recognized and minimized, or avoided altogether, well before the stage of labor when an episiotomy would have appeared to be indicated. Although the resulting data might suggest that the frequency of prolapse had been reduced by the routine use of episiotomy, we do not believe such a direct relationship should be assumed.

If the obstetrician knew the primagravida would eventually bring five, six, or more pregnancies to term, there would be reason to question the advisability of repeatedly "adequate" episiotomies. One comprehensive repair, skillfully completed as an objective worthy of the gynecologist's time and the patient's period of disability, would be a reasonable alternative to multiple and not always carefully repaired episiotomies. However, neither the patient nor her obstetrician know what parity the primigravida will eventually achieve. It is difficult, therefore, to deny the reasonableness and the desirability of providing what may be regarded as the best care of each immediate problem. In the minds of many the question remains: Should the best care involve or require "routine" episiotomy?

For the purposes of this discussion we do not consider it desirable to attempt a definitive evaluation of the relative merits and disadvantages of one type or site of episiotomy as compared with another. The objective of an episiotomy, whether mediolateral or midline, is the same in each instance. The result of either, when repaired in an anatomically correct manner, seems satisfactory to those who prefer one over the other. We have had little personal experience in the use or the repair of any type of episiotomy that does not begin at the midline of the fourchette (at the six o'clock position). The difficulties being experienced by others in developing a realignment of the severed tissues after a "lateral" episiotomy (beginning at the four or eight o'clock position) have been sufficiently memorable to account for our lack of interest in that possibility. With increasing experience, we have become convinced of at least two advantages to be realized that make the midline episiotomy worth the admittedly greater risk of a third degree laceration through the anal sphincter or even a fourth degree laceration extending into the anal canal. First, the anatomic realignments are simpler, the "two sides always match"; and second, after a patient has had repeated episiotomies for pregnancies at term, perineal scarring is much less and dyspareunia is rarely related to the thin midline raphe that tends to develop when repeated incision and repairs have involved only the same midline site. We are also convinced that when extension of the episiotomy into the anal canal does appear imminent, adequate incision cleanly through sphincter and anal wall will assure circumstances in which the repair can be accomplished without the difficulties of trying to realign the tissues separated and irregularly edged by a laceration (that could have been avoided by adequate extension of the midline episiotomy into the anal canal). We have found midline episiotomy, anatomically closed with fine polyglycolic acid or chromic catgut and usually "running sutures," to cause very little discomfort and need very little attention during the puerperium.

We believe the advantages of virtually routine episiotomy greatly outweigh the frequently heard objections to making every delivery an operative procedure. We believe we cannot predict which patient will suffer a significant degree of soft tissue injury if all patients are permitted, and this usually means encouraged, to deliver spontaneously without episiotomy. If episiotomy is done routinely, seldom will there be extensions into sphincter or rectum, and, when such extensions do occur, we are convinced the injury is more readily repaired than the lacerations that most certainly occur during deliveries when episiotomy has not been performed.

We recognize the basis of the opinion that routine episiotomy is not indicated, simply because it can be shown not always to be necessary. Many obstetricians have voiced conviction that an episiotomy need not be performed, because vaginal and outlet dilation may be satisfactorily accomplished by the forces of spontaneous labor, after which involutionary changes restore the vagina and vulva to an undamaged parous state. Admitting that life can be that beautiful, we are not convinced that virtually every parturient will achieve spontaneous delivery without evident, regrettable, and largely preventable soft tissue injury. A sizeable proportion (in Gainey's studies, not less than one in four primigravida) were found to have suffered significant soft tissue damage at the outlet of the type many believe can be largely avoided by routine employment of regional anesthesia for relaxation of the musculature of the pelvic floor and perineum, plus an adequate prophylactic episiotomy, with delivery completed by outlet forceps or a breech assist. It is difficult to evaluate the effects of adequate regional anesthesia without episiotomy, for the two are amost invariably employed together. We are convinced particularly that regional anesthesia contributes significantly to the reduction of soft tissue outlet trauma and is not used merely to avoid the pain that would otherwise be experienced during the incision and repair of an episiotomy. To realize the maximal benefit of an adequate block or regional anesthesia, it should be employed before descent of the presenting part has subjected the pelvic floor to maximal distention, well before damage would be occurring to the perineum and to the soft tissues of the vaginal outlet. We believe episiotomy is chiefly of value in minimizing damage to the support of the lower urethra and the musculature encircling the introitus. The combination of regional anesthesia and episiotomy is more effective and protective than either alone. The disadvantage of anesthesia is the degree of interference with the effectiveness of uterine contractions, but we are also convinced that perhaps the major factor accounting for the decreased expulsive effort is the fact that the patient is more comfortable and no longer contributing the maximal type of voluntary effort that would be made by the unanesthetized patient in her determined effort to complete her delivery.

Many have emphasized personal conviction that delivery of both the presenting vertex or an aftercoming head can be better controlled and maternal soft tissue injury minimized by outlet forceps and delivery of the head between pains. How frequently this would be true would be difficult to determine because the effect of anesthesia often decreases expulsive effort to a point that the second stage of labor would be undesirably prolonged if outlet forceps were not used. Whenever the pros and cons of episiotomy and the prophylactic use of outlet forceps are being discussed, however, we would emphasize that the anesthesia used is not employed primarily to permit the use of episiotomy and forceps, but rather that regional anesthesia is used because of its effectiveness in decreasing maternal soft tissue injuries; and it is primarily the desirability of gaining that advantage that would alone warrant the use of outlet forceps. Admitting that the use of outlet forceps is made necessary because of the effects of anesthesia, we also recognize there are other appreciable advantages to be gained by the use of prophylactic forceps. It is, therefore, the combination of regional anesthesia, episiotomy, and outlet forceps that is of established and significant value in minimizing the extent of maternal injuries due to childbirth.

Only the inexperienced, or the hurried, callous attendants that obstetricians may, at times, appear to have become, can adopt a routine management of vaginal delivery that involves the degree of operative interference inherent in regional anesthesia, episiotomy, and prophylactic forceps without remaining aware of the ever-present risk of iatrogenic injury, which may require prompt objective appraisal and the best of reparative skills. For instance, at one time we employed a midline episiotomy extended in the midline of the vaginal wall to the margin of the posterior fornix in an effort to spare the lower half of the vagina (and particularly the anterior vagina and urethral supporting tissue) from the consequences of having to adequately distend, which distention so often results in detachment of both vaginal wall and urethral supports. Although such a generous midline episiotomy done early enough to have provided adequate protection of the vaginal and urethral supporting tissue did accomplish that protection, it also at times proved to have left the rectal wall inadequately protected. When an episiotomy extended up the midline of the posterior vaginal wall has been done before the presenting vertex had distended the lower vagina, pelvic floor, and perineal musculature, this prophylactic procedure was occasionally complicated by laceration of the anterior rectal wall as the vertex and fetal face descended to the outlet. The anterior wall of the anal canal and the sphincter may even remain intact while such a split in a segment of anterior wall occurs. This type of rectal damage occurred not only in our practice but also in the experience of others who employed a vaginal extension of a midline episiotomy in an effort to better protect the vaginal and urethral supporting tissues. It became evident that we should view the vaginal wall not only as liable to injury, but also as a layer appreciably protective of the underlying rectal wall.

It soon becomes evident that the advantages as well as the risks of prophylactic measures must be weighed before we assume that our efforts will prove to be as helpful as our intentions. We remain convinced that Gainey's observations are reliable, and his conclusions remain valid insofar as the obstetrician's abilities to decrease soft tissue injuries are concerned. The employment of episiotomy, however, is but one measure of the obstetrican's efforts to minimize the damages for which the forces accounting for vaginal delivery must be held responsible. Other equally effective measures should be more widely recognized.

Management of the third stage of labor has been subjected to relatively little consideration insofar as possible effects on the site or degrees of the injuries related to childbirth are concerned. During the centuries when manual exploration of the uterine cavity and manual removal of the placenta were simply not considered, efforts to aid in the expulsion of the placenta consisted almost exclusively of pressure and/or "massage" applied to the uterine fundus through the thickness of the abdominal wall. The forces applied to the fundus probably were rarely of a magnitude comparable to a myometrial contraction plus voluntary bearing-down effort. It is possible, however, that the virtually frantic efforts of an occasional attendant to "Crede out the placenta" could result in added trauma (disruption) of uterine and cervical supporting tissues. In more recent years, if the placenta does not separate promptly, the third stage of labor is usually terminated (within a relatively few minutes after birth of the baby) by manual intrauterine removal of the placenta. At that time the lower uterine segment and cervix are not likely to offer any significant resistance to manual exploration of the uterine cavity and removal of the placenta. As a result today there are very few, if any, circumstances that would justify sufficient pressure on the uterine fundus to provide additional traumatic stretching of the ligamentous support of the fundus and cervix. We would admit that it could be done and, at the same time, expect that it would not occur.

The several hours immediately after delivery of the placenta have been referred to by some as the fourth stage of labor. During that potentially critical period repeated observations by alert attendants should provide assurance that myometrial contraction is being maintained and blood loss is not excessive. During that period we would also recognize the possibility that overly vigorous massage of the fundus in ill-advised attempts to keep the uterus contracted could add to further injury of the then relatively loosely arranged connective tissues of the cardinal and uterosacral ligaments and disruption of the thin-walled, poorly supported, and engorged venous channels in the parametrium. Such additional trauma could, but obviously should not, occur during the fourth stage of labor.

During the altered and increased physical activities of many women during World War II, particularly in industry and transportation, earlier ambulation became a matter of increased interest and virtually a universal practice. Older obstetricians in particular were skeptical, and many were opposed to early ambulation following delivery. There seemed reason to consider that the puerperal uterus, only 12 to 48 hours postpartum, would be heavy enough to add further to the strain on uterine supports, and the result would at least be a delay in parametrial involution and aggravation of any tendency to the descensus that might later become evident. Four decades later, however, there seems no documentation to suggest that early ambulation is anything but beneficial to the parturient. We do not believe that early ambulation has or will increase the frequency or the degree of uterine or vaginal wall prolapse.

Throughout the past two decades those advocating natural childbirth have often tended to regard the obstetrician as a professional obviously threatened by women's awakened awareness that human parturition can occur safely without professional guidance and help. Generally improved maternal health and adequate nutrition during pregnancy are certain to result in better babies being born. An informed and confident parturient will often deliver normally and satisfactorily without professional aid of any kind. Time and experience are certain to bring the same truths to the attention of both the public and the profession. It would be remarkable if the problems and the risks of childbirth, which generations ago created the profession, would not again appear when childbirth occurs naturally and at home. As the need for professional help became evident, it would be well if the skills expected of the obstetrician would be directed not only toward safe delivery of the child but also toward minimizing the occurrence of those maternal injuries that not infrequently result when the forces of an effective labor, unmanaged and unaided, succeed in the completion of a spontaneous delivery.

The art of obstetrics is primarily evidenced in the attendant's understanding of the parturient's need. Assurance and instruction to "relax and let your pains do the work" are indicated at least as often as encouragement to "bear down with your pains." Each bit of advice and encouragement can be helpful, but either cliche can be offered to the wrong patient or at the wrong time. Nontraumatic labor and delivery are not rewards realized by the stoic who laboriously punishes herself with determined efforts. The muscular, perfect physical specimen type may experience a hard time and suffer much greater soft tissue damage than the less aggressive and less "ambitious," virtually lazy type who often proves to be surprisingly relaxed, confident, and effective throughout her labor.

Considering the usual etiology of vaginal wall and/or uterine prolapse, there is need to emphasize several points. First, the most efficient and nontraumatic first stages of labor will be assured when an experienced obstetrician exercises good clinical judgment in an appraisal of the parturient's needs. Analgesics or sedation to help the patient's morale or measures to improve the effectiveness of her uterine contractions can be so employed as to either help or to hinder the progress of labor. Clearly the type and degree of maternal tissue damage is related, not so much to the patient's parity as to the presentation and the position of the presenting part near completion of the first stage of labor. Of virtually equal importance is the character, duration, and frequency of uterine contractions.

It is our conviction that the conduct of labor can, to a significant degree, determine the site and the extent of soft tissue injury. We believe this to be true whether the course of labor be the accomplishment of a confident and intelligent believer in the advantages of natural childbirth or the accomplishment of a cooperative parturient supported and aided by understanding attendants and an obstetrician's management of either dystocia or precipitous labor. In either instance, if the factors during labor that make for later prolapse of the uterus and/or detachment of vaginal wall supports are recognized when they begin to develop and, by good fortune or by good advisement, the forces capable of damaging maternal tissues are decreased, soft tissue damage can be reduced to a minimum. This we believe should be a very major objective in the conduct of every labor and delivery. When the obstetrician is so motivated and so effective, or the woman delivering unaided is so fortunate, there will be less frequent need for intelligent assessment and vaginal repairs skillfully performed by the gynecologic surgeon.

### References

1. Curtis AH, Anson BJ: Perineal birth injuries: Pathogenesis and surgical correction. *Q Bull Northwest Univ Med Sch* 16: 275–284, 1942.
2. DeLee JB: The prophylactic forceps operation. *Am J Obstet Gynecol* 1:34–44, 1920.
3. Gainey HL: Postpartum observation of pelvic tissue damage. *Am J Obstet Gynecol* 45:457–466, 1943.
4. Gainey HL: Postpartum observation of pelvic tissue damage: Further studies. *Am J Obstet Gynecol* 70:800–807, 1955.
5. Gustafson GW: The prevention and treatment of cystocele in the reproductive age. *Urol Cutaneous Rev* 144:160–161, 1940.
6. Magdi I: Obstetric injuries of the perineum. *J Obstet Gynaec Br Emp* 49:687–700, 1942.
7. Power RMH: The pelvic floor in parturition. *Surg Gynecol Obstet* 83:296–311, 1946.
8. Randall CL: Forword: Prolonged and difficult labor. *Clin Obstet Gynecol* 2;271–360, 1959.
9. Randall CL: Childbirth without fear of interference. *Clin Obstet Gynecol* 2:360, 1959.

# CHAPTER 3

# Types of Genital Prolapse

Genital prolapse may result when normal pelvic supports are subjected to chronic increases in intra-abdominal pressure or when congenitally defective genital support responds to even normal intra-abdominal pressure. In consideration of a particular prolapse, it is important for the surgeon to estimate which of the above mechanisms are operative, so that the planned reconstruction and overall medical management of the patient can remedy the specific defect. For example, the genital prolapse and urinary stress incontinence coincident with ascites or large ovarian tumors may be relieved by the restoration of normal intra-abdominal pressure alone if the degree of pelvic strain has not yet become irreversible.

A main deficiency in the usual anatomic or morphologic classification of degrees of genital prolapse is that such a classification does not take into account the significant differences in the various etiologies of prolapse. These etiologic differences must be recognized because they are concerned with the rate and likelihood of progression of the displacement and the chances of surgical cure or recurrence. Therefore, the surgeon must take the various etiologies into consideration if postoperative results are to be optimal.

The effects of either forces or inherent weaknesses may result in varying degrees of genital prolapse and in extreme degree virtually turn the vagina inside out. These forces may work singly or in combination and at quite different times in life. Recognition of primary weakness and identification of the components involved in secondary damage are both essential in the surgeon's evaluation of the patient's problem. The most important single step in surgical treatment is to recognize and correct, or at times overcorrect, the primary weakness or damage. Unless adequate correction of the primary factor is accomplished, recurrence from continued progression is to be expected and will likely occur in spite of initially successful surgical repair of the more obvious damage.

Basically, genital prolapse falls into either of two large groups: prolapse of the upper vagina or eversion of the lower vagina. These may occur separately or together, simultaneously or at different times, but they are produced by quite different etiologic factors, the significance of which was recognized by Victor Bonney (2) in 1914.

Bonney pointed out that the relationship of the vagina to the peritoneal cavity is in the same position as the inturned finger of a rubber glove which may be out-turned by closing the mouth of the glove and compressing air locked within it. (In the instance of the rubber glove, he pointed out, the pressure is purely gaseous and depends upon the amount of force supplied by the hand compressing it. Intra-abdominal pressure is more complicated, however, depending partly on the intestinal gas pressure, which acts equally in all directions, the contraction of muscles surrounding the abdominal cavity, and partly on the weight of the movable viscera that being dependent upon gravity, acts downward.) Why does the rubber glove evert so readily, whereas the vagina does not (Fig. 3.1)?

Vaginal vault prolapse (Fig. 3.2) is primarily the result of a weakening of the supports of the upper half of the vagina. This usually will be noted to have followed the forces and damages of labor and delivery but may be the result of chronically increased intra-abdominal pressure.

The upper vagina may gradually evert within itself. There is usually an enterocele present and generally some degree of cystocele; but an accompanying rectocele is uncommon insomuch as the pelvic and urogenital diaphragms often remain intact.

The cardinal and uterosacral ligaments function as the "stays" and provide the principal suspension of the upper vagina and cervix, holding them over the levator plate. The pelvic diaphragm and its levator plate may be intact, but if the "stays" have become permanently stretched or elongated, this permits the cervix a degree of mobility sufficient for it to slide or fall through the levator hiatus and over the edge of the levator plate, with consequent prolapse of the upper vagina. When, in addition, the patient is observed while straining or bearing down, it will be noted that, although the upper vagina prolapses, the lower vagina is not involved, and neither moves nor tends to evert so long as there is demonstrable integrity of the pelvic and urogenital diaphragms. Because the damage is anterior to the rectum, rectocele is not necessarily associated even though the cul-de-sac is being pulled downward, producing a traction type of enterocele (Chapter 15).

Eversion of the lower vagina (Fig. 3.2) results from loss of its support from damage to the soft tissues attaching it to the pelvic and urogenital diaphragms and, although usually the result of obstetric trauma, may occur as part of a general postmenopausal atrophic weakening of the pelvic supporting tissues or of coincident neuropathy. A third possibility is that of the two conditions being simultaneous, in which case the vagina will be prolapsing above and rolling out or everting below (Fig. 3.2). Which of these two mechanisms is the dominant or initial one can usually be determined by manual replacement of the prolapsed organs and, without touching the patient, asking her to bear down and then observe which segment of vagina seems to prolapse first. If a cystocele and rectocele appear first, followed by the cervix and vaginal vault, the primary site of damage is probably the lower supporting tissues and lower vaginal eversion is dominant. If, on the other hand, the cervix and vaginal vault appear first, followed by the cystocle and rectocele, the primary site of damage in that circumstance is probably the upper vaginal suspensory tissues. Unrestrained progression of either eversion of upper or lower vagina or both may continue so that the result may be a vagina turned completely inside out (Fig. 3.2). When the cervix and uterus extend completely outside the bony pelvis, the condition is termed procidentia (Fig. 3.3). As organs drop, traction is applied to previously uninvolved supporting tissue attached to neighboring organs, and extensive secondary damage will result.

The rate of progression has a great deal to do with the symptomatology and the opportunity for recognition of the etiology. When prolapse is rapidly progressive, acute discomfort or concern is likely to bring the patient promptly to the physician for evaluation, whereas degrees of descensus that are static, chronic, or slowly progressive are more likely to be first noted without the strong complaint of the patient at the time of a routine pelvic examination. In the latter situation, pertinent symptoms may have developed so slowly that the patient has accepted them matter-of-factly without recognizing their relevance. The rate of progression may help to distinguish types of prolapse, which in reality differ both in etiology and in prognosis, i.e., slowly progressive

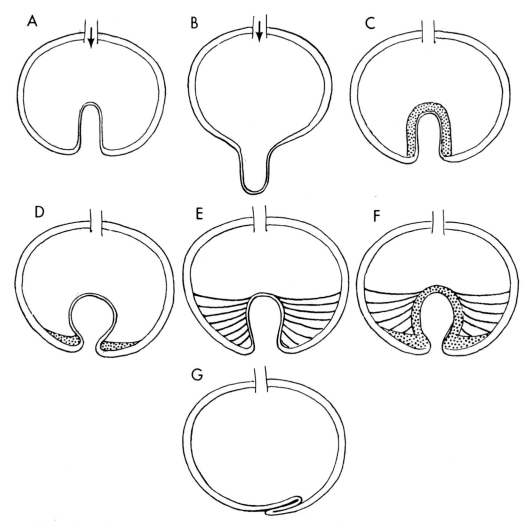

**Figure 3.1.** As an approach to the problem let us first take the case of an artificial cul-de-sac intruding into an artificial, closed gas-containing cavity (*A*) and consider what steps could be taken to prevent the cul-de-sac from turning inside out when the pressure in the closed cavity is raised (*B*).

1. Because the ease with which a cul-de-sac can be turned inside out depends largely on the resistance of its wall and the relation between the thickness of the wall and caliber of the lumen, turning inside out could be prevented either by making the wall of the cul-de-sac rigid or by thickening it so much in relation to the caliber of its lumen that turning inside out would be impossible, as in the case of a piece of pressure tubing (*C*).

2. If the outlet of the cul-de-sac were sufficiently narrowed, complete turning inside out would be rendered impossible for, although the cul-de-sac might collapse down as far as the constriction, it could not pass through it. This is really a special case of the general principle enunciated under 1 (*D*).

3. If the cul-de-sac, instead of being straight, were sharply bent, the effect of raising the pressure in the closed cavity would be to increase the bend and make turning inside out more difficult or impossible (*G*).

4. The out-turning effect could be combated by attaching the wall of the cul-de-sac to the wall of the closed cavity, either directly or by some intermediary structure, as for example a series of threads (*E*) or by a combination of the devices mentioned (*F*). When we come to consider that which obtains in the case of the vagina and uterus we find that nature has anticipated us in all of these devices. (After Bonney V: The sustentacular apparatus of the female genital canal, the displacements that result from the yielding of its several compoments, and their appropriate treatment. *J Obstet Gynaecol Br Emp* 45:328, 1914.

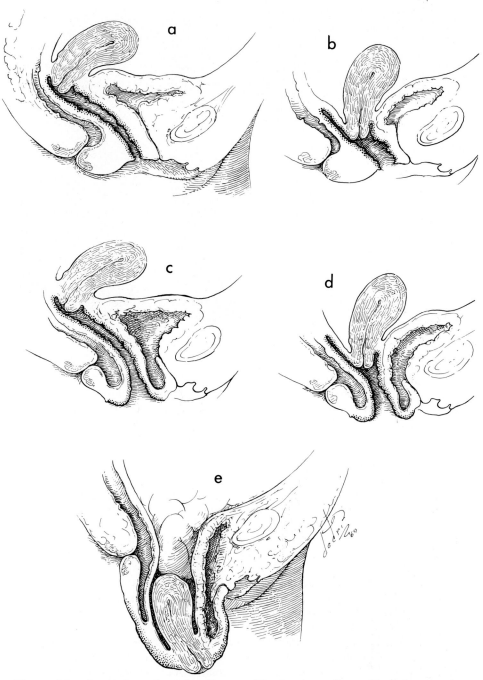

**Figure 3.2.** Sagittal section after Bonney (2) of a normally positioned vagina is seen in (a). Prolapse of the upper vagina (b) may result from weakening of the upper vaginal supports, the cardinal and uterosacral ligament complex. Eversion of the lower vagina (c) results from damage to the pelvic and urogenital diaphragms. Simultaneous vault prolapse and eversion may occur, as depicted in (d). Procidentia (e) may evolve as the result of unrestrained progression of any of the above types of prolapse. (Reproduced with permission of McGraw-Hill from Nichols DH: Types of genital prolapse. *Postgrad Med* 46:183–187, 1969.)

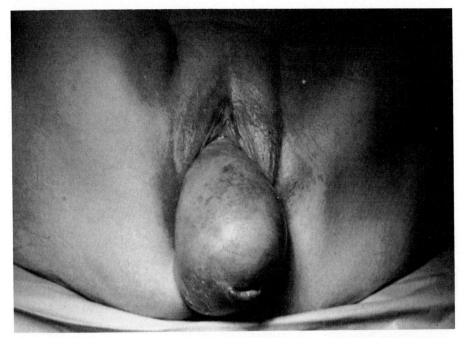

**Figure 3.3.** Procidentia is demonstrated with coincident cystocele and rectocele.

uterovaginal prolapse is usually due to damage to the lateral supports of the cervix and upper vagina, whereas rapidly progressing prolapse is due in all probability to primarily atrophic failure of all of the supporting tissues, including the pelvic floor. Relatively asymptomatic progression of a noted degree of prolapse is far more ominous than is a static condition, because the progression suggests a transient phase inevitably advancing toward more complete prolapse. Detection of prolapse progression from one annual visit to another is more likely when such periodic examinations have involved the same examiner and is less apparent when there has been a different examiner on each visit. The extent of each component of a prolapse will be more convincingly demonstrated by examination of the relaxed and then straining patient in the standing position, which adds the effects of gravity (preferably at least 6 months postpartum, when involution should be complete) (see Fig. 15.4).

The fascial strands maintaining the position of the vagina in the pelvis become stretched and elongated longitudinally in the direction of the force applied to them. Progressive normal labor usually results in thinning and stretching but not disruption of the strands of fascial support. Obviously precipitous force is more likely to disrupt the attachments and continuity of fascial fibers than would be likely with more moderate and repeated stress. Precipitous descent into the vagina resisting rapid dilatation is also likely to result in disruption of connective tissue support, with or without laceration of the vaginal wall.

Involution does not reattach fascia to the sites of original attachment, and if such damage has occurred, it may be evident postpartum. Whenever an examiner first notes the loss of the normal concavity of the vaginal fornices there is reason to expect that vaginal eversion will eventually develop.

Types as well as degrees of genital prolapse may be evident singly or in combination as a result of damage to any one or more of the following seven separate supportive systems: (a) the bony pelvis to which the soft tissues ultimately attach, (b) the subperitoneal retinaculum and smooth muscle component of the broad ligaments, (c) the cardinal and uterosacral ligament complex, (d) the pelvic diaphragm and levator ani and its fibromuscular attachments to the pelvic organs, (e) the urogenital diaphragm, (f) the perineal body, and (g) the walls of the vagina, with essential loss of tone and evident weakness as a result of both pathologic stretching and the attenuating changes of aging.

## NULLIPAROUS PROLAPSE

In North America approximately 2% of the women who develop prolapse are nullipara. An occasional case of congenital origin associated with defective musculature or innervation becomes evident in infancy or childhood. Often nulliparous prolapse will be associated with a lifestyle of heavy physical labor producing marked increases in intra-abdominal pressure. When prolapse becomes evident before the menopause, the primary etiology appears to be pathologic elongation of the cardinal and uterosacral ligament complex of the upper suspensory support system so that such patients typically display a prolapse of the upper vagina and coexistent elongation of the cervix. This may bring with it some traction-produced cystocele and enterocele. In the postmenopausal patient, however, the effects of atrophic changes may be superimposed upon a generalized muscular and connective tissue hypoplasia. The presence of such a common denominator may to some extent be predicted by a relative absence of rugal folds, particularly evident in the vaginal epithelium covering the bladder. Local underdevelopment of the pelvic floor is often associated with noticeable hypoplasia of the uterus, occasionally related to and made worse by postmenopausal atrophy. Such a patient, on straining, may still display bulging of the tissues at the outlet even after extensive repair. Stallworthy (18) has pointed out that a small percentage of those persons in the general population with congenital defects of their supporting tissues may marry and later reproduce. The fact that some subsequently develop prolapse does not prove that it was the pregnancy or delivery that caused the prolapse.

## NEONATAL GENITAL PROLAPSE

Genital prolapse in the newborn has been reported, although it is rare. It may be associated with a congenital pelvic neuropathy affecting the pelvic muscles.

Treatment is by manual reduction and, if the prolapse recurs, the wearing of a tiny pessary, the latter made from a rolled and tied 1-inch Penrose drain. The pessary, removed only for cleaning, may be worn for several weeks (17). If vaginal and uterine edema is so great as to preclude manual replacement of the prolapse, the latter may be covered with hypertonic saline packs for several days, followed by temporarily sewing together the posterior half of the labia minora and majora (1). The stitches are removed after they have been in place for 2 weeks. Initial treatment by replacement is usually without recurrence if there is no significant associated primary neuropathy.

## RACIAL DIFFERENCES IN GENITAL PROLAPSE

There may be individual and racial differences in connective tissue strengths noted by the relative infrequency with which black women sustain lacerations from spontaneous delivery and their relative immunity from uterine prolapse. Magdi (10 ) coined the term "elastic index" of a patient suggesting that when striae gravidarum are broad and coarse, there is less integrity of elastic tissue and the tendency toward prolapse is greater: Conversely, when the striae are fine and narrow, both stretch and involution are adequate and neither laceration nor loss of tone are as likely to occur.

## Genital Prolapse In Bantu Women

Heyns (8) maintains that excess intra-abdominal pressure is a primary cause of genital prolapse in women and has observed the absence of prolapse in Bantu women as a fundamental racial difference. The Bantu woman, by not wearing corsets and by eating but one meal per day, has developed accommodation to a wide range of day-to-day changes in intra-abdominal pressure, even during pregnancy.

The racial incidence of genital prolapse and its significance were reported by F.G. Geldenhuys (3, 4) of the Department of Obstetrics and Gynecology, University of Pretoria, South Africa, who observed that during a 5-year period, from January 1945 through December 1949, 6,302 European gynecologic inpatients were admitted to the Pretoria General Hospital. Of these patients, 410 underwent operations for genital prolapse, an incidence of 6.5%. During the same period, 3,478 Bantu gynecologic patients were admitted, of whom only 21 were operated on for prolapse, an incidence of 0.6%. Direct communication with other institutions in South Africa indicated prolapse to be equally uncommon among other institutions treating Bantu women.

In Switzerland, the incidence of genital prolapse among gynecologic admissions was 12% at the Kanton Hospital in Zurich, and at the Clinique d'Gynecologie et Obstetrique, Geneva, the incidence was 5.7% during the same period of time. In Hamburg, it was 5.4%; in Rome, 6.4%. Prolapse was common in India and in North America. Heyns also reported prolapse to be common in Brazil and in Egypt, but less common among Indonesians and Chinese.

In summary, it appears that prolapse occurs rather frequently among the white races, the Egyptians, and the women of India. It occurs less frequently among Orientals and American Negroes and is particularly uncommon in the South African Bantu as well as in the Negro of West Africa.

The most common single etiologic factor of genital prolapse is parturition, and it may be related to increased intra-abdominal pressure and softening of the pelvic connective tissues and smooth muscle as a result of hormonal influences. The trauma of labor and the increased weight of the uterus during the period of involution may also be contributing factors. The return of the pelvic floor to normal is faster in the Bantu woman than in the European, and subinvolution of the uterus is uncommon in the Bantu.

Although episiotomy is common in America, it seems to have been followed by a lesser incidence of prolapse. A routine episiotomy is not performed in the Bantu inasmuch as they are delivered for the most part at home under primitive conditions. The incidence of forceps deliveries is similarly much lower among the Bantu than among Europeans.

The size of the Bantu infant at birth is comparable to that of the European, and the Bantu is often prone to premature bearing down long before full dilation of the cervix. Grand multiparity is common among the Bantu. In two-thirds of Bantu births, the fetal head is unengaged before the onset of labor. The average age of the Bantu primipara is not much different from that of the European primipara, and retroversion of the uterus is as common in Bantu women as in the European. Early rising after delivery is widely practiced by Bantu women.

## Chronically Increased Intra-Abdominal Pressure

The Bantu woman differs from her European counterpart in that she makes more frequent use of the squatting position for defecation. They do, however, perform about the same hard manual labor as their men, much as do European peasant women. It has been suggested that the mesoderm of Negroes differs in a number of respects from that of the Europeans, as is evidenced by the proliferation of connective tissue. For example, neurofibromatosis is common among Negroes, keloids develop more rapidly, the corium of the skin is thicker and has more sweat glands, the lips are thicker as a result of fibroelastic tissue, and uterine leiomyomata are nine times more common than among the Europeans. The same observation seems to apply to the Bantu. Some believe that the woman with a wide, flat pelvis is more liable to develop prolapse, in contrast to the woman with a contracted pelvis where the bony supports of the pelvic diaphragm are relatively small in comparison to the area of stress and strain. There is little doubt that the Bantu pelvis is comparatively small in relation to that of the European.

Postmenopausal atrophy is difficult to evaluate among the Bantu, considering that the decade from 60 to 70 years of age was the most common period for a patient to be operated upon for genital prolapse at Pretoria General Hospital. The European women more frequently reached this age than the Bantu, because the average life expectancy of the former was 63 years. However, those Bantu women who do reach an advanced age do not often show genital prolapse.

Malnutrition is common among the Bantu and deficiency diseases are frequent, but they do not appear to predispose these women to genital prolapse.

## Posture

The Bantu woman has more pronounced lordosis than does the European woman.

## Conclusion

Geldenhuys believed it was not so much environment which influenced the occurrence of prolapse but rather inherent racial constitutional factors, such as the size and form of the pelvis, the quality of the connective tissue and pelvic supports, and the tendency to fibrosis.

Zacharin (20) has studied possible causes for the relative infrequency of both genital prolapse and urinary stress incontinence among Orientals. His dissections of Chinese cadavers at the University of Hong Kong revealed that their primary urethral suspensory mechanism was almost vestigial, in contrast to magnificent development of their levator ani complex—the opposite situation of the usual occidental female. Unanswered, yet, is whether this better development of the levator ani is an inherited characteristic or one acquired from their traditional way of life and lifelong habit of sitting and of defecation in the squatting position.

Malpas (11) has described a nonprogressive postobstetric genital prolapse characterized by mild degrees of relaxation, in which the lateral supporting tissues of the vagina and uterus, although stretched and torn, apparently become refused to the lateral walls of the pelvis but at a lower level. This refusion is sufficiently stable in most instances to relieve the patient of troublesome symptoms, provided the urogenital diaphragm remains relatively well preserved. If the pelvic diaphragm is not damaged, the lesion may remain nonprogressive and not require operative repair. Absence of progression between periodic examinations tends to identify this type of genital prolapse.

The resultant types of prolapse may exist in a pure state or, more commonly, seem to be mixed or combined with one another in varying degrees. If optimal surgical results are to be obtained, it is essential for the surgeon to interpret the various components correctly and employ appropriate reconstruction.

## ELONGATION OF THE CERVIX

Elongation of the cervix is most commonly seen in association with anterior segment damage and was characterized by Paramore ( 12) as "expansion of the escaped cervix." The apparent enlargement of the cervix is secondary to congestion within the tissues of the cervix under circumstances in which the cervix has dropped anterior to the genital hiatus. Although unable to maintain support of the cervix, the levator plate still exists as a supporting tissue posterior to the cervix. The edge of the genital hiatus in that circumstance acts as a mechanical barrier to the return circulation of the cervix, favoring venous stasis and apparent hypertrophy of the cervix itself. Persisting constriction causes not only edema and lymphagiectasia but later fibrosis, and the circulatory changes may at times result in ulceration of the surface of the cervix.

## PSEUDOPROLAPSE

During diagnostic dilation and curettage, with the patient under general anesthesia, the cervix of a movable uterus can easily be brought to the vaginal outlet, but this may or may not represent observation of genuine prolapse. There is significant difference in the findings suggesting prolapse when the evaluation involves an anethestized patient. Under anesthesia, the levator ani is in effect paralyzed, the patient is not straining but is recumbent and relaxed, and there is no increased intra-abdominal pressure. However, direct traction on the cervix is an abnormal pull in an abnormal direction. Under such circumstances the pulled-upon cervix acts as a driving wedge through the levator hiatus, which has already partly been separated by the speculum distending the introitus and retracting the pelvic floor (14). A patient evaluated in this way may have no genuine genital prolapse, particularly when pelvic relationships are being evaluated with the tone of the muscular and connective tissue supports paralyzed by anesthesia. The best assessment of the true degree of genital prolapse and the weakness of support can be determined with certainty by examination of the unanesthetized patient, first recumbent and then standing, using neither speculum nor tenaculum. It is helpful to ask the patient to bear down in order to see which organ appears first, as this will provide a reliable suggestion as to the site of primary damage. Insertion of speculum and traction with a tenaculum will provide reliable help determining the technical features of a planned repair. Although it is easy to describe cystoceles and rectoceles on an entirely anatomic or degree basis, this concept does not take into account some significant variations in areas of specific weakness due to differences in the basic etiology from one cystocele and rectocele to another, which explains why identical techniques of repair may result in surprisingly different results.

## SEGMENTAL DAMAGE

There are certain natural cleavage planes (also noted in Chapter 1) about the female pelvic organ systems that, under certain stressful situations, permit segmental avulsion and pathologic sliding of one or more organ systems upon another. These concepts are of the utmost practical significance and, for clinical purposes, may be summarized as follows:

1. A retropubic plane between the pubis and urethra is brought into clinical significance when the pubourethral ligament portion of the urogenital diaphragm has become avulsed or stretched, permitting the proximal urethra to rotate from its usual situation with consequent "wheeling" and rotational descent of the bladder neck (Fig. 1.29). This is usually the result of the shearing trauma of the descending fetal head beneath a wide-angled gynecoid pubic arch (Fig. 2.3). An equally undesirably close fit of the fetal head may also be due to a relatively small fetal head or to a short precipitous labor or arrest in the second stage.

2. The posterior vaginal plane of cleavage exists between the posterior vaginal wall and the anterior wall of the rectum, i.e., in the rectovaginal space. The organ systems anterior to this space are to a large extent interconnected by common attachments, especially in the upper two-thirds of the vagina. Here the anterolateral attachments of the cardinal ligaments (hypogastric sheath) bind the vagina and cervix firmly together to such an extent that the cervix functions almost as a part or extension of the anterior vaginal wall. The length of the anterior vaginal wall plus the diameter of the cervix normally equals the length of the posterior vaginal wall. The most cranial portion of the rectovaginal space terminates at the most caudal portion of the cul-de-sac of Douglas, which of itself has both flexibility and mobility, and with the rectovaginal space forms a more or less frictionless midline plane down which the structures anterior to the rectovaginal space can slide under certain circumstances without disturbing those primarily rectal structures posterior to the rectovaginal space. Classic procidentia (Fig. 3.3), therefore, with prolapse of the upper vagina may permit the entire uterus and much of the bladder to protrude outside the introitus, with coexistent enterocele (sliding hernia), frequently without accompanying rectocele (15). Such a condition, especially involving the bladder, may be called primary anterior segment damage and it often results from chronically increased intraperitoneal pressure or from damage sustained during the first stage of labor as a result of bearing down or attempted delivery before full dilation of the cervix. Anterior segment damage, per se, does not include damage to the levator ani or its sheath.

3. The perineal and anterior rectal segments reflect damage to the support and attachments of the perineum, and to the posterior structures of the rectovaginal space, including the anterior wall of the rectum and its fascial envelopment. It is commonly associated with avulsion of the vaginal and perineal attachments to the levator ani (fibers of Luschka) as a result of unrecognized or unrepaired obstetric trauma to these attachments during the second stage of labor. The central portion of the rectovaginal septum (the fascia of Denonvilliers) can be traumatically detached from the cranial margin of the perineal body. The damage will be evident as a mid- and lower vaginal rectocele and can be expected when there is a narrow pubic arch. This type of relaxation will often be seen without significant degree of cystocele, uterine prolapse, or enterocele, because the latter structures may all be adequately supported in their normal and usual relationships.

4. The lower or retrorectal segment is, fortunately, the least common site of damage but, when present, is usually associated either with acquired major damage to the levator ani or to its innervation. Occasional congenital neuropathy may be coexistent with a spina bifida. Defects in the lower perineal segment permit perineal prolapse or descent of the anus, so that the

patient with a flat perineum may actually sit upon her anus, a most distressing situation.

Forcing defecation may be a factor in the production of rectal prolapse. A distended freely mobile segment of rectal wall may virtually intussuscept into the previously normal caliber of the anal canal.

Tipping of the attenuated pelvic diaphragm and levator plate produces funneling of the pelvic basin causing almost ribbon-like stools that become increasingly narrowed the harder the patient strains. The condition may be relieved surgically by retrorectal levatorplasty (see Chapter 13).

Prolapse of the rectum is of overwhelming clinical importance to the patient so afflicted and, fortunately, is not often coincident with genital prolapse and is the result of a different etiology (Fig. 3.4). Unless the surgeon has had special training and experience in rectal surgery, he should enlist the cooperation of an appropriate surgical consultant when effecting the necessary reconstruction. Consultation and cooperative planning enhance the design and accomplishment of a good result.

## RECTAL PROLAPSE

This occurs predominantly in women who are thin and elderly and is more common in nulliparous than multiparous patients. It is probable that aging has produced a diminished tone of the pelvic muscles, and chronic constipation and laxative abuse are seen. There is sometimes a coincident uterine prolapse (16).

The symptoms are primarily those of rectal protrusion with straining or lifting, incomplete bowel movements, and rectal incontinence. As the condition becomes more advanced and the prolapsed rectum remains outside a greater portion of the time, bleeding develops. The physical examination is often clear

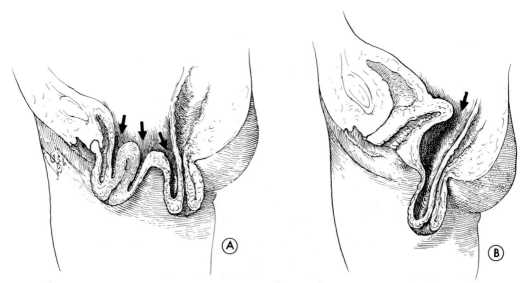

**Figure 3.4.** Rectal prolapse associated with enterocele. *A*, rectal prolapse is coincident with genital procidentia. *B*, the rectal prolapse is posterior to the vagina, which is not involved. (Reproduced with permission of Harper & Row from Nichols DH: Types of enterocele and principles underlying the choice of operation for repair. *Obstet Gynecol* 40:257–363, 1972.)

but the bowel protrudes when the patient strains as by a Valsalva maneuver. Its walls are thick, especially anteriorly, and there may be an enterocele sac containing small bowel. The anus is usually patulous up to three or four finger breadths in diameter, and the condition is surprisingly painless (17).

Etiology of rectal prolapse is probably the result of a rectorectal intussusception, rather than a sliding hernia. The anatomic abnormalities that are noted are probably the result and not the cause of the prolapse.

Of the treatments that have been offered, the most successful are transabdominal (19). Others are transperineal and some are combined. Simple obliteration of the cul-de-sac on the thought that this represented a sliding hernia has not been consistently effective, there being a 63% recurrence rate. Intra-abdominal and transperineal plication of the levator muscles have been employed but the greatest lasting successes have been reported using the transabdominal rectal and sigmoid suspension operations with or without the use of foreign materials. Retrorectal levatorplasty may be used for the early stages, and for the elderly or poor risk patient, perineal anal encirclement as by the Thiersch technique has been recommended although this does insert a foreign body around the anus and there is a resultant small anal diameter and risk of ulceration.

Because rectal prolapse is often associated with anal incontinence, a knowledge of the causes and treatments of rectal prolapse requires some thoughtful appreciation of the normal mechanisms of lower bowel function and some consideration as to how this may be pathologically altered.

## LEVATOR ANI FUNCTION IN DEFECATION

Bowel function is to a large extent the product of habit. Defecation of sigmoid colon content is achieved by first voluntarily relaxing the pelvic diaphragm, unlocking the colic valve, and relaxing the external anal sphincter. Modest increases in intra-abdominal pressure, as by bearing down, then force the stool content downward. Rectal filling opens the internal sphincter. The gastrocolic reflex pattern regularly assists by promoting intestinal peristalsis. A disorder of any of these steps predisposes to or causes constipation. Regular and excessive bearing down may stretch the anatomic integrity of the pudendal nerve and consequently weaken the muscles it innervates, occasionally resulting in a permanent loss of muscle tone in the now denervated pelvic diaphragm and external anal sphincter. The neuropathic loss of the tone of the anal sphincter permits it to relax at inopportune times producing rectal incontinence that may be most difficult to treat surgically. The Parks group has suggested that this loss of voluntary muscle tone within the pelvic diaphragm may be associated with coincident urinary stress incontinence as well (7).

## RECTAL CONTINENCE

The levator ani and the external anal sphincter differ from other striated muscles of the body in that they maintain a constant state of tone inversely proportional to the quantity of the rectal content. Because intestinal peristalsis continues around the clock, although at apparently various degrees of intensity, this aforementioned tone is responsible for our normal rectal continence when we are both awake and asleep. Were it not for the effectiveness of this tone, we would be regularly soiled during sleep when the rest of our voluntary muscle system is relaxed.

Contraction of the levator ani and puborectalis muscles exerts pull upon the genital hiatus toward the pubis creating an angle in rectal inclination that functions effectively as a valve, according to the observations of Parks (13), and there is reflex reciprocity with the tone of the external anal sphincter. These muscles are innervated by the pudendal nerve and its accessory branches, and they function in synergism. The innervation of the puborectalis is less certain, possibly coming from a sacral plexus component.

Neuromuscular pressure receptors within the intrinsic striated muscular content of the levatores ani are responsible for mediating this tone and apparently communicate with the central nervous system by way of the pudendal nerve on each side of the body arising generally from S3 and S4. Either congenital or acquired pathology of the pudendal nerve can alter the efficiency of its work and thus influence the ability and efficiency of these neuromuscular receptors to influence pressure and maintain this responsive muscular tone. Acquired damage may result from the trauma of stretching of the pelvic floor during childbirth and quite possibly from the chronic habit of excessive straining at stool.

Constipation, then, is *not* commonly caused by the presence of *rectocele*, although it may coexist. The primary symptoms of rectocele are aching after a bowel movement and incomplete bowel movements often requiring manual expression to achieve evacuation. Effective posterior colporrhaphy should relieve these primary symptoms but will not necessarily relieve constipation other than that produced by stool being caught in a pocket of rectal wall precluding complete emptying of the bowel. There are many women with rectocele who are not constipated, and there are many more constipated women without rectocele.

In the patient with perineal descent, constipation may appear as an early symptom due to loss of integrity of an intact pelvic diaphragm producing levator funneling during defecation bearing down. As this phenomenon of bearing down becomes more regular and intense, the pudendal nerve may be further damaged by stretching, disturbing the innervation of both the pelvic diaphragm and the external anal sphincter with resultant partial paralysis and atrophy of these muscles, contributing to anal *incontinence* as a later symptom.

Henry (6) has suggested the relationship between rectal prolapse and anal incontinence as follows:

"I think the primary pathology is one of neuropathy affecting the pelvic floor—in many patients a consequence of damage to the pudendal nerve damage inflicted by traumatic childbirth. Incontinence may not develop initially if the internal anal sphincter is functioning normally. Pelvic floor denervation initiates rectal prolapse because of disruption of the anorectal flap valve. The prolapse starts with descent of the anterior rectal wall and at a later stage a circumferential complete prolapse intussuscepts through the anus. The dilatation of the internal anal sphincter caused by the prolapsing rectum then destroys the only mechanism protecting anorectal continence and a major functional problem results. Because the internal sphincter recovers, many patients recover a reasonable degree of control after successful repair of the prolapse. If continence is not recovered within six months we will offer the patient a transperineal post-anal repair (of the puborectalis and the pelvic diaphragm)."

Few types of segmental relaxation develop independently. More frequently the patient presents combinations of segmental damage. With the exception of severe generalized prolapse developing in postmenopausal years, the degree of damage of one particular segment is usually more evident than is the damage to other segments. Most of the reconstructive effort should be directed to the primary site of the most significant damage.

When a perineal defect suggesting injury of the retrorectal segment is accompanied by a high residual urine volume, particularly in the nulliparous patient, a urethrocystometrogram and neurologic evaluation should be considered to evaluate the possibility of defective pelvic innervation and resulting incompetence of the levator ani. There may be a coexistent spina bifida occulta, or a low spinal disc syndrome productive of constipation and difficulty in emptying the bladder.

High rectocele is associated with pathologic overstretching of the vaginal and rectal supporting tissues, and there is often coexistent enterocele that must be identified and repaired. Reconstruction that will assure restoration of a horizontal axis to the upper posterior vagina will lessen the chances of recurrence. Jeffcoate (9) recognized posterior colporrhaphy as a frequent cause of dyspareunia or apareunia among Liverpool patients and stated that the need for posterior colporrhaphy in a particular patient should be determined by examining the *unanesthetized* patient. Only if the examination shows a need for posterior vaginal repair should the procedure be included in a particular patient's surgical reconstruction.

Although various cleavage planes may be developed within the pelvis, which suggest the lines along which genital prolapse has developed, the most significant is clearly that provided between the interfaces of the rectovaginal space. As will be noted in Figure 3.5 significant increases in intra-abdominal pressure may be exerted on tissues anterior to the rectovaginal space, resulting in a prolapse of the upper vagina and elongation of the cardinal-uterosacral

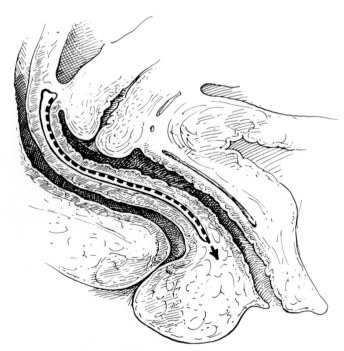

**Figure 3.5.** Sagittal section of the pelvis showing the rectovaginal space. Significant increases in intra-abdominal pressure may force the cervix and the posterior vaginal wall along this natural cleavage plane, as indicated by the *dotted line.*

ligament complex. Because of the attachment of the base of the bladder to the upper vagina and cervix by the supravaginal septum, descent of the cervix is likely to be accompanied by a traction descent of the bladder. The same findings may be observed after obstetric damage to the upper suspensory structures of the birth canal. In this situation, the descent of the cervix brings the anterior wall of the pouch of Douglas with it, and a traction type of enterocele is produced (Chapter 15). Traction to a tenaculum applied to the posterior lip of the cervix permits demonstration of the length of the latter, the location and width of the posterior cul-de-sac, and the length and strength of the usually hypertrophic uterosacral ligaments (Fig. 3.6). The posterior peritoneal wall of such an enterocele is attached to the anterior surface of the rectum, which usually does not become involved in this type of prolapse. Because the uterine cervix and anterior vaginal wall function and are supported as a unit, weakness and subsequent hypertrophy of the connective tissue in this area is the greatest. Elements of the cardinal-uterosacral ligament complex are long and hypertrophic. Enterocele is (as stated) invariably present, whereas rectocele may be absent or of a minor degree (Figs. 3.7 and 3.8). This type of traction enterocele occurs not only as a result of traction upon the anterior cul-de-sac but may also follow damage to the subperitoneal fibromuscular connective tissues.

With prolapse of the vagina and its consequent vaginal telescoping, the length of the vagina is shortened, and the width of the anterior vaginal wall is increased.

With eversion, the length and the width of the vaginal wall increase, and appropriate modification of the technique of colporrhaphy may be required (Chapters 11 and 12).

It would be helpful to abandon once and for all the concept of a single cause of genital prolapse. Rather, we should recognize that there are many different causes that may be more or less evident, acting singly or in combination to account for a particular clinical situation.

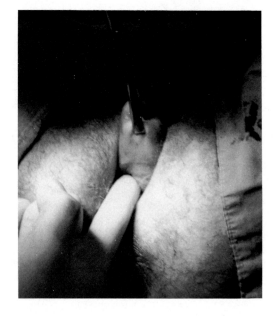

**Figure 3.6.**  The length and strength of the uterosacral ligaments as well as the location of the lowermost tip of the cul-de-sac of Douglas are determined by applying traction to a vulsellum applied to the posterior lip of the cervix. The elongated cervix and the long, strong uterosacral ligaments are shown. The lowermost extent of the cul-de-sac of Douglas is seen as the transverse shadow above the index finger.

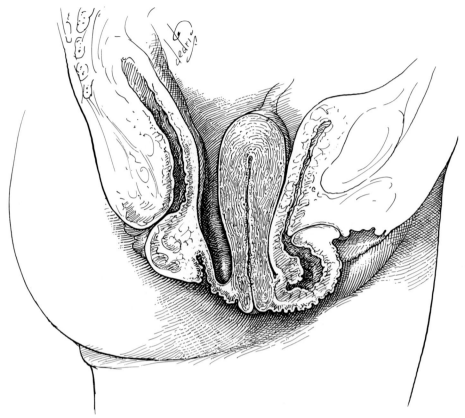

**Figure 3.7.** Uterovaginal or sliding prolapse is depicted. There is enterocele but no rectocele present. The uterosacral ligaments are long and strong. Note the position of the uninvolved anterior rectal wall. (After Halban J, Tandler : *Anatomie und Atiologie der genitalprolapse beim Weibe. Braumuller, Wien, 1907.*

## SUMMARY AND CONCLUSIONS

Genital prolapse is usually a manifestation of either prolapse of the upper vagina or eversion of the lower vagina. Although these are phenomena of different etiologies and prognosis, they may occur separately or in combination. The surgeon must recognize and differentiate primary sites of weakness from resulting secondary changes, for the optimal results of treatment will depend upon adequate repair of the primary damage. Progression of residual prolapse as a result of unrecognized and unrepaired weakness can be expected when a repair has failed to correct the primary problem.

It is possible that genital prolapse is more common among clinical diabetic patients because of weakness induced by high glycosylation of connective tissues coincident with hyperglycemia. This attractive thesis is discussed further in Chapter 23.

When genital prolapse and massive rectal prolapse coexist, they should each be treated, although by different surgical procedures. The genital prolapse should be treated first and, in most instances, by transvaginal colpopexy and

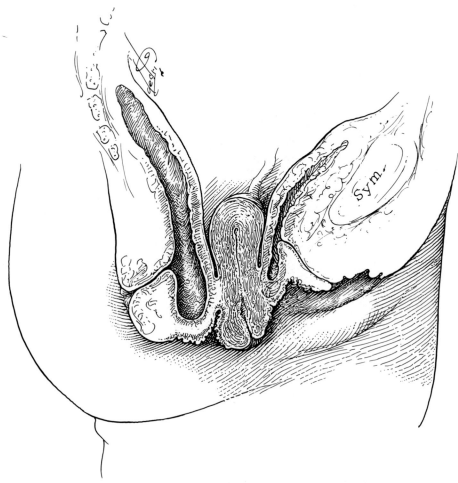

**Figure 3.8.** General postmenopausal genital prolapse resulting from atrophy and weakening of all of the endopelvic supporting tissues. A rectocele is present but no enterocele. The uterosacral ligaments are weak and hard to define by palpation. Note the defect in the support of the anterior rectal wall. (After Halban J, Tandler J: *Anatomie und Atiologie der genitalprolapse biem Weibe.* Braumuller, Wien, 1907.

colporrhaphy. The rectal prolapse generally should be treated by transabdominal rectopexy.

For discussion of the specific types of cystocele, rectocele, perineal prolapse, and enterocele, the reader is referred to Chapters 11–13 and 15 respectively. Postpartum chronic eversion of the uterus is discussed in Chapter 4.

### References

1. Ajabor LN, Okojie SE: Genital Prolapse in the Newborn. *Int Surg* 61:496–497, 1976.
2. Bonney V: The sustentacular apparatus of the female genital canal, the displacements that result from the yielding of its several components, and their appropriate treatment. *J Obstet Gynaecol Br Emp* 45: 328–344, 1914.
3. Geldenhuys FG: Genitale prolapse by die Bantoe. *S Afr Med J* 24:749–751, 1950.
4. Geldenhuys FG: On the Etiology of Genital Prolapse. MD Thesis, South Africa, University of Pretoria, 1951.
5. Halban J, Tandler J: *Anatomie und Atiologie der genitalprolapse beim Weibe.* Braumuller, Wien, 1907.

6. Henry MM: Personal communication, September 2, 1987.
7. Henry MM, Swash M (eds): *Colpoproctology and the Pelvic Floor*. London, Butterworths, 1985.
8. Heyns OS: Genital prolapse. In Charlewood GP (ed): *Bantu Gynaecology*. Johannesburg, Witwatersrand University Press, 1956.
9. Jeffcoate TNA: Posterior colporrhaphy. *Am J Obstet Gynecol* 77:490, 1959.
10. Magdi I: Obstetric injuries of the perineum. *J Obstet Gynaecol Br Commonw* 49:687–700, 1942.
11. Malpas P: The choice of operation for genital prolapse. In Meigs JV, Sturgis SH (eds): *Progress in Gynecology*. New York, Grune & Stratton, vol 3, 1957.
12. Paramore RH: *The Statics of the Female Pelvic Viscera*. London, HK Lewis, vol 2, 1925, p 273.
13. Parks AG: Anorectal incontinence. *Proc Roy Soc Med* 68:681–690, 1975.
14. Porges RF: A practical system of diagnosis and classification of pelvic relaxations. *Surg Gynecol Obstet* 117:769–773, 1963.
15. Ricci JV, Thom CH, Kron WL: Cleavage planes in reconstructive vaginal plastic surgery. *Am J Surg* 76: 354–363, 1948.
16. Schoetz DJ Jr, Veidenheimer MC: Rectal prolapse—pathogenesis and clinical features. In Henry MM, Swash M (eds): *Colpoproctology and the Pelvic Floor*. London, Butterworths, 1985, pp 303–307.
17. Shuwarger D, Young RL: Management of neonatal genital prolapse: Case reports and historic review. *Obstet Gynecol* 66: 615–635, 1985.
18. Stallworthy J: Personal communication.
19. Watts JD, Rothenberger DA, Goldberg SM: Rectal prolapse—treatment. In Henry MM, Swash M (eds): *Colpoproctology and the Pelvic Floor*. London, Butterworths, 1985, pp 308–339.
20. Zacharin RG: A Chinese anatomy—the pelvic supporting tissues of the Chinese and Occidental female compared and contrasted. *Aust NZ J Obstet Gynaecol* 17:11, 1977.

# CHAPTER 4

# Choice of Operation for Genital Prolapse

For the patient for whom nonemergency gynecologic surgery is recommended, a careful physical examination and work-up must precede the recommendation passed on to the patient. The patient must then be given adequate time to think about it and express any questions or concerns that she may have. This is sometimes best done at a revisit. If the patient has questions or difficulty about accepting a recommendation, a second opinion can be offered. The patient must also be told that her questions and concerns can be addressed again not only preoperatively but also during the hospital postoperative phase and full convalescence. It is helpful for the surgeon to ancitipate the usual questions that a patient may have regarding a particular procedure and, lest they be forgotten, answer them before they have been asked. These might include considerations as to her future sex life, her future fertility, and the disposition of her ovaries.

The surgeon should identify in each case the site, etiology, and extent of damage to the supporting tissues of the birth canal in order to define the objectives and to select the procedure necessary to assure a satisfactory repair. Questions relevant to decision making include: (*a*) What are the symptoms and do they correlate with the anatomic damage? (*b*) Has there been demonstrable progression of the prolapse? (*c*) What are the chances of restoring a vagina to normal with minimal chance of recurrence of prolapse?

Every operation must be tailored to the needs of each individual, taking into consideration the patient's reproductive potential, her marital state, age, habits, occupation, work, and activities, as well as the effect of any incidental diseases that may be present. If there is a desire for future pregnancy, it is usually better to postpone reconstructive surgery until childbearing has been completed.

For those who cannot wait, the surgical treatment of symptomatic genital prolapse requires some resourcefulness for the patient who cannot retain a pessary and wishes to have more children. If there is marked elongation of the cervix, cervical amputation with the Manchester-type repair can be useful in which that portion of the cardinal ligament that has been separated from the amputated portion of the cervix can be crossed in front of the remaining cervix. For the patient without cervical elongation, a transabdominal sacrocervical colpopexy, using fascia lata, is useful (20).

Coital interest must be respected. It is important to avoid excessive shortening or narrowing the vagina of a sexually active patient. Planned massive weight loss should be accomplished preoperatively, because the removal of ischiorectal fat from beneath the pelvic diaphragm may decrease the effectiveness of its support.

An individual with chronic respiratory disease, such as asthma, hay fever, chronic bronchitis, or a smoker's chronic cough usually has subjected her pelvic supporting tissues to major and pathologic surges of increased intra-abdominal pressure. These will continue after any type of surgical reconstruction, predisposing to an early recurrence of her prolapse. The type of activities and work to which the patient has been accustomed must be considered; for instance, increased intra-abdominal pressure from frequent heavy lifting has considerable influence on the strains to which the pelvic supporting tissues are subjected after an indicated repair.

Keeping in mind that most forms of symptomatic genital prolapse are progressive, one must determine which damage is primary and which is secondary, because, unless the primary cause is identified and corrected (or, as Bonney [3, 4] wrote: "necessarily overcorrected"), recurrence and progression are to be expected.

The convenient but simplistic concept of thinking of genital prolapse in terms of the position of the cervix in relation to the introitus fails to take into account the significant differences in the etiology of each component of an individual's genital prolapse. For example, pathologically increased intra-abdominal pressure may not only have produced damage but may directly influence the incidence of recurrence. Because the uterus is but passively involved, the primary defect with prolapse will be found in the uterovaginal supporting tissues, and it is to these supporting tissues that appropriate repair must be directed (Fig. 4.1). In many instances, vaginal removal of a prolapsed but otherwise normal uterus will be appropriate in order to mobilize the supporting tissues of the cervix and uterus adequately for use in the vaginal vault reconstruction (Fig. 4.2).

If the patient wishes to retain a mildly prolapsed uterus with cervical elongation, the lower cervix can be amputated and the now shortened cardinal

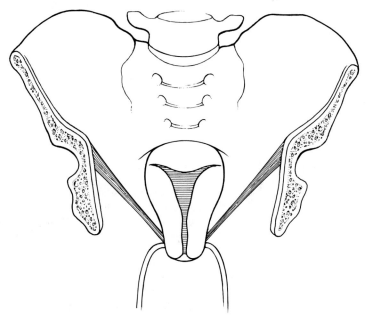

**Figure 4.1.**   Uterine prolapse with elongation of the cardinal-uterosacral ligament complex is noted.

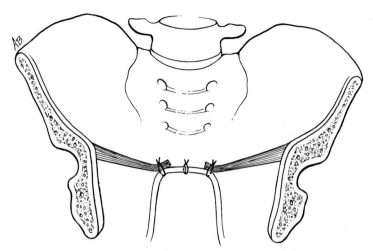

**Figure 4.2.** Hysterectomy has been performed and the now shortened cardinal-uterosacral ligament complex has been fixed to the vaginal vault on either side.

ligaments reattached to the remaining uterus by crossing them in front of the uterus, aiding in its support (Fig. 4.3).

We believe it unwise to evaluate a genital prolapse for repair while the tissues of a postpartum patient are still undergoing involution. Postponing such an evaluation for another 3 to 6 months, until involution is complete, will assure a more reliable appraisal.

Although genital damages may appear superficially similar, various combinations of possible etiologies may be present. These distinctive differences are of great importance, as they have to do not only with the rate and likelihood of progression of the disease, but also with the prognosis for surgical success. Variations in the technique of repair are indicated when significant damages have been produced by (*a*) "normal" supporting tissue that has been stretched

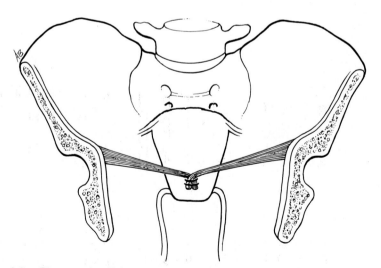

**Figure 4.3.** The cervix, if long, has been amputated, and the now shortened cardinal-uterosacral ligament complex crossed and sewn to the anterior surface of the remaining cervix and lower uterine segment.

or attenuated by chronically increased intra-abdominal pressure; (*b*) congenitally attenuated supporting tissues but with normal intra-abdominal pressure;
(*c*) congenitally attenuated supporting tissues coexistent with chronically
increased intra-abdominal pressure; and (*d*) any of the above to which may be
added the postmenopausal degenerative changes in pelvic supportive tissues.

The surgeon must take such factors into consideration if operative results are
to be uniformly good. Thus, there should be no standard technique for all
repairs because there is no standard damage to the supporting tissues.

To repair less than all the demonstrable weakness is analogous to repairing
all but a portion of an incisional hernia, for, in a sense, genital prolapse is
comparable to other types of hernia. For purposes of comparison, let us
imagine that the damaged vagina has been opened along each lateral wall and
displayed in a linear fashion (Fig. 4.4). Liken such segment to a ventral or
incisional hernia. Would it make good sense to repair only one-third or
two-thirds of a hernia and not the remainder? Would not the unrepaired
segment remain still a hernia, reduced to a weak spot of concentrated weakness
that must now bear the full brunt of changes in intra-abdominal pressure and, as

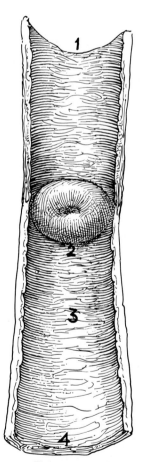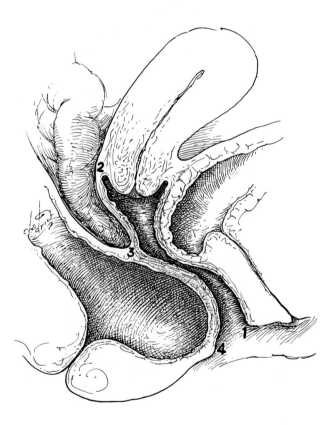

**Figure 4.4.**  Sagittal section of a pelvis showing segmental relaxation is on the
right. The anterior vaginal segment is indicated between *1* and *2*, the superior
between *2* and *3*, and the posterior between *3* and *4*. The damaged vagina has been
imaginatively opened and displayed in a linear fashion, in the drawing to the *left*.
The numbers correspond to the sites of segmental damage.

a result, tend to enlarge even faster? All genital thirds, or segments, if demonstrably weakened, should be repaired at the same operation, correcting the entire hernia. Anterior colporrhaphy generally should reconstruct the full length of the anterior vaginal wall including the urogenital diaphragm and all supports of the urethra and vesicourethral junction. Because the anterior vagina sits upon and derives considerable support from an adequate posterior wall, this procedure should be followed by repair of any demonstrable damage to the posterior wall. Failure to repair obvious cystocele often requires reoperation in later years. If a surgeon's patients experience a noticeable incidence of dyspareunia or apareunia due to vaginal narrowing, ridges, or an overly tightened perineum due to careless "routine" posterior colporrhaphy, the surgeon should change his or her technique. The development of a more careful repair should seek to avoid tender ridges while maintaining an adequate introitus and vaginal depth. One should not abandon posterior colporrhaphy and perineorrhaphy when it is indicated.

Since a dropped uterus is the result and not the cause of a genital prolapse, hysterectomy without repair is an exercise in futility. In his classic paper indicting posterior colporrhaphy as a cause of dyspareunia and apareunia, Jeffcoate (9) stated that the need for posterior colporrhaphy in a particular patient should be determined by examining the unanesthetized patient. If this examination shows a need for posterior vaginal repair, the procedure should be included in the surgical reconstruction.

It is paradoxical that, although the symptoms of various components of genital prolapse are generally associated with specific and demonstrable anatomic weakness, the anatomic defects may, at times, be present without symptoms. Whether this is a fact of evolution of the weakness or, to some extent, may represent accommodation and forbearance on the part of the patient is unknown. It is unlikely that one can make an asymptomatic patient feel better by electively operating upon her, and one should be equally cautious in recommending surgery when symptoms are present without evident or substantiating pathology.

A genital prolapse should be repaired when it is significantly progressive or sufficiently distressing for the patient to have complained of it to the gynecologist (22).

Bonney (3, 4) suggested that three levels of damage to pelvic supports should be considered, which might have been injured singly or in any combination (Fig. 4.5A). There is obvious need to develop skill in three-dimensional thinking in the assessment of pelvic damage. Successful surgical reconstruction requires identification of each level of damage with appropriate repair.

1. Damage to the upper steadying apparatus (Fig. 4.5B), the round and broad ligaments, may result in excessive mobility of the uterine fundus and is commonly associated with retroversion. Uncomplicated damage to this level of support is usually nonprogressive and asymptomatic and does not, of itself, indicate surgery.

2. Damage to the middle holding group (Fig. 4.5C), the cardinal-uterosacral ligament complex, results in a gradual but progressive eversion of the upper vagina, often with coincident elongation of the cervix. If the upper supports are strong or the fundus is pathologically adherent, the uterine body may remain in its usual intra-abdominal location while the cervix elongates and descends. The cervix and anterior vagina often function as a single unit, however, and often share in the response to damage by the development of cervical elongation and a cystocele. Both changes are basically due to obstetric trauma, both are slowly progressive, and together they comprise the most common type and appearance of prolapse. Because the pelvic diaphragm is usually intact in this

situation, rectocele does not characteristically accompany this type of prolapse. Extensive posterior colporrhaphy is not often necessary. Satisfactory treatment includes vaginal hysterectomy, excision of any enterocele, and shortening and reattachment of the transected cardinal-uterosacral ligament complex to the posterior vaginal vault. To preserve length, the vaginal vault may be approximated in the sagittal plane (i.e., the six to twelve o'clock positions), and a noticeably widened posterior fornix should be narrowed by appropriate wedging or resection.

3. Damage to the lower group of supporting tissues (Fig. 4.5D), the pelvic and urogenital diaphragms, the perineum and muscles contained therein, usually results in eversion of the vagina with development of a cystocele and a low or midrectocele, both of which should be corrected by appropriate anterior and posterior colporrhaphy.

When the vaginal rugae covering the bladder are flattened more than those preserved in the lateral vaginal walls or when there is demonstrable progression in the size of the cystoceles, anterior colporrhaphy is indicated. Anterior repair is indicated if there is bladder symptomatology; a bearing-down sensation, urinary incontinence, urinary stress incontinence, high residual urine with frequent episodes of cystitis, or overflow incontinence in the absence of a nonreversible neuropathy (as may be produced by multiple sclerosis, diabetes, or advanced lues). The technique of colporrhaphy varies according to whether the prolapse is uterovaginal or general and whether the urogenital diaphragm has been damaged. The common midline defects should be repaired. If there is demonstrable lateral detachment of the supports of the vagina from the arcus tendineus, they should be reunited, preferably transvaginally. This can be determined at the preliminary physical examination in which a lateral wall defect that comes down when the patient strains does not go back when she contracts or "holds" the muscles of her pelvic diaphragm (1).

One should differentiate between rotational descent of the bladder neck (anterior pseudocystocele) and true or posterior cystocele. The presence of vaginal rugal folds helps considerably in making the differential diagnosis, and any coexistent descent of the vaginal vault is important. When rugal folds are absent with cystocele there is a significant midline defect, the full length of the vaginal wall should be reconstructed, including the support of the vesicourethral junction. The presence of rugae and rotational descent of the bladder neck indicate that support of the vesicourethral junction should be a primary objective of a repair. Demonstrable urethral funneling should be corrected but the most important goal is to re-elevate the vesicourethral junction. The junction should be elevated so that it is once again within the influence of changes in intra-abdominal pressure and no longer is the most dependent portion of the bladder.

Whereas the work of Green (6) has called attention to the posterior urethrovesical angle and urethral inclination, Ball (2) has emphasized the significance of urethral funneling; an anatomic defect that physiologically "shortens" the effective urethral length by permitting the transmission of bladder pressure directly to the urine inside the funnel. If the effective vesicourethral junction (i.e., the point at which the distal neck of the funnel joins the remaining urethra) is caudal to the area responsive to changes in intra-abdominal pressure, the increase would be transmitted only to the bladder, and if intravesical pressure exceeded intraurethral pressure, urinary stress incontinence would result.

When does one plicate the urogenital diaphragm? If a rotational descent of the bladder neck is found during anterior colporrhaphy, this is evidence of damage to the urogenital diaphragm, which should be surgically restored even

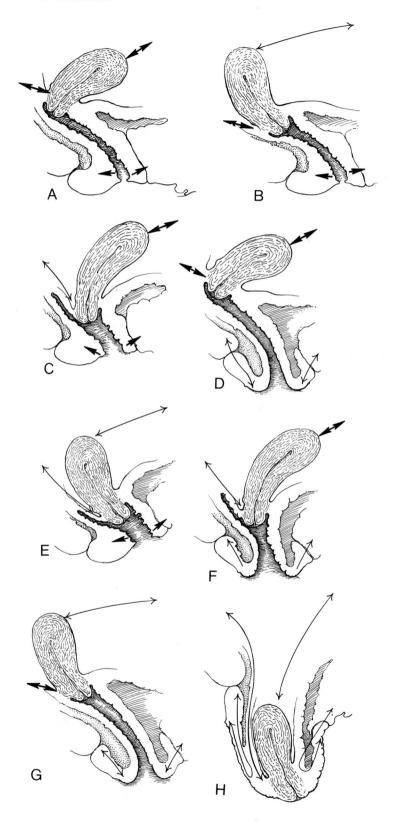

if the patient is continent, lest correction of the cystocele alone risk flattening of the posterior urethrovesical angle, risking stress incontinence (21).

Dislocation cystocele coincident with vaginal eversion results from damage to lateral connective tissue supports. Under such circumstances there may be preservation of vaginal rugae in the premenopausal patient. This finding is in contrast to the cystocele produced by overdistension with destruction of the fibromuscular elasticity in the vaginal wall itself, often with increase in the total length and width of the vaginal wall and fornices. The former condition is corrected primarily by restoration of vaginal depth, axis, and support; the latter is corrected primarily by reduction of vaginal width by excision of an appropriately shaped wedge of vaginal mucosa including the area of maximum thinning, usually midvaginal.

In perhaps one-quarter of instances of symptomatic genital prolapse, eversion of the vault coexists with that of the lower vagina, and the surgeon must take each of these etiologic differences into account in planning the technique of repair, which will differ from one patient to another.

The surgical repair of coexistent cystocele and urethral detachment is necessarily quite different from that of cystocele alone. Symmonds and Jordan (21) have called attention to the importance of a history of previous stress incontinence, now relieved, in certain patients now presenting with an enlarging cystocele. The stress incontinence disappeared, because, as the cystocele became larger and the bladder dropped more than the urethra, a posterior urethrovesical angle reappeared. The surgeon must accomplish a reconstruction that will provide adequate support of both the urethra and the bladder

---

**Figure 4.5.**  The three levels of normal genital support (upper, middle, lower) are indicated by *thick short arrows. Thin long arrows* indicate weakened support. *A,* sagittal section through normal female pelvis shows good support of all levels. The upper level contains round and broad ligaments. Uterosacral and cardinal ligaments are contained in middle level. The lower supporting group includes the pelvic and urogenital diaphragms, and the perineum and muscles contained therein. The uterine fundus is situated anteriorly. The vagina is not everted. *B,* damage is to the upper supports with consequent retroversion of uterus. The positions of vagina, bladder, and rectum are normal. *C,* damage is shown to middle supporting group alone. Because intra-abdominal position of uterine fundus is maintained by strong upper level support, the upper vagina becomes everted with descent and elongation of cervix. Strong lower support resists formation of cystocele or rectocele, but middle support damage is often accompanied by enterocele. *D,* loss of lower supports is illustrated. The lower vagina is everted with cystocele and rectocele, but normal upper and middle supports hold the upper vagina and uterus in position for the present. *E,* defective middle and upper supports, retroversion and descent of the uterus, and inversion of the upper vagina is shown. Strong lower supports resist eversion, and true cystocele and rectocele are not present. *F,* defective middle and lower supports, eversion of upper vagina, descent of cervix, and eversion of lower vagina with cystocele and rectocele is shown. Strong upper supports retain uterine fundus in its usual position, permitting elongation of cervix. *G,* damage is to the upper and lower, but not the middle, supports. Retroversion of uterus and eversion of lower vagina with cystocele and rectocele but no eversion of upper vagina or descent of cervix. *H,* damage to all three levels of support is illustrated. Vagina is turned inside out and entire uterus lies outside the pelvis. Eversion is complete. (By permission from McGraw-Hill in Nichols DH: The choice of operation for genital prolapse. *Postgrad Med* 47:163–167, 1970.)

neck. Failure to restore urethral support may result in a return of the stress incontinence.

To be effective, the posterior colporrhaphy must be carried to above the most cranial point of the rectocele (see Chapter 12). The uterus and cervix may remain in the same position for years until the supporting tissues weaken with aging, causing a prolapse of the middle or upper portions of the vagina.

4. Actual damage to the upper and middle, but not lower, supports (Fig. 4.5E) is quite frequent, however, and the resulting eversion of the upper vagina often develops with descent of a normal-sized, usually retroverted uterus but with no eversion of the lower vagina. Effective treatment would include vaginal hysterectomy with shortening of the uterosacral ligaments and excision of any enterocele, as in number 2 above.

5. Damage to the genital supports of the middle and lower but not to the upper (broad ligament and fundus) vagina is also often seen (Fig. 4.5F). This produces simultaneous elongation of the cervix with eversion of both upper and lower vagina with development of both cystocele and rectocele. Because the uterine fundus remains supported at a normal intra-abdominal level, elongation of the cervix will continue until it protrudes beyond the vulvar orifice. A uterine sound introduced into such a uterus will reveal a surprising depth of the uterine cavity, largely accounted for by the length of the cervical canal. The gynecologic surgeon should anticipate technical changes peculiar to the increased length of the cervix. Surgical technique should be modified to take into account the higher lateral attachment of the uterosacral and cardinal ligaments, and the higher reflections of the anterior and posterior peritoneal folds. The incision circumscribing the cervix is made appropriately further away from the external cervical os. Although good vaginal depth may be obtained in this circumstance by cervical amputation plus an anterior and posterior colporrhaphy (Manchester procedure), the incidence of subsequent uterine disease has made vaginal hysterectomy with repair the treatment of choice when the fundus is freely movable and the patient has completed her family, and the surgeon is experienced and comfortable with the techniques of vaginal hysterectomy for the uterus which, though movable, is not prolapsed. In fact, most reconstructive surgery is deferred until after the period of desired childbearing. Because vaginal hysterectomy involves opening the cul-de-sac, any coexistent enterocele is readily evaluated and treated.

6. The treatment of damage to the lower vaginal and upper uterine, but not the middle, supports (Fig. 4.5G) is usually the same as for number 3, essentially an anterior and posterior colporrhaphy, although the presence of uterine pathology might indicate either vaginal or abdominal hysterectomy.

Rectocele, of course, may occur at various levels of the vagina, and the entire defect should be repaired whenever an anterior colporrhaphy has been performed. A posterior vaginal repair is particularly indicated if the rectocele is associated with incomplete bowel movements that require digital manipulation for completion or when the patient complains of a sensation of postevacuation rectal pressure or fullness.

If a symptomatic rectocele enlarges progressively during a period of observation, or is large enough to alter the normal vaginal axis, or is associated with enterocele, a repair is indicated. Repair should also usually be considered when the patient herself requests it.

Because the presence and strength of the pubovaginalis muscle is inconstant, apparently being better developed among Negroid peoples than among Anglo-Saxons, the need for so-called "levator stitches" as a feature of perineorrhaphy is subject to wide variation. In the reconstruction of a torn or defective perineal body, the levator *fascia* of each side (pubococcygeus-pubovaginalis component) may be approximated at the apex of the proposed perineal body reconstruction some 2 to 2 1/2 inches above the hymenal margin. If these stitches, when necessary, are properly placed, they should constitute a first step in the reconstruction of a wedge or plane of perineum and should not result in a palpable ridge beneath the posterior vaginal wall. Indeed, after each stitch is placed and before it is tied, the operator should apply traction to the ends of the crossed sutures and, if a ridge is found, the suture should be removed and replaced less deeply and closer to the rectum. If permitted to remain, it may become a subject of distress for the patient, her husband, and her surgeon, for it may represent a cause of future dyspareunia or apareunia, as emphasized by Jeffcoate.

Stitches should be tied only as tightly as is necessary to approximate the tissue. Stitches that are too snug will probably strangulate the tissue, with the destruction of basic substrate and replacement by tender areas of rigid inelastic fibrosis. Because the perineal body is composed of a number of different structures, which vary from one individual to another, there are a variety of deficiencies that can develop.

In the patient without laceration of the external anal sphincter, rectal incontinence as evidenced by chronic soiling and often preceded by loss of sensory discrimination between solid, liquid, and gaseous rectal content may identify the patient who is at increased risk for future rectal prolapse. Careful examination may disclose a perineal descent syndrome with elongation of the levator ani. If voluntary contractions of the pubococcygei and external anal sphincter are of poor quality, a pudendal neuropathy may be related( 8, 17, 18). In this circumstance, the internal anal sphincter may be all that provides the remaining degree of continence. When this final vulnerable protective function is gone, the patient's rectum may become totally incontinent. Specific symptoms include obstipation, diminished diameter of passed stool, and often, chronic rectal soiling. If perineal descent is symptomatic or visibly progressive, it should be strongly considered for repair either by retrorectal levatorplasty (14, 15) or by the Parks postanal repair (17 ).

The configuration of the patient's pelvis is a determining factor in whether the uterus can be removed safely from below by the experienced operator. In the examination preceding surgery, the operator should be able to insert his or her fist gently between the ischial spines when palpating the perineum. Helpful information can also be obtained from the vulvar slant, which will help distinguish between the ample measurements of the gynecoid pelvis, in contrast to the restricted size of the pelvic outlet as identified with the android pelvis (see Chapter 10).

When vaginal hysterectomy is performed on a patient with an asymptomatic cystocele and rectocele, it is our view that these latter abnormalities should be repaired at the time of the original surgery to correct an abnormal vaginal depth and axis. This step will diminish significantly the opportunity for future vaginal eversion.

Krige (10) has written:

"The choice of a case for vaginal hysterectomy may be easy if the chief indication for operation is definite second or later degree of prolapse. The more enterprising surgeon has learned from experience that certain cases prove to be deceptively difficult, consequently he exercises great care in picking his cases. There are times when a case of large cystocele and rectocele well outside the introitus call for treatment from below, but excision of the uterus may be a real trial and struggle for the surgeon. However, with increasing experience he learns to assess the laxity of the vault, mobility of the cervix and viability of the uterus, by manual and speculum examination. A significant bulge in the posterior fornix may indicate high rectocele or potential enterocele and calls for vaginal hysterectomy with repair. Confidence in technique enables one to tackle a different case knowingly. It is a peculiar fact that the struggle in a really difficult vaginal hysterectomy is often not reflected in the patient's uneventful recovery. The surgeon's list of indications not only reveals his or her mental attitude toward the operation, but also confidence or lack thereof in personal operative ability and technique. If training has been inadequate, the correct decision on the indicated operation becomes a problem. There are times when he or she feels the patient should have a vaginal hysterectomy, but courage fails and giving in to the doubt created, the surgeon falls back on archaic abdomino-vaginal operations. Justification for this failure is found in the tradition and conservatism of senior gynecologists and their apparent satisfaction with such procedures, an attitude that has depressingly retarded developments. Under present conditions, the young surgeon has few opportunities to improve personal technique. With proper instruction, vaginal hysterectomy becomes a safe and simple operation."

Of 1393 vaginal hysterectomies performed by Krige, 90% involved simultaneous anterior and posterior colporrhaphy. Of 889 vaginal hysterectomies by Navratil (13) for benign disease of the uterus, 73% included simultaneous vaginal repair. Gray (5) reported 97% repair in 1410 cases, and Hawksworth and Roux (8) reported 90% repair in 1000 vaginal hysterectomies.

Richter (19) reported 3468 hysterectomies between 1956 and 1971, of which 2611, or 75%, were done vaginally. More than 87% (87.4%) of the vaginal hysterectomies were combined with a pelvic floor repair. In such experienced hands, vaginal hysterectomy has clearly replaced abdominal hysterectomy in all cases in which a vaginal repair is indicated.

## VAGINAL HYSTERECTOMY INDICATIONS AND CONTRAINDICATIONS

Primary indications for vaginal hysterectomy are symptomatic or progressive genital prolapse and uterine abnormality, either dysfunction or neoplasia.

Inclusion of hysterectomy in an indicated vaginal repair can be considered if the cul-de-sac of Douglas is free, not obliterated by inflammatory adhesions or endometriosis, and the uterus is movable and not too large. Provided that the uterus is freely movable and not too large, most can be removed safely by the vaginal route. When there is no prolapse, the anatomic relationships are remarkably similar in all cases, making the technical details of hysterectomy often easier than in the patient with advanced prolapse. When hysterectomy is required in the obese patient, the vaginal route is usually accomplished by less morbidity than the abdominal (16).

The indications for abdominal hysterectomy are those that represent the contraindication for vaginal hysterectomy. Relative contraindications that merit consideration are adnexal disease, inflammatory or neoplastic, conditions producing obliteration of the cul-de-sac, unusually large size of the uterus, and certain types of invasive malignant disease. Very few surgeons who have once mastered a safe vaginal hysterectomy technique will later abandon it in favor of the abdominal route. As the operator's confidence and experience in vaginal hysterectomy increase, one's indications for the operation will become more liberal.

With uterovaginal prolapse, the fundus, of course, may occupy a relatively normal position within the pelvis, although the cervix may be markedly elongated. The operator should have experience performing vaginal hysterectomy upon the nonprolapsed uterus before choosing to treat prolapse of the cervix by hysterectomy instead of a Manchester procedure. When the uterus is not prolapsed, ventral fixation or uterine suspension is of no value as treatment for an elongated prolapsing cervix. When the fundus of the uterus has remained at a normal position, removing it or fixing it anteriorly will not remove an elongated cervix from the vagina.

Because abdominal wall relaxation is not required for transvaginal surgery, the depth and duration of anesthesia are decreased. Postoperative respiratory excursions are more adequate because the abdomen is not immobilized by incisional tenderness and pain, and the attendant complications of atelectasis and pneumonia are decreased. There is no risk of abdominal wound infection or incisional hernia. There will be less postoperative ileus and less need for postoperative parenteral feeding because of minimal handling of bowel. Ambulation is more comfortable because of the absence of abdominal incisional pain. Most important, unsuspected enterocele can be diagnosed and corrected as part of the primary surgical process, along with correction of any symptomatic or progressive vaginal relaxation, all during the same operative procedure, without the delay of repositioning and redraping the patient.

Pelvic examination under anesthesia should immediately precede hysterectomy. This confirms the uterine size and mobility, the location of the posterior cul-de-sac and the length and strength of the cardinal-uterosacral ligament complex. Any question as to the condition of the adnexal or other intraabdominal pelvic pathology may be resolved by coincident preliminary laparoscopy. If there is some uncertainty about the feasibility of the vaginal route for hysterectomy, the operator, nevertheless, can still begin the operation. Should progress prove unexpectedly difficult or should the operator be unable to find and open either cul-de-sac, vaginal efforts to remove the uterus can be discontinued. Vaginal reconstruction can be completed while a new surgical set-up is being prepared so the hysterectomy can be completed abdominally.

When hysterectomy is performed because of intrinsic pathology within the uterus itself, the operation is fundamentally destructive, and, as long as it has been accomplished safely, it makes very little difference whether the uterus is removed upside down, sideways, or inside out, as long as removal is safe and without damage to adjacent organs. But when the operation of hysterectomy is part of a reconstruction, the principles pertinent to the two approaches are entirely different. In extirpation for primary uterine disease, the specific technique is unimportant as long as the uterus is removed safely. But when hysterectomy is part of a planned reconstruction, each step must be planned, purposeful, and in accord with the primary objective of using, preserving, and strengthening pelvic support tissues.

The indication for hysterectomy coincident with vaginal reconstruction relates to the degree of the patient's discomfort and inconvenience. When there is a history of prolonged bleeding and one finds a significantly lowered blood count, and other reasons for anemia have been excluded, the chronic blood loss itself, although it may be acceptable to the patient, may well indicate a hysterectomy.

Vaginal oophorectomy may be performed if the ovaries are found surgically accessible or low in the pelvis (Chapter 10).

Vaginal hysterectomy may be essentially extrafascial and, therefore, can be safely employed as the treatment by hysterectomy in a patient with adenocarcinoma of the endometrium if it is of low grade and stage and particularly if the patient is obese or elderly. Coincident transvaginal salpingo-oophorectomy is desirable (5). If postoperative examination of the hysterectomy specimen shows unexpected tumor envolvement of the middle or outer third of the myometrium, postoperative external radiation therapy can be planned.

All things being equal, the choice of an abdominal over a vaginal route for hysterectomy might be a little like taking tonsils out through an incision in the side of the neck, an analogy suggested by Moir in discussing the choice of approach for the repair of vesicovaginal fistula.

Occasionally, the appendix will be found in the operative field and may be removed, unless a valid reason exists for not performing appendectomy. When vaginal appendectomy has been accomplished, the operator must remember to inform the patient, so the absence of an abdominal scar will not mislead those responsible for her future medical care.

7. The result of damage at all three levels of support is likely to be a vagina turned completely inside out (Fig. 4.5H). Most women with procidentia are unable to retain a vaginal pessary for an extended period of time because of the damage to and the relaxation of the pelvic diaphragm. As a result, the treatment of choice will usually be vaginal hysterectomy and extensive colporrhaphy, with corresponding reduction in vaginal width and depth. Success in such a case will need all the technical virtuosity, skill, and good fortune a surgeon can summon, but the prognosis for a usable vagina is guarded, unless sacrospinous colpopexy or sacrocolpopexy is employed (see Chapter 16, "Massive Eversion of the Vagina"). Enterocele, when present, must always be resected, even in those uncommon instances when the surgeon feels obliged to resort to vaginectomy or colpocleisis.

There are two principal types of colpectomy, subtotal and total. The subtotal operation is especially useful if the uterus is present, atrophic in size, without elongation of the cervix, and when one desires not to open the peritoneal cavity. The total colpectomy is more advisable when the above conditions are not present.

When eversion of a vagina coexists with congenital enterocele, it is essential that the operator open the peritoneal cavity and resect or occlude the necessary enterocele sac to eliminate a residual postoperative enterocele (Chapter 15).

Such "recurrence" will often be progressive, continuing to dissect between the obliterated vagina and the rectum until it appears as a symptomatic bulge in the perineum. This carries with it all the symptoms of falling out that were present with the original vault eversion, and it is now technically more formidable to repair.

Malpas (11) points out that only the anterior wall of the enterocele descends with the uterus in uterovaginal or sliding prolapse. This kind of enterocele, is, in his opinion, incidental to the prolapse but not the prime anatomic feature, the latter being the elongated cardinal-uterosacral ligament complex. It is, of course, desirable to excise the sac and then perform a high ligation of the neck along with a cul-de-plasty in order to minimize the risk of postmenopausal reoperation.

An enterocele may sometimes coexist with general prolapse, but more commonly, there is with this type a descent of the cul-de-sac without dissection or formation of a sac between the rectum and the vagina. There is equal descent of both anterior and posterior walls of the cul-de-sac, the latter bringing with it the anterior wall of the rectum. It is essential to mobilize the peritoneum laterally as well as anteriorly and posteriorly and to excise the entire sac since it is often a prominent anatomic feature of the prolapse itself. If strong cardinal-uterosacral ligaments are not available nor even palpable, as is so often the case, an alternative method of supporting the vault must be incorporated as part of the initial procedure. Sacrospinous colpopexy is an example of such a method. Removal of the peritoneal sac is best accomplished after the hysterectomy.

Although uncomplicated uterine retroversion often precedes prolapse, there is no reason to conclude that retroversion causes genital prolapse. Because prolapse and retroversion may coexist, the surgical correction of one should be recognized as having no influence on the cure or progression of the other.

Consequently, uterine suspension or fixation is not a treatment directed to the primary cause of coexistent or eventual prolapse. The progressive development of prolapse will be only temporarily slowed as a result of uterine suspension, and apparent improvement will have been accomplished at the expense of increasing the complexity and difficulty of subsequent definitive repair. In the management of most instances of early progressive genital prolapse, vaginal hysterectomy and repair should be performed rather than uterine suspension and tubal ligation.

The place of the vaginal pessary in presurgical evaluation is principally to determine whether a patient's symptoms of backache and falling out are of pelvic or orthopaedic origin. If there is question as to which of these factors accounts for the complaing, a properly fitted vaginal pessary should be inserted as a therapeutic test and observation made as to whether the patient's symptoms are relieved. The pessary should be removed after a few weeks and the patient observed for another period to determine whether the symptoms recur. If the symptoms are significantly relieved while wearing the pessary and recur after its removal, the patient's complaints probably are of intrapelvic origin and correctable by appropriate reconstructive gynecologic surgery. If the symptoms are unrelieved by the pessary and unaffected by its removal, they are probably due to problems unrelated to weakness of pelvic connective tissues, in which case therapy should be directed more appropriately toward proper orthopaedic and hygenic measures. A differential point in the history of such patients is that backache which is present on arising and tends to improve as the day goes on is likely to be a symptom of orthopaedic weakness, whereas a backache that comes on after the patient is on her feet for a time and is rather promptly relieved when lying down is the type of complaint probably related to genital prolapse. As a diagnostic aid, this characteristic discomfort may be reproduced at examination by traction upon the cervix, which will stretch the retroperitoneal pelvic nerve supply contained in the uterosacral ligaments.

When symptoms are relieved by the use of the pessary, the gynecologist should be prepared to resist the patient's request for reinsertion of the pessary as a substitute for the indicated surgery. She should be advised that the pessary is only palliative, not curative, and acts by continuing a stretch in the opposite direction of tissues that have already been pathologically elongated. Silent progression of the prolapse and widening of the levator hiatus usually will continue until a pessary can no longer be retained. At that time, the now older patient will be a less favorable operative risk, and with fewer remaining years in which to enjoy the comfort that surgery should provide.

Vaginal vault prolapse after either abdominal or vaginal hysterectomy usually is the result of insufficient surgical attention to identification and treatment of enterocele or of the primary sites of weakness in the individual's pelvic supporting tissues. The management of this important problem is the subject of Chapter 16.

In the event that rectal prolapse coexists with genital prolapse, the surgery and repair for the genital prolapse should be accomplished as the first of a two-stage single operation, to be followed by a transabdominal Ripstein-type suspension of the rectum (12). In a patient with symptomatic perineal descent, the transvaginal reconstruction should precede the retrorectal levatorplasty (see Chapter 13).

## SUMMARY

The surgeon should think of prolapse in terms of the sites of damage to the musculoconnective tissue supports of the birth canal rather than giving sole consideration to the positions of the uterus and cervix relative to the vulvar outlet. The primary site of damage should be identified and emphasized in the repair, with effort to preserve an adequate vagina whenever possible. One must be ever mindful of the importance of the patient's posture and the effects of asthma, bronchitis, hay fever, tight girdles, and corsets as factors increasing intra-abdominal pressure and stress on pelvic supporting tissues. The patient with genital prolapse who manifests any of these additional symptoms and findings is a good candidate for postoperative recurrence. Whenever possible the surgical intent should be to overcorrect the primary site of damage while making every effort to preserve vaginal length and a normal vaginal axis. A wide vaginal vault should be narrowed.

Generally speaking, the more severe the prolapse, the more difficult the operation, but the greater will be the patient's appreciation. There is no other field in surgery in which the gratitude of the patient and her husband for a good result is so genuine and the surgeon's efforts so truly appreciated.

The surgeon should have and exhibit enthusiasm, knowledge, and confidence about the specific procedure that is planned. Although a surgeon may have performed countless surgical reconstructions, to each particular patient her own surgery is the most important operation of all. It is the surgeon's obligation to choose the operation carefully, explain it thoroughly to the patient, and perform it well. The surgeon's thoughtful and unhurried daily rounds during the postoperative hospital stay add immeasurably to the patient's recovery, both physiologically and psychologically.

As TeLinde (22) has emphasized, there is much to be gained when the gynecologic surgeon follows the results of his surgery by periodic pelvic examination over a number of years, correlating any recurrent disease, and especially late recurrence, with the choice of operation and the surgical technique employed for a particular patient. Such evidence is objective, positive, and purposeful and will help influence one's future choice of procedure, either by reinforcement or change, as circumstances require. Equally significant analysis is practically impossible in a clinic-type or short-term practice where the patient is not actually followed for a long period of time by the surgeon who was responsible for the choice and technique of repair.

## References

1. Baden WF, Walker TA: Evaluation of the Stress Incontinent Patient. In Cantor EB (ed): *Female Urinary Stress Incontinence.* Springfield, IL, Charles C Thomas, 1979.
2. Ball TL: Anterior and posterior cystocele: cystocele revisited; Of some antifacialists and facilists as I knew them. *Clin Obstet Gynecol* 9:1062–1069, 1964.
3. Bonney V: The sustentacular apparatus of the female genital canal, the displacements that result from the yielding of its several components, and their appropriate treatment. *J Obstet Gynaecol Br Commonw* 45:328–344, 1914.
4. Bonney V: The principles that should underlie all operations for prolapse. *J Obstet Gynaecol Br Emp* 41:669–683, 1934.
5. Gray LA: *Vaginal Hysterectomy.* Springfield, IL, Charles C Thomas, ed. 3 1983.
6. Green TH: Development of a plan for the diagnosis and treatment of urinary stress incontinence. *Am J Obstet Gynecol* 83:632–648, 1961.
7. Hawksworth W, Roux JP: Vaginal hysterectomy. *J Obstet Gynaecol Br Commonw* 63:214–228, 1958.
8. Henry MM, Swash M: *Colpoproctology and the Pelvic Floor.* London, Butterworths, 1985.
9. Jeffcoate TNA: Posterior colporrhaphy. *Am J Obstet Gynecol* 77:490, 1959.
10. Krige CF: The repair of genital prolapse combined with vaginal hysterectomy. *J Obstet Gynaecol Br Commonw* 69:570–583, 1962.
11. Malpas P: *Genital Prolapse in Allied Condition.* New York, Grune & Stratton, 1955.
12. McMahan JD, Ripstein CB: Rectal prolapse. *Am Surg* 53:37–40, 1987.
13. Navratil E: The place of vaginal hysterectomy. *J Obstet Gynaecol Br Commonw* 72:841–846, 1965.
14. Nichols DH: Retrorectal levatorplasty for anal and perineal prolapse. *Surg Gynecol Obstet* 154:251–254, 1982.
15. Nichols DH: Retrorectal levatorplasty with

colporrhaphy. *Clin Obstet Gynecol* 25:939–947, 1982.

16. Nichols DH, Randall CL: Techniques to decrease morbidity in the obese patient. In Ludwig H, Thomsen K (eds): *Gynecology and Obstetrics*. Berlin, Springer-Verlag, 1986, pp. 619–620.

17. Parks AG: Anorectal incontinence. *Proc Roy Soc Med* 68:681–690, 1975.

18. Parks AG, Swash M, Urich H: Sphincter denervation in anorectal incontinence and rectal prolapse. *J Br Soc Gastroenterol* 18:656, 1977.

19. Richter K: Ekrankungen der Vagina. In Schwalm Doderlein: *Klinic der Frauenheilkunde und Geburtshilfe*. Munchen, Urban & Schwarzenberg, vol. VIII, 1971.

20. Stoesser FG: Construction of a sacrocervical ligament for uterine suspension. *Surg Gynecol Obstet* 101:638–641, 1955.

21. Symmonds RE, Jordan LT: Iatrogenic stress incontinence of urine. *Am J Obstet Gynecol* 82:1231, 1961.

22. TeLinde RW: Prolapse of the uterus and allied conditions. *Am J Obstet Gynecol* 93:444, 1966.

# CHAPTER 5

# Choice of Operation for Urinary Stress Incontinence

Because urinary incontinence is a symptom complex that includes etiologic components of varied relationships, it constitutes a mixture of symptoms that compete and combine to account for varying degrees of disability. Some components are inflammatory; some are the result of neurologic disturbances affecting the voiding mechanism; others are the result of congenital deficiency or of iatrogenic disease. Specific anatomic deficiencies may have so altered normal bladder physiology as to make it difficult for the patient to retain her urine at times of increased intra-abdominal pressure. When dominant, this component is referred to as urinary stress incontinence and may vary between such wide extremes as an occasional almost incidental occurrence to a major and very real social disability.

The different anatomic and physiologic factors involved in the development of urinary incontinence should be separately identified, because they play a most important role in the selection of appropriate, individualized therapy for the woman. The hydrodynamics of micturition and stress incontinence have been summarized by Crisp (8) as follows:

1. The intracystic pressure is equal to, or slightly greater than, an intra-abdominal pressure under normal conditions, regardless of the degree of filling. It measures approximately 2 mm Hg.
2. Intracystic pressure rises immediately and directly as the intra-abdominal pressure increases. This occurs whether the bladder is in normal position or in marked prolapse, since the law of hydrostatics (Pascal's law) states that when an external pressure is applied to the wall of a container of fluid, this pressure is transmitted equally in all directions.
3. Under conditions of rest, the pressure within the urethra is greater (2 to 6 mm Hg) than the intracystic pressure. The pressure within the urethral segment rises proportionately to the increase in intracystic pressure. These observations confirmed by Beck, Hsu, and Maughan (6), show that stress incontinence cannot occur without some incompetence of the urethral segment. Urethral pressure depends not only on the involuntary resistance, which includes the urethral mucosa, periurethral tissues, and vasculature, but also on the voluntary resistance of the midportion of the urethra and the pubourethral ligaments. The patient will not be incontinent as long as the voluntary muscular segment functions normally, maintaining the combined pressure of the urethra greater than the intravesicle pressure with or without additional intra-abdominal pressure that is associated with stress of coughing, etc.

Many investigators have stated that the problem of stress incontinence is centered around the loss of the posterior urethrovesical angle. These authors give the impression that in order to be continent, the female must have an angle of obstruction that prevents incontinence but that she may lower to void. The loss of the posterior vesical angle is only a sign of, not the cause of, stress incontinence. Resistance of flow in any tubular structure is inversely proportional to the diameter of the pipe, and directly proportional to its length. Angulation of the pipe does not significantly change this principle. There is, of course, a degree of back-thrust of the urinary stream at the point of angulation, but it is probably insignificant.

To reiterate, intraurethral pressure is dependent upon good support of both segments of the urethra. Keeping in mind the many variables that occur during micturition, involuntary loss of urine occurs when intravesical pressure is greater than intra-urethral pressure.

In the presence of a large cystocele, increases in intra-abdominal intravesical pressure will be transmitted largely to the most dependent portion of the cystocele (at the vaginal introitus), rather than against the attenuated urethrovesical junction. In addition, progressive development of prolapse of the bladder tends to angulate or to kink the urethra to some extent. Sometimes this action will "cure" the patient's incontinence or even overcompensate for the leakage, in that the bladder must be manually elevated before the patient is able to void. Careful search of the history of many patients who have maximal prolapse (who are continent, as a rule) will disclose a past history of stress incontinence, now relieved.

As part of the preliminary physical examination, the patient with a genital prolapse should be examined in the office while standing, her bladder *unemptied*. The gynecologist should replace the prolapse within the pelvis, and while holding it there ask the patient to cough or strain. If, at this time, an otherwise continent patient leaks urine, this patient will require some coexistent surgical support of the vesicourethral unction during reconstructive surgery, or a postoperative urinary stress incontinence (USI) can be predicted and almost assured. Operative correction of the uterine prolapse and repair of the cystocele not only corrects the urethral angulation, but also directs any increases in intravesical pressure upon the atonic funneled neck of the bladder and urethra. When a patient has this condition, the same attention should be given to the urethra as in a patient with severe stress incontinence, lest she be very wet and unhappy after repair of the cystocele and correction of the prolapse have been accomplished. At least 3 to 6 months should lapse before re-operative surgical correction. Mere repetition of a vaginal procedure or simple vaginal operation may not help. As a rule, a suprapubic or combined approach will be required. Primary operation is not indicated per se for an asymptomatic cystocele.

Much interest has been evidenced in comparison of the reported success rates with the varied operative procedures for the relief of USI. For purposes of comparative study, the symptom complex of USI might well be divided into at least two major groups: first, severe and socially disabling USI; and second, minor degrees of incontinence often coexistent with other more significant pelvic pathology for which surgery is indicated. In the latter group, treatment of the USI may be of relatively secondary importance, but failure to include indicated repair may be followed by a result that will be unsatisfactory from the patient's standpoint.

To compile and report in terms of a single percentage figure, the "cure rate" of patients with varying causes and degrees of urinary incontinence, as has so frequently been done in the past, only contributes to the confusion. Different reported series containing widely divergent percentages of each of the possible types and degrees of incontinence must be supported by data reflecting success rates with each of the clinical and anatomic problems recognized. Otherwise, a meaningful comparison between the relative successes with the different surgical procedures becomes difficult if not impossible.

Obviously the criteria of "cure" and the duration of that cure are important, but the period of observation after surgery is of major importance. It would appear that the long-term successes of repeated procedures have been somewhat inversely proportional to the postoperative period of observation. A follow-up period of not less than 2 years seems adequate and reliable if one is to report conclusive and meaningful results. Follow-up re-evaluations after more than 2 years can be misleading, however, as some of those being followed will begin to be affected by normal aging processes. Postmenopausal atrophic changes alone will confuse the evaluation of the operative procedures themselves by the addition of still another variable. The effects of the aging process upon USI are quite different from a comparison of results of various operations. One must not only compare peaches with peaches and apples with apples, but young peaches with young and old with old.

To a considerable degree, the symptoms of USI are subjective, and of somewhat variable intensity according to the type of the individual's activities, social as well as physical, degree of social acceptability, and the extent to which the patient will tolerate the situation. Because these factors are not necessarily interdependent, there is need to employ diagnostic methods of measuring the improvement due to the surgery employed, in addition to subjective description.

## DIAGNOSIS

The preoperative investigation of urinary incontinence need not be formidable and certainly should be individualized for each patient. There is no substitute for a careful, thoughtful, and detailed history. Questions should be meaningful and close attention should be given to the patient's responses. One seeks to establish both the nature and the severity of the disability, as well as its duration. One wishes early on to identify various contributing components to the symptoms of incontinence, including urgency, detrusor instability, frequency, and stress. Because so many drugs have as side effects sympathetic, parasympathetic, or detrusor response (32), a detailed recitation of what medications the patient is taking is relevant, including a description of the effect on the patient's urinary symptoms.

Although the filling out of a questionnaire may be offered, reciting the questions verbally provides a broader opportunity for patient response and elaboration than a simple yes or no answer.

Suitable leading questions may be found among the following:

1. Do you lose your urine when you laugh, cough, or sneeze?
2. Is the loss immediate, or is it 30 to 45 seconds after you laugh, cough, or sneeze?
3. Do you lose urine when you are lying down?
4. Do you have to get up at night to pass your urine? Can you make it to the bathroom?
5. Have you a history of any bladder or kidney infections? Were they accompanied by chills, fever, or backache?
6. Does the sound of running water make you want to pass your urine?
7. When you put your foot in the bath to see if the water is too hot before

you get in, does it give you a sudden urge to pass your urine? Do you pass it?

8. Have you had any change in bowel habits coincident with your change in bladder habits?
9. How often do you pass your urine during the day? During the night?
10. How much tea, coffee, cola drinks, or chocolate do you consume?
11. Did you have trouble with bedwetting as a child?
12. Did other members of your family have problems in holding their urine?
13. Did you have any trouble holding your urine during pregnancy?
14. Did you have any trouble passing or holding your urine after delivery?
15. What medications are you taking regularly?
16. Do you have any burning when you pass your urine?
17. After you have passed your urine and stand up, does it sometimes feel as though you have to go a second time? If you try to go a second time, do you find there was really no need? Is there any urinary dribbling after voiding?
18. Have you had any operations on the vagina, uterus, or bladder, and did they affect bladder function at all?
19. How long have you been having your problem?
20. Was the onset gradual or sudden?
21. Are you beyond the menopause?
22. Was your problem worse at the time of menopause?
23. Are you taking any hormone supplements? Have the hormone supplements helped your bladder function?
24. Do you ever lose urine during intercourse?
25. How many times can you stop and start the stream?
26. When the urine involuntarily begins to leak, can you stop the stream?
27. How much sanitary protection do you wear? Only when you have a cold or respiratory infection, or must you wear something all the time?

Green (13) has characterized the disorders responsible for the *symptom* of USI follows:

1. True Anatomic USI (75% to 85% of cases): There is abnormal configuration and location of the urethrovesical junction, with the proximal urethra displaced outside the intra-abdominal field of force. Urethra, bladder, detrusor function, and neuropharmocologic control are normal.
2. Detrusor Dyssynergia (15% to 20% of cases). A hyperirritable detrusor reflex is involuntarily triggered by a sudden increase in intra-abdominal pressure or by a critical volume of bladder urine. Incontinence is of an "involuntary voiding" type and occurs despite a normal urethrovesical support and anatomic configuration.
3. Combination of True Anatomic USI and Detrusor Dyssynergia (5% to 10% of cases).
4. Miscellaneous Disorders (5% to 10% of cases):
   (a) Rigid, Frozen, "Pipe-stem" Urethra. There is low resting intraurethral pressure, and any sudden increase in intra-abdominal pressure is not transmitted to the proximal urethral lumen sufficient to equal and offset the pressure increase. This occurs despite normal urethrovesical anatomy and support. The disorder is seen most often in patients who have had multiple surgical procedures in the region of the bladder neck.
   (b) Urethral Diverticulum. It may fill during voiding and then be emptied by a sudden cough or change in position.
   (c) Short Urethra Syndrome (or total urinary incontinence). The urethra is too short (0.5 to 1.5 cm) to maintain adequate intraurethral pressure, either at rest or with sudden increases in intra-abdominal pressure.

Although the patient experiences a stress-type leakage, actually she has total urinary incontinence and leaks constantly.

Green has listed symptoms of true anatomic USI:

1. Urgency, frequency, and urgency incontinence are usually absent. (Minimal urgency and frequency are occasionally seen in patients with marked funneling of the vesical neck.)
2. Leakage of urine occurs at the instant of physical stress.
3. A variable but limited volume of urine is lost instantaneously and simultaneously with the physical stress.
4. Leakage will occur with stress even though the bladder has recently emptied and contains only a small volume of urine.
5. Leakage occurs only in the upright position (usually only in the standing position). Usually simple changes in position are not accompanied by leakage. Incontinence never occurs at night in bed.
6. Most often, leakage is caused by coughing, sneezing, laughing, vigorous athletic activity, and similar stresses that produce sudden large increases in intra-abdominal pressure. Ordinarily, the sound of running water or normal walking or running activity do not cause loss of urine.
7. Patients usually can stop their stream while in the act of normal voiding.
8. There is no associated psychosomatic disorder.
9. There are no spontaneous remissions or exacerbations, although there may be progressive increase in the frequency and severity of USI with the passage of time.
10. Usually, there is no past history of functional disorders of bladder control. There may be a history of transient stress incontinence during and for a short time after one or more earlier pregnancies. Then the symptom fails to clear up after a subsequent pregnancy and persists and often worsens over the years.

And, Green has identified contrasting symptoms of uninhibited involuntary detrusor contraction:

1. Urgency, frequency (nocturnal as well), and painless incontinence are usually prominent.
2. Usually there is a considerable latent period or lag of several seconds between the physical stress and the onset of leakage.
3. A large volume of urine is lost, often in gushes, a steady stream, or prolonged dribbling, and the leakage occurs over a protracted interval of several seconds. (Actual uninhibited involuntary voiding is occurring.)
4. Leakage is more likely to occur when the bladder is moderately full; each patient seems to have her own critical volume at which frequency, urgency, and stress-induced incontinence are most likely to be experienced.
5. Leakage may occur in any position and often is triggered by a change in position. Leakage may occur even in bed.
6. Walking or running or the sound of running water often trigger incontinence, whereas coughing, sneezing, or laughing do so less consistently.
7. Patients usually find it difficult to halt the stream during normal voiding.
8. An underlying, generalized anxiety or depressive state is often discernible.
9. Often there are spontaneous remissions and exacerbations in relation to changes in the total life situation. Usually, fluctuations involve weeks, months, or even several years, but in some patients there may be daily variations, with symptoms tending to disappear at night.

10. There is often a history of voiding and bladder difficulties, including enuresis, dating back to early childhood.

The Marshall- or Bonney-type test is an important and simple diagnostic procedure for the demonstration of stress incontinence. It is readily performed in the office and can easily be combined with a simplified cystometric evaluation (36).

The patient is asked to void before examination and then is catheterized to measure residual urine volume. The urine sample is put aside for analysis, and the glass or plastic funnel of a sterile 60-ml Asepto syringe is attached to the catheter. The bottom of the syringe is held about the level of the patient's pubis, and sterile saline in increments of 50 ml is poured into the syringe (Fig. 5.1). The patient is asked to identify the first urge to void. The volume of saline instilled is recorded, after which increments are added until maximal patient discomfort is approached, at which time the total volume used is again noted. All but 250 to 300 ml of saline is permitted to run out, and the catheter is removed. The saline volumes and subjective feelings give not only a fairly valid estimation of bladder tone, helping to identify either hypertonia or hypotonia, but spontaneous uninhibited bladder contractions also can be identified by a rise in the column of saline in the glass syringe. (An observation of abnormality suggests the need for more sophisticated urodynamic study of such a patient.) The patient is then asked to cough; if no urine is lost, the perineum should be depressed and the cough repeated (18). If urine is lost, the vesicourethral junction should be elevated by the examiner, care being taken not to occlude the urethra by pressure, and the patient is asked to cough again. If no urine is lost with coughing when the patient is in the lithotomy position, she should be asked to stand and to cough again. The test is considered positive if no additional urine is expelled by coughing when the vesicourethral junction is so elevated.

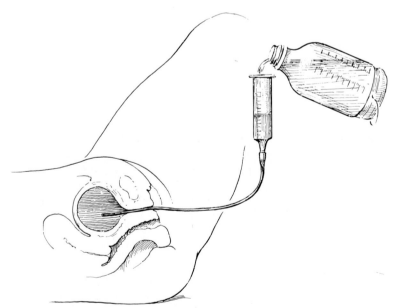

**Figure 5.1.**   After the residual urine volume has been measured, sterile saline is instilled in increments of 50 ml, and the bladder capacity is measured. The catheter and all but 250 to 300 ml are removed, and a Marshall or Bonney test is done with the patient first in the recumbent, then in the standing position.

In evaluating a presumably positive Marshall test, one should note carefully the time interval between the cough and the loss of urine. If the condition is truly one of urinary stress incontinence, the loss will be immediate and usually can be stopped by the patient's coluntary pubococcygeal contraction. If there is a delay of several seconds between the cough and the loss of urine, the patient is probably experiencing a provoked detrusor contraction, which is a form of bladder instability and not stress incontinence. The patient may be unable to stop the stream. In this instance, the investigation should be centered around a probable diagnosis of detrusor instability, for which the treatment is generally nonsurgical (9, 11, 20). A surgeon should be most cautious about recommending surgery to correct USI in the presence of a negative Marshall test without first obtaining a confirmatory urethrocystometrogram. If there has been a history of pyelonephritis or previous chronically recurrent cystitis, urine cultures and an intravenous pyelogram are indicated. The results should be considered carefully and appropriate treatment given.

Comparison of pre- and postoperative bead-chain urethrocystograms of urethrocystocolpograms, when now used, is primarily as part of the investigation of certain individuals with recurrent incontinence, or when the patient is part of a special study group. A urethral chain may be introduced inside a split rubber catheter or through the convenient device of Thaddigsmann (Fig. 5.2). A modification of urethrocystography in which the urethra is opacified without a chain has been described by Morgan (26). The advantage of his modified technique is that there is no chain or catheter to splint or, by its weight, depress the urethra artificially, altering the view of the relationship with the bladder.
*Technique*

1. A 5% solution of sodium iodide and 30 ml of lipiodol are instilled into the bladder.
2. Barium paste (5 ml) is instilled into the urethra.
3. If coincident colpography is desired, 5 ml of barium paste may be instilled into the vagina.

Without the splinting of the catheter, this technique demonstrates the S-shaped curve of the urethra and any funneling or changes in luminal size at different levels within the urethra, and may provide visualization of any urethral diverticulum or an occasional urethrovaginal fistula.

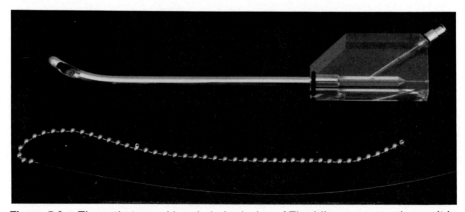

**Figure 5.2.** The catheter and bead-chain device of Thaddigsmann are shown. It is available on order from: Research Engineering and Development Industries, 11002 Ranier Avenue South, Seattle, WA 98178.

If the Marshall test in the supine position is negative, one should determine whether, by depressing the perineum and asking the patient to laugh, cough, or sneeze, it becomes positive (18). It should also be determined whether the patient can voluntarily contract her pubococcygeal muscles and external anal sphincter. (Failure to be able to do so may correlate with anal incontinence and possibly a pudendal neuropathy, as suggested by the studies of the Parks Institute in London.)

If the patient is incapable of effective voluntary contraction of her pubococcygeal muscles, ask her to start on a period of daily perineal resistive exercises, employing isometric contractions, 15 to 20 in a row, 3 seconds per contraction, repeated as a sequence six times a day, starting when first arising, then midmorning, lunchtime, midafternoon, suppertime, and bedtime. Some estimate of the effectiveness of the patient's pubococcygei in controlling urinary incontinence may be obtained by determining how many times the patient can stop and start the stream during the process of voiding. If the muscles are effective and strong, a patient should be able to stop and start the stream six to eight times when voiding from a full bladder. When the muscle is weak and ineffective, the patient may be unable to stop the stream at all or, at most, once or twice; this gives some evidence of the value that might be obtained by a course of isometric contraction exercises. Developing strength from perineal resistive exercises requires about 3 months of daily effort to bring about a significant improvement and the patient should be cautioned not to expect vast improvement overnight.

If the Marshall test is positive, ask the patient to tighten her levator muscles and repeat the cough. See if she is now dry. If she is dry when coughing in the presence of voluntarily contracted pubococcygei, teach her this safeguard as an almost "automatic reflex" so that whenever it is necessary for her to laugh, cough, or sneeze, she must contract her pelvic muscles ust *before* the stress rather than just after. In many cases, this may be all the treatment the patient requires (30).

These interpretations may be correlated with pre- and postoperative endoscopy and with direct simultaneous intraurethral intravesical pressuremeasurements.

Simultaneous measurement of intraurethral and intravesical pressures (1, 3, 6, 15, 16, 31) (urethrocystometry) should be strongly considered when the stress incontinence is recurrent or when there is a history of enuresis, spontaneous voiding, inability to stop the stream, suspected neuropathy involving bladder function (disk, spina fida, multiple sclerosis, diabetic neuropathy, central nervous system lues, etc.), or the finding of a high postvoiding urinary residual volume without evident outlet or urethral obstruction. This testing should be performed with the patient both supine and standing (38). Urethral instability is not uncommon, and should be diagnosed and treated (40). Gleason et al. (12) suggested that the results obtained from a water-filled system for urethrocystometry have less false positive results than those using gas or air, despite the obvious convenience of the latter. However, direct urethroscopy in a gas medium is of great help in evaluation of the urethra and of the competency of the vesical neck (37).

The greater the number of previous operative failures in a particular patient, the more detailed and extensive should be the work-up.

## TREATMENT

Adequate preoperative incontinence study requires suspicion, evaluation, definition, and elimination of the dissimilar but occasionally coexistent etiologies of urinary incontinence (19) and the incontinence resulting from poor voiding habits. If pre- and postoperative comparisons are not carried out in these individuals, there will be confusion concerning the degrees of surgical success attributed to a specific technique for the relief of stress incontinence. Coexistent detrusor instability or urgency incontinence is so often present that when unrecognized and untreated it, too, will affect the rate of surgical cure. The patient does not know why she is losing her urine, but she wants relief. The burden of investigation is upon the doctor who must recognize and treat correctly each of the various factors accounting for her symptoms.

The presence of urethral funneling may stimulate detrusor contractibility reflex by the presence of urine in the proximal urethra at a time when the patient is not voiding. This appears to be associated with funneling or vesicalization of the urethra that may, thus, not only lower the physiologic vesicourethral unction but may activate this detrusor reflex, particularly when the patient is in a nonsupine position and gravity has pulled even small amounts of urine into this pathologically dilated urethra (4). For this reason, the presence of funneling, once diagnosed, should be corrected surgically as a part of any surgical procedure designed for the treatment of a patient's urinary stress incontinence.

Urethral funneling is even more significant when associated with rotational descent of the bladder neck.

Urethral funneling may be diagnosed by: (a) a lateral cystogram—look also for flattening of the posterior urethrovesical angle at rest; (b) physical examination of the patient standing, with the examiner's finger placed lightly under the lower anterior vaginal wall, seeking the palpagle transmission of a cough impulse into the proximal urethra; (c) direct urethroscopy is not necessarily diagnostic, though it may help diagnose urethral smooth muscle sphincter insufficiency-the latter and funneling appear to be two different entities, although they may coexist; (d) urethral pressure profilometry may demonstrate an unexpectedly low slope starting at the proximal urethra; (e) visualization at surgery.

The prudent surgeon will not offer a surgical relief for someone's incontinence until certain of the etiology. One must consider the possibility of a small but undiagnosed fistula especially in a patient with a history of previous pelvic surgery.

One must be cautious of making sweeping recommendations and assurances of good postoperative prognostic results in a patient with a history of coincident rectal incontinence because this suggests the problem of pudendal denervation, usually from childbirth or chronic straining that may not be surgically remedial and may follow a long history of constipation and obstipation with stretching of the pudendal nerve resulting in partial denervation of the structures thus innervated by it, i.e., the levator ani and the external anal sphincter. Onset of constipation coincident with urinary incontinence, particularly after a fall, suggests the possibility of herniation of an intervertebral disk. This should be diagnosed from appropriate neurologic examination and study, but one must be mindful that if this occurs within the cauda equina it may not appear on a myelogram.

Nonsurgical treatment of urinary stress incontinence, which also is useful often as both a preoperative and postoperative supplement, includes (a) planned courses of perineal resistive exercise; (b) estrogen supplementation, when appropriate; (c) avoidance of tight abdominal garments that unnecessarily increase intra-abdominal pressure; and (d) correcting chronic respiratory illness, stopping smoking, etc.

Before deciding upon the best operation for a specific patient's stress incontinence, the surgeon must decide first if it is stress incontinence that is to be treated, or whether the patient's complaint is really urgency or even simply the result of poor voiding habits. When urgency and stress incontinence coexist, it is generally best that the urgency component be treated first because it is well known that infection, when present, increases detrusor irritability. Once the urgency has been relieved, many patients will no longer be incontinent. Conversely, the swelling and trauma of surgery can make an untreated urgency component worse for several months; the patient will not be likely to make the subtle distinction between the two types, and she is likely simply to conclude that she is worse than before surgery.

Judging by the number of cases of urgency incontinence treated unsuccessfully by inappropriate surgery, it is apparent that the subtle distinction is not always being made between detrusor instability and USI. The operation will be recorded as a surgical failure when, in fact, it should not have been performed in the first place. An inappropriate operation compounds the patient's problem. A proper choice of the initial operation properly performed offers the best chance for cure and should be made by the surgeon who is to do the procedure. The surgeon who depends on someone else to tell what to do should generally not be the one to do it.

Choices for surgical treatment seem to be among three types: transvaginal, suprapubic, and combined vaginoabdominal. Often a procedure seems to be selected on the basis of considerations more political than logical. One possible reason giving rise to apparent discrepancy between the cure rates reported by the gynecologist and the urologist is the obviously dissimilar distribution of the etiologic factors among cases of USI as a primary urologic symptom, as compared to the etiology accounting for a majority of patients among whom incontinence has developed as a secondary gynecologic symptom. For one school of thought always to choose a suprapubic pin-up operation is as inappropriate an individualization as for another discipline always to perform a transvaginal procedure.

There are halfway or partial degrees of success in surgical relief. Anything less than 100% successful result in a particular patient is not necessarily a failure if her disability has been reduced from a major and socially unacceptable degree of incontinence to a minor and acceptable problem.

Some correlation with patient diathesis in type is important as well. Irrespective of her urethrovesical configuration, an obese woman may have different problems with intra-abdominal pressure than a thin patient, affecting the long-term success after surgical treatment for USI. Similarly, a chronic asthmatic or a patient with hay fever, bronchitis, or chronic cough is prone to have much less long-term success after certain procedures than would result from the same operation performed on an individual without the respiratory contribution.

A statement that operation A is better than operation B will only be meaningful if it is qualified by description of (a) which condition, (b) with what coexistent related symptoms and findings, (c) with what degree of disability the patient had experienced, (d) by which specific surgical approach, and (e) for how long the result has been observed.

When USI is quite mild, often inconstant, and not of itself sufficiently disturbing to have motivated the patient to seek a repair, that degree of incontinence alone is not likely to warrant the disability and risks of surgery; but when a similarly mild degree of incontinence coexists with other indications for repair (e.g., rectocele, genital prolapse), adequate coincident transvaginal surgical reconstruction should indeed be advised.

The surgeon responsible for the treatment must not only recognize the need for and interpret adequate preoperative studies, but also must be skilled and experienced in the full range of operative procedures than can be employed and choose the best one suited for a particular patient. No competent gynecologist will restrict all choice to a single procedure or recommend only the procedure which that surgeon may be best able to perform. The choice of an inappropriate operation usually compounds the patient's problem. One can hope to achieve a 2-year cure rate of urinary incontinence, approaching 95% only by well-considered appraisal of a patient's problem and selection of the proper operation for that problem. Without making such effort and exercising such judgment, both patient and surgeon needlessly settle for an overall failure rate of not less than 20%.

An operative procedure should so improve urethral tone and pressure that it may exceed intravesical pressure both at rest and when intra-abdominal pressure is increased. This will be favored by elevating the vesicourethral junction to a point once again above the bottom of the hydrostatic column of water. As a result, changes in intra-abdominal pressure will be transmitted to the proximal urethra as well as the bladder.

Hawksworth and Roux (14) suggested that most successful operations for the correction of USI are, in fact, "sling operations," elevating the urethrovesical unction by using the patient's own tissues in situ, transplanting them from another site, or using a foreign material. The effect is similar because they all elevate the vesicourethral junction to a point within the pelvis where the proximal urethra and bladder are simultaneously subject to increases in intra-abdominal pressure. A comparison is shown in Figure 5.3.

When urethral funneling or vesicalization is present, Kelly-type mattress stitches (see Chapter 11) will restore the urethral lumen to normal size and improve the effectiveness of local muscular tone in re-establishing a mechanism for closure of the vesical neck.

Urethral detachment, or rotational descent of the bladder neck, however, implies damage to the ligamentous or fibromuscular support of the urethra. When this is coincident with a drop in urethral tone so that intraurethral pressure no longer exceeds intravesical pressure, involuntary incontinence may take place (5). Treatment consists of surgically elevating the vesicourethral junction so that it is once again within the range of effective response to increases in intra-abdominal pressure. This may be accomplished by transvaginal techniques, as detailed in Chapter 11.

Pubourethral ligament plication as part of an anterior colporrhaphy is ideal when used with surgical treatment for a coexisting genital prolapse, and this plication may be used to prevent urinary incontinence as a result of the straightening out of a posterior urethrovesical angle during the course of an anterior colporrhaphy (Chapter 11). The White (42) or Figuranov (10) transvaginal reattachment of paraurethral tissue to the pubic end of the arcus tendineus (2, 43) is useful when one finds either insufficient tissue strength for midline plication or evidence of lack of forniceal support. Pathologic damage to the levator plate may be measured indirectly by urethrocolpography (Chapter 23) and appropriate surgical remedy should be instituted. Because of infection of the bolster requiring its removal and failure to increase intraurethral pressure significantly and failure to repair other sites of weakness of pelvic support, we do not use the Stamey modification (39) of the original Pereyra (34) operation. If a reason is present for coincident primary laparotomy (ovarian tumor, large uterine leiomyoma, etc.), a primary suprapubic procedure may be elected, though any posterior cystocele should be corrected separately. Coincident transabdominal obliteration of a deep or wide cul-de-sac is desirable to prevent the future development of a postoperative enterocele such as might result from a change in the vaginal axis, leaving a cul-de-sac unprotected.

## RECURRENT URINARY STRESS INCONTINENCE

When the patient's primary symptom is recurrent, severe, and socially disabling USI, one should give special consideration to a combined procedure. A combined approach may be of special interest if urethral vesicalization or funneling is present that will permit plication of both anterior and posterior urethrovesical angles followed by a Marshall-Marchetti-Krantz (23) procedure, a Burch (7), or a "sling"-type of repair. In the absence of demonstrable funneling, plication of the vesicourethral junction or bladder neck may be omitted in order to lessen the chance of a subsequent stricture.

Using the pubourethral ligament plication stitch (Fig. 11.16) with a complementary perineorrhaphy (18, 22, 27), we have approached rotational descent of the bladder neck (urethral detachment) by a primary vaginal procedure that elevates the vesicourethral junction. If midling urethral support is lacking the alternative of paravaginal attachment (2, 10, 42, 43) is available, and depending upon the extent of damage, both may be employed. Because this relocates the vesicourethral junction at a higher level within the pelvis and it is supported by an appropriate perineorrhaphy, it accomplishes more than simple urethral plication. When there is flattening of the posterior urethrovesical angle without rotational descent of the bladder neck, one may choose either a vaginal, suprapubic, or combined approach, depending on the severity of the patient's symptoms, the presence of coexistent medical disease such as asthma or hay fever, or coexistent vaginal or intra-abdominal pathology, which requires simultaneous correction. If the vaginal operation is chosen, the operator's attention is directed to the requirement that the repair emphasize plication and support of the vesical neck and the proximal urethra with its supporting tissues, with less emphasis on cystocele repair posterior to the vesicourethral junction.

When the cystocele and lateral fornices but not the vault of the vagina come down when a patient strains but the lateral fornices do not go back when the patient contracts her pubococcygei, this is good evidence of a lateral vaginal attachment defect that might be made a part of the patient's surgical repair (2). Very little if any vaginal membrane should be resected in this circumstance, but complementary perineorrhaphy is usually indicated with each anterior colporrhaphy.

There are specific but uncommon circumstances in which the operator might wish to combine a vaginal hysterectomy and appropriate colporrhaphy with a retropubic suburethral sling procedure, e.g., symptomatic and progressive genital prolapse in a patient with recurrent severe and socially disabling USI, often accompanied by a chronic respiratory disease. The technique of the combined operation should begin with an incision in each groin through the rectus aponeurosis, bluntly through the rectus muscle and the transversalis fascia, and extraperitoneally to the obturator foramen in the space of Retzius on each side. Then, the vaginal hysterectomy and excision of any enterocele are accomplished and the anterior colporrhaphy begun. Our choice of sling material may be either from transplanted fascia or single-layered Mersilene mesh or 1 mm Gore-Tex. The suburethral sling is tacked beneath the vesicourethral junction and pulled through the tunnel on each side into the space of Retzius to appear at the wound in the groin, and the anterior colporrhaphy is finished. Any necessary posterior colporrhaphy is done, the vagina is packed, elevating the vesicourethral unction, and the operator's attention is redirected

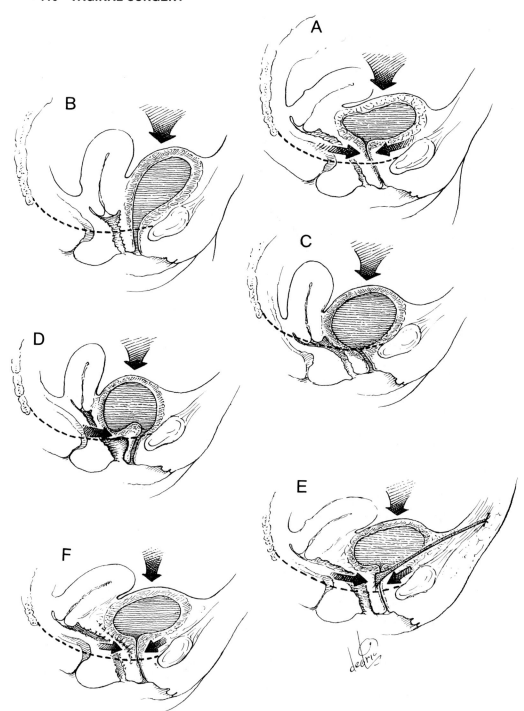

**Figure 5.3.** Illustrating the relationship between increases in intra-abdominal pressure to intravesical and intraurethral pressures. *A*, the continent state of the anatomically normal patient is represented. An increase in intra-abdominal pressure is noted by the *large arrow* being applied directly to the bladder. Increases applied to the proximal urethra are indicated by the *smaller arrows*. The lower limit of the physiologic "body cavity," or usual position of the pelvic diaphragm, is

to the abdominal groin incision where the ends of the sling are fixed on each side to the rectus aponeurosis.

A suprapubic operative procedure for the relief of severe and socially disabling USI might be considered when either or both of the following criteria are present: (*a*) The incontinence is secondary to failure of a previous repair. (*b*) There is coexistent contributing medical disease: emphysema, asthma, hay fever, heavy smoking, chronic bronchitis, obesity, etc.

Although adequate performance of the Marshall-Marchetti-Krantz procedure does relieve a rotational descent of the bladder neck, it does not treat a distention cystocele. The sling procedure, on the other hand, does require a vaginal portion of the operation, which opens the vaginal wall at the time the sling is to be fixed and this exposure permits the operator to treat any coexistent cystocele surgically while fixing the sling in place.

When pubourethral ligament support is poor or the tissues are excessively thin or scarred, a suprapubic procedure is especially attractive. Although the Marshall-Marchetti-Krantz pin-up procedure, or any one of its various modifications, "pulls" the urethrovesical junction back into the pelvis, it does not necessarily restore the integrity of a damaged bladder base plate, nor does it treat coincident distention-type cystocele. The vesicourethral junction is now permanently fixed in a retropubic position from which it will no longer descend physiologically during voiding.

A suprapubic sling procedure "pushes" the vesicourethral unction back into the pelvis and tends to restore the competence of a damaged base plate. As the

---

indicated by the *dotted line*. B, there is loss or straightening of the urethrovesical angle, and increases in intra-abdominal pressure are being applied to the bladder but not to the urethra. In this situation, intravesical pressure will exceed intraurethral pressure, and incontinence may result. C, there is loss or lengthening of urethral support with rotational descent of the urethrovesical junction at rest, and the urethra is effectively displaced to a point below the physiologic "abdominal cavity." Increases in intra-abdominal pressure are transmitted primarily to the bladder and not the urethra; and at these moments, intravesical pressure will exceed intraurethral pressure, and incontinence may result. D, the effect of a Marshall-Marchetti-Krantz procedure or any of its modifications is shown. In this instance, the tissues lateral to the urethra have been fixed to the posterior surface of the pubis and the urethrovesical junction restored to a point within the body cavity. Increases in intra-abdominal pressure are applied to the bladder (as noted by the large arrow above) and to the posterior surface of the proximal urethra (as noted by the *smaller arrow*). E, the effect of a sling procedure is demonstrated. The urethrovesical junction has been elevated with prompt restoration of this junction to a point within the body cavity. Integrity of the bladder base plate has been restored. Increases in intra-abdominal pressure are applied to both the bladder (as noted by the *large arrow*) and the anterior and posterior surfaces of the urethra (as noted by the *smaller arrows*). F, the effects of appropriate anterior colporrhaphy which has included plication and elevation of the urethrovesical unction. The large arrow indicates the transmission of intra-abdominal pressure to the bladder, and the smaller arrows indicate similar transmission of the increase in pressure to the proximal urethra. Transmission of intra-abdominal pressure to the proximal urethra as well as the bladder is noted in A, D, E, and F, preserving a positive ratio between intraurethral and intravesical pressure when the bladder is at rest, restoring urinary incontinence. (Reproduced with permission of Williams & Wilkins from Nichols DH: Anatomic considerations in stress urinary incontinence. In Slate WB (ed): *Disorders of the Female Urethra and Urinary Incontinence*, ed. 2, 1982.)

rectus muscles and the levator ani relax during voiding, the vesicourethral unction may descend to some extent.

The techniques of the pin-up operation are well known (8, 23) and need not be detailed here. An intraoperative choice between a Marshall-Marchetti-Krantz operation, which sews periurethral tissue to the back of the pubis, and the Burch, which sews perivaginal tissue to Cooper's ligament, may be made according to whether the pubic periosteum can securely hold the sutures placed into it. Anterior plication of the urethra may be added if urethral funneling is evident (21).

## SLINGS

Hawksworth and Roux (14) long ago wrote that most of the surgical means of supporting the vesicourethral junction are sling procedures of one type or another whether by plication of the lateral walls of the vagina or urethra of tissues normally found in that area, whether the vagina is attached to the back of the pubis as in the pin-up operation, or whether a material is used as a transplantable sling actually to elevate the vesicourethral junction. The latter can be in the form of abdominal fascia that has been relocated or in grafts such as fascia lata or a foreign material such as Mersilene mesh or Gore-Tex.

The sling procedure as we know it, using a transplantable material, has been one of several methods used to treat severe and socially disabling urinary stress incontinence. The mechanical effect of a sling is shown in Figure 5.4.

Having decided to use one, there is need for a choice of materials to use, as special circumstances will dictate certain advantages of one over another.

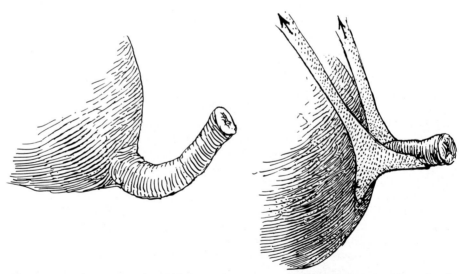

**Figure 5.4.** A preoperative deficiency in support of the vesicourethral junction is shown on the left which permits flattening of the vesicourethral angle, often resulting in urinary stress incontinence. A diagrammatic representation of the effect of the suburethral sling is shown on the right after it has been sewn in place. The vesicourethral junction is elevated over a wide area, reducing any tendency toward strangulation and pressure necrosis. (Reproduced with permission of the The American College of Obstetricians and Gynecologists from Nichols DH: The Mersilene mesh gauze hammock for severe urinary stress incontinence. *Obstet Gynecol* 41:88–93, 1973.)

### Vesicourethral Sling

When one has decided to use a suprapubic vesicourethral sling procedure for the treatment of severe or recurrent socially disabling urinary stress incontinence (16, 17, 33, 35), our choice of material from which the sling is made has often been between Mersilene mesh (never Mersilene tape) or 1 mm Gore-Tex or fascia lata (25, 28, 29, 41).

Macrophotography of the unstretched weave Mersilene mesh (Fig. 5.5) shows by the configuration of the spaces between the threads why it will stretch in one direction more than the other. The gauze hammock must be cut from the sheet of mesh in the direction of least stretch. Mersilene mesh, by its thinness and flexibility, seems to be superior to Marlex as a choice of synthetic sling material. Zoedler's nylon net (44) and lyophilized dura are not readily available in the United States.

The vaginal incision should be closed in two layers using absorbable sutures; one buried, insulating the mesh, and a second layer of everting mattress stitches. Alternatively, the vaginal lapping operation may be used if there is a wide belly of mesh or Gore-Tex to be buried, or the bulbocavernosus fat pad transplant may be used if the synthetic belly is narrow (see Chapter 18).

The vaginal incision must be closed without tension; lateral vaginal relaxing incisions are made should it be evident that tension is present. By the use of Mersilene mesh or Gore-Tex, the length and width of the sling or hammock can be predetermined and cut to size. The tension under which it is fixed in place is not as critical as that of the fascial sling, as Mersilene has a little flexibility. Also, the use of these materials does save the patient the uncomfortable leg that follows the technique of obtaining a strip of fascia lata.

Particularly in situations where there is risk of postoperative vaginal necrosis, i.e., atrophic vagina, previous radiation, or extensive scarring from previous repair, the surgeon might wish to select a sling made of fascia lata, as

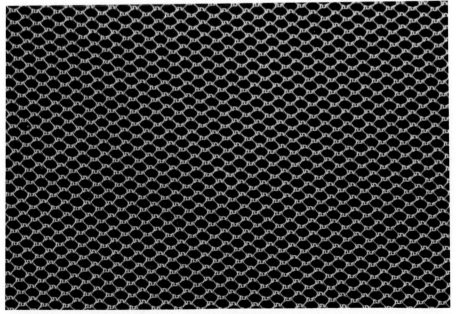

**Figure 5.5.** Macrophotograph of Mersilene mesh is shown. It is single layered, porous, and very flexible.

championed by Ridley (35, 36), as a modification of the Goebell-Frankenheim-Stoeckel procedure. This material is a homograft and not likely to be rejected or to harbor prolonged infection even if deliberately exteriorized in the vagina, as might be planned when the vaginal wall is particularly thin (35, 36, 41) (Fig. 5.6).

Rectus fascia obtained through the conventional midline or Pfannensteil incision is less than optimal, because the direction of fibers in the strip so obtained is oblique and, therefore, not of maximal strength. To obtain a suitable long strip from an abdominal incision would require a crescent-shaped incision that would be cosmetically unattractive. Furthermore, cutting strips cut from the midline rectus fascia is associated with an increased risk of postoperative wound hernia.

A strip of fascia lata is obtained by the technique suggested by Ridley (35) and shown in Figure 5.7. Its overall width may be increased somewhat by increasing the distance between the parallel incisions shown in Figure 5.7B and curving the strip inside the Masson stripper. When too narrow, the suburethral pressure of the strap may be concentrated in too small an area, increasing the risk of pressure necrosis of the urethra. If the central belly of the sling is still too narrow, it may widened by central incisions.

The suburethral sling may further be prevented from rolling or postoperative migration by fixing it in a permanent position to the periurethral tissue and to the bladder capsule using a number of interrupted stitches.

When too short, there is risk that the tension of the strap may be sewn to the rectus aponeurosis too tightly with resultant inability of the patient to void or to completely empty her bladder.

The tension under which a sling of inelastic fascia lata must be placed is more critical than that of the more flexible and slightly elastic Mersilene mesh. Although the length may be increased by aplicing two strips of fascia together,

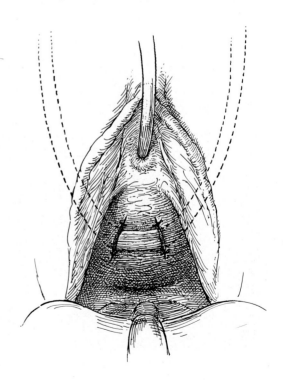

**Figure 5.6.** When the vaginal wall is unusually thin, the belly of a fascial sling may remain exteriorized and exposed in the vagina as shown. The *dotted lines* indicate the retropubic path of the tails of the sling. Epithelialization is complete in about 6 weeks.

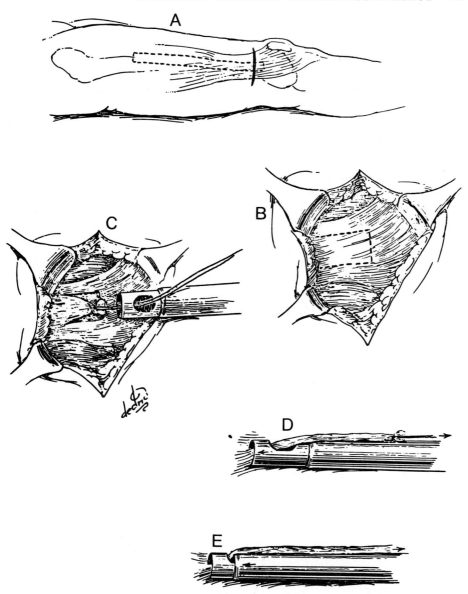

**Figure 5.7.** The location and technique for obtaining a fascia lata homograft is depicted. A skin incision in the right thigh above the patella is shown and the piece of fascia to be excised is indicated by the *dotted line* in A. The incision in the distal portion of the fascia lata is identified in B; and this is threaded into the distal end of a Masson fascia stripper as shown in C. The stripper is passed subcutaneously as far as it will go while countertraction is made at the distal end of the fascial strip, which is held by a Kocher hemostat, D. When the stripper can proceed no further, the outer sleeve is unscrewed and slid distally as a guillotine over the central barrel, E, transecting the fascia at its proximal end. The fascia and fascia stripper are removed, the visible remaining fascia lata defect can be closed with a few interrupted polyglycolic acid-type sutures, and the skin incision is closed. (Reproduced with permission of Charles C Thomas from Nichols DH: The sling operations. In Cantor EB (ed): Female Urinary Stress Incontinence, 1979.)

an alternate method of lengthening the strip is shown in Figure 5.8, which does not require joining two spearate strips together beneath the urethra at their most vulnerable point. In this modification, a stitch is required to hold the folded strip until scarring fuses it.

## GAUZE OR GORE-TEX HAMMOCK OPERATION IN REPAIR OF SEVERE OR RECURRENT URINARY STRESS INCONTINENCE

The synthetic plastic hammock is not a cure-all, but appears more advantageous than the Marshall-Marchetti-Krantz operation by virtue of permitting variation in intraurethral pressure, as the sling is tightened coincident with rectus muscle contraction associated with coughing, etc. This is in contrast to the fixed, relatively inflexible rigidity resulting from the Marshall-Marchetti-Krantz procedure. Both operations tend to restore or elevate a dropped urethrovesical junction to within the pelvis where it is responsive again to changes in intra-abdominal pressure which, thus, can affect equally both intraurethral and intravesical pressures. Even in the presence of sudden changes in intra-abdominal pressure, as with coughing or sneezing, continence will be maintained if the resting or nonvoiding intraurethral pressure remains greater than the intravesical pressure.

A challenging situation may arise with the development of stress incontinence in a patient previously subjected to colpectomy or colpocleisis. Because exposure of the vesicourethral junction is difficult in these instances, one can consider a divided sling technique (35), wherein, through a transabdominal incision, each urethral end of a half sling may be attached to the paraurethral fibromuscular tissue on each respective side and fixed to the rectus aponeurosis. Blind tunneling beneath the urethrovesical junction, as is necessary with

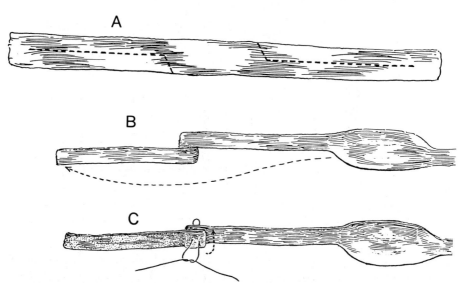

**Figure 5.8.** A means of increasing the length of the fascia strip is shown. Incisions are made along the path of the *dotted lines* shown in *A*; then back as depicted in *B*; and folded over as indicated in *C*. A single stitch is placed as shown, to fix the folded fascia in place. The same procedure is accomplished on the opposite end of the fascial strip. (Reproduced with permission of Charles C Thomas from Nichols DH: The sling operations. In Cantor EB (ed): *Female Urinary Stress Incontinence*, 1979.)

the Millin sling procedure (24), is not recommended because of the increased risk of urethral or vesical penetration.

## Technique of the Sling Operation

The anesthetized patient is placed in modified lithotomy position (Fig. 5.9), and the abdomen, vulva, and vagina are scrubbed, painted with antiseptic solution, and draped. The operation is commenced suprapubically with a 5-cm incision through the skin overlying each groin, parallel to the inguinal ligament. The incision is medial to the pubic tubercle and extends laterally toward the anterior iliac spine. For the patient with a previous Marshall-Marchetti-Krantz procedure (23), these incisions are lateral to the site of retropubic scarring that need not be disturbed. If the patient has previously experienced a Burch-type (7) suspension of vagina to Cooper's ligament, a conventional Pfannensteil incision is made through the skin and fascia, and the stitches of the Burch procedure are identified and cut, and the vesicourethral junction is freed by sharp dissection from the back of the pubis. Any cystotomy here should be closed in two layers, if possible. Each incision is deepened to the rectus sheath, which is opened by a 3-cm incision parallel to the skin incision. Each rectus muscle is penetrated by the tips of the curved Mayo scissors, with the curve directed toward the pubis, and the operator's index finger or the closed scissor tips are advanced extraperitoneally through the transversalis fascia into the

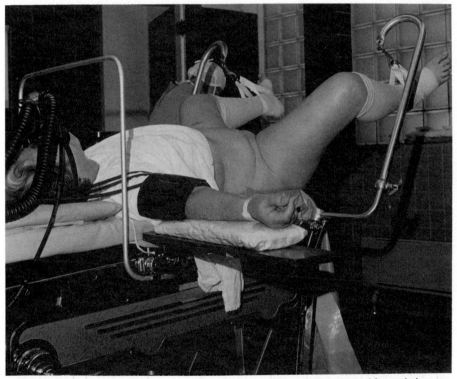

**Figure 5.9.** Elastic stockings have been applied to each leg. After abdomen, vagina, and perineum have been prepared and draped, further redraping and repositioning of the patient on the operating table later in the procedure becomes unnecessary. Even in the markedly obese patients, the inguinal incision can be made below the panniculus. The arrangement of operating table, patient, and stirrups is not unlike that used for laparoscopy.

space of Retzius. If scissors are used, the tips are opened somewhat and withdrawn, enlarging the deeper incision. Blunt finger dissection continues to the posterior surface of the obturator foramen. A sterile pack is placed in each wound, the operator and assistants reposition themselves, and the vaginal portion of the operation commences. By using the stirrups in the position chosen for laparoscopy, it has not been necessary nor desirable to reprepare and redrape the patient between the different phases of the operation. A transurethral no. 16 silicone-coated Foley catheter is inserted into the bladder, and 50 ml of sterile evaporated milk or commercial infant formula are instilled to identify better any unrecognized penetration of the bladder during the course of the procedure. Prompt appearance of the milk will be obvious, but it does not stain the surrounding tissue for the duration of the case as would be true were methylene blue or indigo carmine used. The bulb on the Foley catheter is identified, and the vaginal wall is picked up between two Allis clamps placed at the three and nine o'clock positions, proximal to the position of the Foley bulb. A longitudinal full-thickness vaginal incision is made between the clamps into the vesicovaginal space and carried anteriorly by sharp dissection, separating vagina from urethra to within 1.5 cm of the urethral meatus. The separation of bladder from vagina is carried posteriorly, well beyond the bulb on the catheter, the full distance to the vault of the vagina if a cystocele is to be repaired, and the dissection is carried laterally as far as the pubic rami. Lateral dissection of the vaginal wall from the vesicourethral junction in previously operated patients may release troublesome scar tissue that may have been holding the internal urethral orifice open. If there is evidence of funneling within the proximal urethra, the tissues surrounding the urethral wall at the vesicourethral unction may be strengthened and supported by imbrication with one or more Kelly-type plication stitches, using fine polyglycolic-type suture. (Moir once commented that the addition of such suburethral plication was analogous to a man's lack of confidence by wearing both a belt and suspenders. However, we see no harm in using these funnel-plication sutures.) The position of the urethrovesical junction is carefully reconfirmed by palpation of the site of the inflated Foley catheter bulb. The tissues of the urogenital diaphragm on each paraurethral side of the vesicourethral junction are perforated bluntly with the tips of the curved Mayo scissors, directed upward and laterally away from the bladder toward the previously established retropubic inguinal tunnel, into the space of Retzius. The scissors are opened 1 to 2 cm and withdrawn, enlarging the opening. It is important to stay close to the pubic rami but to avoid the periosteum. Some venous bleeding is occasionally seen and responds readily to gauze-sponge tamponade. The sterile packs are removed from the abdominal incisions and an abdominal approach is resumed. The surgeon inserts the tip of the left index finger through the abdominal incision on the patient's right and introduces the tip of a uterine dressing forceps, concave side toward the operator, into the transvaginal tunnel through the urogenital diaphragm on the patient's right, until it meets the left index fingertip posterior to the obturator foramen. The uterine dressing forceps is advanced, keeping contact with the surgeon's left index finger so as to avoid unwanted penetration of bladder or peritoneum, until the tip appears at the skin surface of the incision in the right groin. here, the tip of the clamp grasps one end of a long heavy silk pilot suture which is withdrawn through the retropubic tunnel. A similar procedure is accomplished on the patient's left (Fig. 5.10). The fascia lata strap, or a precut Gore-Tex hammock, or a Mersilene mesh hammock (available from Ethicon, Inc., Sommerville, NJ, catalog no. RM 43 or RM 54) measuring no more than 2.5 cm maximum width at the center of its belly and tapering to 1.5 cm at each end of the hammock, measures 32 cm in length. It is important

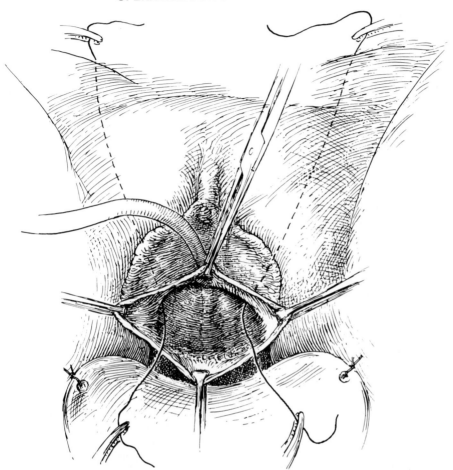

**Figure 5.10.** A short abdominal extraperitoneal incision has been made through each rectus aponeurosis into the space of Retzius. The anterior vaginal wall has been opened and the urogenital diaphragm penetrated. A silk pilot suture has been placed through this tunnel on each side. (Reproduced with permission of the American College of Obstetricians and Gynecologists from Nichols DH: The Mersilene mesh gauze hammock for severe urinary stress incontinence. *Obstet Gynecol* 41:88–93, 1973.)

that the maximum width of the plastic hammock be no greater than 2.5 to 3 cm to aid in optimum positioning beneath the vesicourethral junction. Any wider diameter would bring the posterior margin of the synthetic hammock too far onto the posterioinferior surface of the bladder, while one much narrower might strangulate the urethra. Moir has stressed the importance of cutting the sheet of gauze in the direction of least stretch. It is held in place transversely beneath the posterior urethra, and the ends are temporarily clamped to the drapes by two hemostats at the threeand nine-o'clock positions. The anterior margin of the wide hammock belly is tacked and fixed to the undersurface of the lateral paraurethral connective tissue by two interrupted 00 nonabsorbable synthetic sutures, and the posterior edge of the belly is sewn to the postero-lateral surface of the bladder capsule. An additional interrupted tacking suture or two is placed in the posterior midline of the gauze hammock belly fixing it to the bladder capsule. This stretches the hammock anteroposteriorly, without tension, but with sufficient pull to remove most of the wrinkles from the belly of the strap. Each silk pilot suture is tied to the respective tail end of the plastic mesh or fascial strap and drawn through its tunnel (Fig. 5.11). If an anterior colporrhaphy is to be accomplished, it is completed now. Thin or defective vaginal walls require that the gauze be covered by a Martius bulbocavernosus transplant, or if the vagina is sufficiently wide, the vaginal lapping operation may be used to advantage as described in Chapter 18. The edges of the anterior vaginal wall, trimmed only if necessary, are approximated in two layers: a deep or buried layer of interrupted 00 polyglycolic sutures followed by a superficial layer of interrupted mattress sutures (also of 00 polyglycolic) (Fig. 5.12). Any tension on the vaginal sutures line should be relieved by lateral vaginal relaxing incisions. Any necessary posterior colporrhaphy or perineorrhaphy is next accomplished, and the vagina is packed overnight with iodoform gauze. The packing itself acts as a bolster in supporting and elevating the vesicourethral junction. When it is in place the operator's attention is redirected to the abdomen and the sling is sewn to the point where it penetrates the rectus aponeurosis, only tightly enough to take up any slack that may be present. It may be presumed that when the patient is subsequently standing the vesi-courethral junction, supported by the properly placed sling, will be at the same position that it occupied when the packing was in place, having restored the proximal urethral to an intra-abdominal position.

After the free ends of the hammock have been securely anchored to the rectus fascia using nonabsorbable synthetic sutures, the excess tails are trimmed and removed from the operative field, and any remaining rectus fascia incision is closed with interrupted sutures. The skin is closed with skin clips or interrupted silk mattress sutures. The wide belly of this sling distributes suburethral pressure over a wide area, and the sling neither constricts the urethra nor decreases its lumen, although it does appear to increase both urethral tone and intraurethral pressure by providing a firm support upon which the urethral may rest. In the rare event of unexpected bladder penetration during placement of the sling, any externally visible opening can be repaired. If good exposure is not available, the sling may be repositioned so as to be away from the penetration, the edges of the penetration permitted to fall together, and the catheter decompression of the bladder maintained a full 14 days, permitting the bladder to heal.

## Altering the Tension of the Sling Postoperatively

If the sling, of whatever material has been used, has been placed too loosely to achieve an increase in intraurethral pressure sufficient to restore continence, this will become evident shortly after the Foley catheter has been removed in the immediate postoperative period. Similarly, if it has been placed too tightly, the patient may not be able to empty her bladder. To lessen the chance of traumatic necrosis of the overlying flap of vagina, the approach of choice to tighten the sling is by a transabdominal approach through one of the groin incisions. This is easiest within the first 7 to 14 days after surgery when there is as yet minimal fibrosis and scarring around the sling. Simply releasing one end of the sling from its attachment to the abdominal aponeuresis is sufficient to relieve the tension of a sling applied too tightly. (Weeks or months later it is more difficult to find the abdominal end of the sling, by this time buried in scar tissue, but it will be found adherent to the underside of the lower edge of the incision through the rectus aponeurosis. Alternatively, it may be severed through a transvaginal incision.) Alterations in tension need be applied to but one end of the sling, thus only one of the groin incisions needs to be reopened.

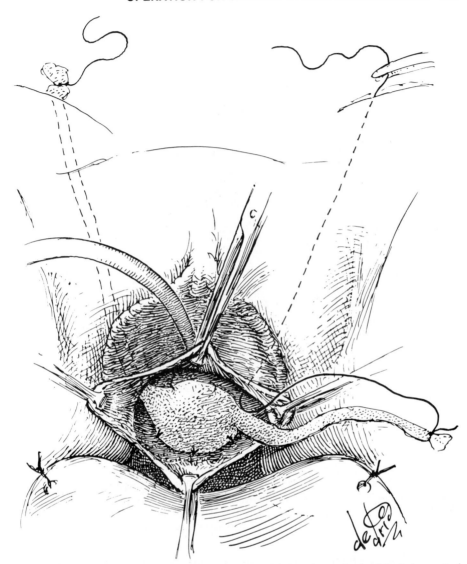

**Figure 5.11.** The belly of the strap or hammock has been tacked by interrupted synthetic nonabsorbable 000 sutures to the undersurface of the periurethral connective tissue anteriorly, and to the bladder capsule posteriorly. The ends of the hammock have been tied to the vaginal pilot sutures, and traction upon the pilot suture on the patient's right has drawn the strap through the preformed tunnel. The end of the strap to which the pilot suture was tied appears in the wound in the patient's right groin. A similar maneuver will be performed on the patient's left, and the vaginal wall closed with two layers of interrupted 00 polyglycolic acid-type sutures, a deeper buried layer and a superficial layer of interrupted mattress sutures. An iodoform-impregnated gauze vaginal pack is inserted. Without repositioning the patient, the ends of the hammock are sewn without extra tension to the rectus aponeurosis, and the incision in each groin is closed. (Reproduced with permission of the American College of Obstetricians and Gynecologists from Nichols DH: The Mersilene mesh gauze hammock for severe urinary stress incontinence. *Obstet Gynecol* 41:88–93, 1973.)

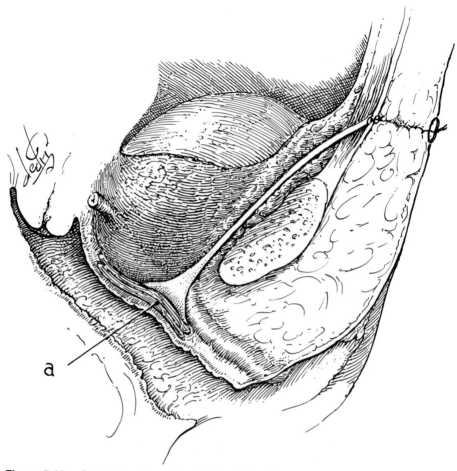

**Figure 5.12.** Sagittal section showing a suburethral sling in place. The vagina has been closed in two layers (a) to insulate the belly of the sling from the vagina. (Reproduced with permission of Charles C Thomas from Nichols DH: The sling operations. In Cantor EB (ed): *Female Urinary Stress Incontinence,* 1979.)

The degree to which the sling should be tightened or loosened can be judged by simultaneous direct urethroscopy in the operating room. After the abdominal end of the sling has been mobilized, the sling is fixed at sucha point under direct visualization that the internal urethral orifice has just closed. This requires a two-team approach: an abdominal operating team and a urethroscopist. Carbon dioxide urethroscopy seems ideal for this procedure. Lacking a urethroscope, a hysteroscope or laparoscope can be used transurethrally. In the absence of urethroscopy, a less precise method of determining sling tension can be elected. One can choose the point at which sudden manual abdominal compression against the full bladder will not produce leaking, or, if the patient is under spinal anesthesia, she can be asked to cough, and the sling tension chosen at which there is no transurethral leakage.

## CONCLUSION

It is evident that when one has chosen to use a suburethral sling procedure for the surgical treatment of severe or recurrent USI, there are various materials and techniques that may be selected to remedy the patient's disability. Several of these have been described, along with the circumstances whereby one might favor one over another. We emphasize that the surgeon should be familiar with and experienced in several techniques in order to be able to select those materials and technical steps that will best serve the needs of each individual patient.

## References

1. Asmussen M, Ulmsten U: Simultaneous urethro-cystometry with a new technique. *Scand J Urol Nephrol* 10:7–11, 1976.
2. Baden WF, Walker TA: Evaluation of the Stess-Incontinent Patient. In Cantor EB (ed): *Female Urinary Stress Incontinence.* Springfield, IL, Charles C Thomas, 1979, pp. 157–158.
3. Bates CP, Loose H, Stanton SLR: The objective study of incontinence after repair operations. *Surg Gynecol Obstet* 136:17–22, 1973.
4. Beck RP, Arnusch D, King C: Results in treating 210 patients with detrusor overactivity incontinence of urine. *Am Obstet Gynecol* 125:593–596, 1976.
5. Beck RP, Hsu N: Relationship of urethral length and anterior wall relaxation to urinary stress incontinence. *Am J Obstet Gynecol* 89:738–741, 1964.
6. Beck RP, Hsu N, Maughan GB: Simultaneous intraurethral and intravesical pressure studies in patients surgically treated for stress incontinence. *Am J Obstet Gynecol* 91:314–319, 1965.
7. Burch JD: Urethrovaginal fixation to Cooper's ligament for correction of stress incontinence, cystocele, and prolapse. *Am Obstet Gynecol* 81:281, 1961.
8. Crisp W: Urinary pressure incontinence in the female. *Ariz Med* 23:513–516, 1966.
9. Fantl JA, Hurt WG, Dunn LJ: Dysfunctional detrusor control. *Am J Obstet Gynecol* 129:299–303, 1977.
10. Figuranov KM: Surgical treatment of urinary incontinence in women. *Akush Ginekol* 6:7–13, 1949 (in Russian).
11. Fliegner JR, Glenning PP: Seven years experience in the evaluation and management of patients with urge incontinence of urine. *Aust NZ J Obstet Gynaecol* 19:42–44, 1979.
12. Gleason DM, Bottaccini MR, Reilly RJ: Comparison of cystometrograms and urethral profiles with gas and water media. *Urology* 9:155–160, 1977.
13. Green TH: Urinary stress incontinence: Differential diagnosis, pathophysiology, and management. *Am J Obstet Gynecol* 122:368–400, 1975.
14. Hawksworth W, Roux JP: Vaginal hysterectomy. *J Obstet Gynaecol Br Commonw* 63:214, 1958.
15. Henriksson L, Ulmsten U: A urodynamic evaluation of the effects of abdominal urethrocystopexy and vaginal sling urethro-
plasty in women with stress incontinence. *Am J Obstet Gynecol* 131:77–82, 1978.
16. Hodgkinson CP: Stress urinary incontinence. *Am J Obstet Gynecol* 108:1141, 1970.
17. Hodgkinson CP, Kelley WT: Urinary stress incontinence in the female III; rounded ligament technique for retropubic suspension of the urethra. *Obstet Gynecol* 10:493–499, 1957.
18. Howkins J, Stallworthy J: In *Bonney's Gynaecological Surgery.* 8th ed. London, Balliere Tindall, 1974, pp 550-551.
19. Jeffcoate TNA, Francis W: Urgency incontinence in the female. *Am J Obstet Gynecol* 94:604–618, 1966.
20. Khanna OP: Disorders of micturition. *Urology* 8:316–328, 1976.
21. Lee RA: Correcting recurrent stress incontinence. *Contemp Obstet Gynecol* 12:33–41, 1978.
22. Malpas P: The choice of operation for genital prolapse. *Progr Gynecol* 3:663–673, 1957.
23. Marshall VF, Marchetti AA, Krantz KE: The correction of stress incontinence by simple vesicourethral suspension. *Surg Gynecol Obstet* 88:509, 1949.
24. Millin T, Reed CD: Stress incontinence of urine in the female. *Postgrad Med J* 24:51, 1948.
25. Moir JC: The gauze-hammock operation. *J Obstet Gynaecol Br Commonw* 75:1, 1968.
26. Morgan JE: Personal communication.
27. Nesbitt REL, Hofmann JC: Management of urinary stress incontinence in the female. *Surg Gynecol Obstet* 132:588–596, 1971.
28. Nichols DH: In Taymor ML, Green TH (eds): *Progress in Gynecology.* Vol. 6, New York, Grune & Stratton, 1975.
29. Nichols DH: The sling operations. In Cantor EB (ed): *Female Urinary Stress Incontinence.* Springfield IL, Charles C Thomas, 1979.
30. Novak F: *Surgical Gynecologic Techniques.* New York, John Wiley & Sons, 1978.
31. Obrink A, Bunne G: Urethral pressure profile at pubococcygeal repair for stress incontinence. *Acta Obstet Gynecol Scand* 59:433–437, 1980.
32. Ostergard DR: The effect of drugs on the lower urinary tract. *Obstet Gynecol Surv* 34:424–431, 1979.
33. Parker RT, Addison WA, Wilson CJ: Fascia lata urethrovesical suspension for re-

current stress urinary incontinence. *Am J Obstet Gynecol* 135:843, 1979.

34. Pereyra AJ: A simplified surgical procedure for the correction of stress incontinence in women. *West J Surg* 67:223, 1959.

35. Ridley JH: Surgery for stress urinary incontinence. In Ridley H (ed): *Gynecologic Surgery: Errors, Safeguards, Salvage*, ed. 2, Baltimore, Williams & Wilkins, 1981.

36. Ridley JH: Urinary incontinence not curable by sphincter plication. In TeLinde RW, Mattingly RF (eds): *Operative Gynecology*, ed. 4, Philadelphia, JB Lippincott, 1970.

37. Robertson JL: *Genitourinary Problems in Women*. Springfield, IL, Charles C Thomas, 1977.

38. Sand PK, Hill RC, Ostergard DR: Supine Urethroscopic and Standing Cystometry as Screening Methods for the Detectio–n of Detrusor Instability. *Obstet Gynecol* 70: 57–60, 1987.

39. Stamey TA: Endoscopic suspension of the vesical neck for urinary incontinence. *Surg Gynecol Obstet* 136:547–554, 1973.

40. Weil A, Miege B, Rottenberg R, et al: Clinical Significance of urethral Instability. *Obstet Gynecol* 68:106–110, 1986.

41. Wheeless CR, Wharton LR, Dorsey JH, et al: The Goebell-Stoeckel operation for universal cases of urinary incontinence. *Am J Obstet Gynecol* 128:546–549, 1977.

42. White GR: Cystocele—A radical cure by suturing lateral sulci of vagina to white lines of pelvic fascia. *JAMA* 53:1707–9, 1909.

43. Word BH Jr, Mongtomery HA: Personal communication.

44. Zoedler D: Die operative Behandlung der Weiblichen Ahnninkontinenz mit dem Kinststaff-Netz-Band. *Actuelle Urol* 1:28, 1970.

# CHAPTER 6

# Preoperative and Postoperative Care

## PREOPERATIVE CARE

The gynecologic surgeon should always be mindful of the whole patient, particularly during preoperative evaluation of the individual and her problem. Despite inevitable concentration of his interest in the pelvis and related reproductive capacity, the gynecologist must know the patient's past and current medical history and be considerate as well of any current systemic problem, particularly any cardiac, blood pressure, or endocrine abnormality. A positive family history including gynecologic disorders should be determined. A history or evidence of pulmonary disease, asthma, emphysema, or excessive smoking would be significant. If the patient has emphysema or significant respiratory symptoms, spirometry and a study of blood gases are advisable. We would urge a preoperative patient to decrease or stop smoking for days or preferably weeks before scheduled surgery. Investigation should include evaluation of any history or "suspicion" of diabetes or phlebitis, or any "tendency" to abnormality in bleeding or probability of an excessive use of alcohol. Preoperative communication with the patient's internist or her family doctor is mandatory, particularly when there is a history of heart disease, angina, or arrhythmia, or if the patient has been taking antihypertensive medication or has a history of rheumatism. A current consultation is equally important if the patient is a diabetic, in which case the duration, severity, and current management of the disease should be known to the surgeon. An invitation should be extended to her internist or family doctor to participate in the managment of the medical aspects of her postoperative care. Medications the patient has taken within the preceding year should be reviewed and their present effect evaluated. The effects of anticonvulsant drugs and diuretics should be recognized, and, in connection with the latter, any potassium or chloride depletion should be recognized and corrected preoperatively. It is important that the use of oral contraceptives be known. Whenever possible, all steroids should be discontinued at least a month before surgery in order to minimize the chance of pulmonary, coronary, or cerebral thrombosis and embolism. The presence of any disease not under current control, including upper respiratory infections, a history of myocardial infarction, or a history of an increasingly progressive angina in which more symptoms are occurring in spite of reduced activity all should warrant re-evaluation and reconjfirmation of the indications and benefits for the scheduled surgery. It is equally important to be aware of a history of mental instability or any adverse experience with previous surgery or anesthesia. It is well to inquire whether the patient remembers an allergy or hypersensitivity to drugs taken previously, sometimes long ago. Allergies, particularly to medications, should be made known to both the surgeon and the anesthesiologist, including a history of allergies all but forgotten. Current or regularly used drugs the patient may have become accustomed to taking may have become such a habit that unless asked, the patient may forget to bring them to the surgeon's attention. As the medical history is developed, the frequent or regular use of aspirin, tranquilizers, antihypertensive agents, antibiotics, birth control pills, or steroids used in the treatment of acne, arthritis, or rheumatism are examples of drugs frequently thought to be of insufficient significance to mention, but each should be reported to the surgeon. The genitourinary system should have been investigated preoperatively with as much thoroughness as the patient's history and symptoms indicate. The surgical dictation of any previous pelvic surgery should be requested and reviewed. If the cervix is still present, preoperative evaluation should include the report of a Papanicolaou smear taken and evaluated within the year preceding surgery. An adequate evaluation of any recently abnormal uterine bleeding is necessary. A preoperative chest x-ray is desirable. With the patient over 50, or if there is any suspicion of cardiac abnormality, an electrocardiogram is advisable, not only for the information it can supply preoperatively, but as a baseline for comparison with any postoperative study that might be required. Preoperative laboratory screening should include a complete blood count, coagulation studies, biochemical profile, and a blood type and screening determination. The reports of all of these procedures should be recorded on the patient's chart and reviewed before she is taken to the operating room. The patient should be carefully and conscientiously examined for any contraindication to what is usually elective surgery. The life expectancy of the patient and the longevity of her ancestors should always be taken into consideration, for to ignore the patient's overall welfare will ultimately discredit both the surgeon and the procedure performed. Abnormal findings should always be personally evaluated and discussed without placing reliance on the previous opinions of others.

We believe it advisable to apply elastic stockings, of graduated compression if available, from the feet to the midthigh preoperatively, particularly if the patient has appreciable varices or a history of previous phlebitis or thrombosis. Alternately they may be applied at the conclusion of an operation when the patient has been in the lithotomy or a marked Trendelenburg position, before the legs are lowered and the head is raised. Whether this practice reduces the risk of embolism is debatable, but it effectively reduces the incidence of thrombosis (22) and the size of the venous bed into which blood will pool as soon as the patient's body is leveled or her feet have been taken down from the stirrups. Under such circumstances the prophylactic use of elastic stockings will appreciably reduce the degree of postoperative hypotension, which will predispose some patients to cardiac or cerebral thrombosis or might at least confuse the recovery room phase of the patient's postoperative course.

We do not recommend the use of subcutaneous minidoses of heparin, fearing an insufficient effectiveness in reducing the incidence of embolization to offset the risk of a significant increase in intraoperative and postoperative bleeding (4).

## Steroids

When a patient is taking cortisone or prednisone, it should, if possible, be stopped 10 days before surgery and not resumed until after the first 4 or 5 days postoperatively. In such patients the surgeon should strongly consider the use of nonabsorbable suture in buried tissue layers subject to tension. If temporary suspension of the drug cannot be safely accomplished, massive doses of vitamin A (50,000 to 100,000 units daily) or anabolic steroids may reverse the inhibition of collagen formation and inflammatory reaction (8).

## Preoperative Psychologic Preparation

In addition to the usual physiologic and anatomic preparations for surgery, there should be an appropriate psychologic evaluation of the patient by the surgeon. It is always good to encourage the patient's expression of her questions and possible fears. Such adequate preparation will add immeasurably to the patient's expectations of a successful outcome, and she will be less dismayed by postoperative discomforts and the time required for complete recovery. It is as important for the surgeon to understand the manner in which the patient conceives of her problem and its treatment (6) as it is for her to understand how her surgeon views her condition and the surgery recommended. The most desirable one-to-one relationship requires a considerate surgeon and an informed, confident patient. When developed preoperatively, the patient's understanding and confidence will assure cooperation, an improved postoperative course, and a more optimistic long-term evaluation of her result. Although both patient and surgeon are aware that he or she has accompanied many other patients down the same surgical pathway, to each particular patient her operation is the all-important one, and her surgeon can do no less than to keep her point of view constantly in mind. This is the poorest of times to appear impatient, hurried, or indifferent, or to suggest the importance of anything other than this patient's current problem throughout pre- and postoperative periods. Advice and restrictions in postoperative activities should not be considered without knowledge and an appreciation of the individual's home situation. A quiet personal conversation will do much to dispel the fear of being abandoned during the stay in an unfamiliar hospital room. The surgeon should emphasize the intention of seeing the patient each day throughout her period of hospitalization and, no matter how busy his daily schedule, time must be found to answer any questions carefully and in an unhurried manner in order to dispel the patient's unnecessary fears. Knowledge of a chronically ill child or parent, a husband's current employment crisis, or the pressing problems of other members of the patient's immediate family will enable the surgeon to understand some patients' apparently unreasonable anxiety. Some appreciation of the patient's relationships with her family and her husband is usually very important. If a genuine neurosis is present, the surgeon must clearly understand and honestly question whether his operative measures will bring about the desired gynecological cure. In such tragic situations, surgery too often provides only an excuse for the patient to blame her marital disharmony upon the effects of her surgery. With continued failure to recognize the shortcomings in her own relationship with her husband, an operative procedure that was indicated and satisfactorily performed may be blamed for having made her worse.

A considerate visit to the patient in the hospital by her surgeon the day or evening before a scheduled operation is of inestimable value in providing her with a chance to bring to light any last minute questions or problems that may have been troubling her and to relate herself more closely with her surgeon. Certainly, at some time before the day of the operation, if the surgeon knows he or she may be away or unavailable during a portion of the patient's postoperative stay, such an explanation should be clearly given to the patient, in order to dispel thoughts of postoperative abandonment. If the surgeon knows he or she will have to be away, such an explanation should also be carefully given to the patient, relating the arrangements that have been made for her care during the absence, clearly indicating who will be responsible, how this individual can be reached, and when the surgeon expects to return to resume personal supervision of her care. It must be recognized that the importance and the quality of the patient's care may be just as significant after discharge from the hospital as during hospitalization. Home calls are seldom necessary, and the apprehensions most frequently accounting for a request for the gynecologist to see the postoperative patient at home during her convalescence will be considerably lessened by assurance before the patient leaves the hospital that her surgeon will be available for telephoned questions and consultation while she is confined to her home. In this way the cooperation and confidence of the patient will be maintained until her recovery is complete and her return to unrestricted activities has been approved. The wise and considerate surgeon will not permit the delicate and, at times, very personal relationship with his patient to extend inappropriately beyond the timeframe of her convalescence. Future dependence upon her surgeon, that was for a time a highly desirable relationship, should be consciously discouraged as the patient resumes her private life and personal responsibilities. To assure a successful transition and termination requires intelligent and purposeful application of practical psychology and good patient care. The details will be different with almost every patient. Much of the success of one's practice is predicated on the development of concepts and practice that elevates the surgeon from the role of mere technical craftsman to the intended and more effective role of the physician. The implications of hysterectomy to the individual patient's psychology should be understood by the physician as he or she considers how a particular patient perceives of her problem and the results of the recommended surgery. These considerations were well summarized by Polivy (17). For some women, an escape from the concerns regarding conception may be entirely offset by the fear the operation will mean a loss of femininity. Being freed of the inconveniences of menometrorrhagia and dysmenorrhea spares many patients predictable and undesirable disabilities. The gynecologist should make certain his patient also understands that the quality of her response to her husband will likely be enhanced by her freedom from the fear of pregnancy.

Hysterectomy in the absence of demonstrable significant pelvic pathology seems more likely to be followed by subsequent emotional depression or milder instability. There are several helpful points to aid in the recognition of a candidate disposed to postoperative psychological difficulties. The surgery addict, often an hysterical neurotic with the scars of many operations, will usually report intense but ill-defined pains and often harbors a need to suffer. The surprisingly indifferent woman should also be a warning, however, because indifference often serves as a simple facade behind which there exists an immature refusal to even think about the operation. Predictably, this degree of rejection is likely to be followed by an infantile type of emotional response to all postoperative discomforts and dysfunctions. When noted preoperatively, apparent indifference should be considered a mask, repressing anxiety and a denial of the trauma to come. In sharp contrast, the overanxious patient evidence worry about technical details, the site and size of her incision, the type of anesthesia, and the postoperative visiting hours. It would be expedient to recognize such concerns as evidence of a good candidate for postoperative unhappiness and perhaps severe emotional instability. Still another problem is the would-be seductive patient, whose fantasies in regard to her doctor-patient relationships may readily transcend the usual bounds of professional responsibility. The desirable degree of insight into the probabilities of the patient's mental and emotional stability after surgery may usually be gained, but only as a result of discussing with the patient before surgery her feelings about the loss of her uterus and her expectations following surgery, as well as her concepts related to previous operations and her reactions to those experiences.

Predisposing factors to postoperative psychiatric disturbances that may prolong the period of disability should be suspected when an operation proves the absence of demonstrable pelvic disease, when there is a history of previous psychiatric care, especially depression, or when there are evidences of marital discord, particularly in a young patient. An attempt should be made to recognize and assess such factors and to place them in proper perspective ahead of time. When accomplished, both the patient and her surgeon will be spared hours of postoperative apprehension, indecision, and lack of progress. When a need for professional psychiatric help is suspected, it will be most effective if such support is made available well ahead of time so that the psychiatrist, too, may have developed a desirable degree of rapport with the patient before the strain of postoperative discomfort is added to any pre-existing psychiatric needs.

Patients who seem neurotic preoperatively are certain to be manifestly neurotic postoperatively. In such instances the surgeon will be well advised to search for and dispel myths and fears that may well and long have been repressed, to reassure the patient particularly of the preservation of her femininity, giving due consideration to possible ethnic attitudes and customs. Often the latter may have traditionally clear-cut and deeply ingrained concepts about the occurrence of menstruation and the importance of preserving the uterus. Inclusion of the psychologic aspects of an adequte preoperative evaluation of the patient will help avoid what might otherwise become a medically unexpected and surgically unwarranted complication, which all too frequently makes a surgical experience a most unhappy and unsatisfactory memory for all concerned.

### Preoperative Hair Removal

We believe that preoperative shaving of the surgical site offers no advantage to the patient and by abrading the skin may precipitate an increased incidence of wound infection (1). Patients are no longer shaved routinely, but long hairs may be clipped, if desired, to keep them out of the surgical field. The unshaven patients are much more comfortable in the later postoperative recovery phase.

### Preventive Antibiotics

Considering the vagina as a site for surgery, one must be mindful that it is chronically contaminated by multiple bacteria. The bacteriology of the vaginal canal of each woman varies, both in bacterial types and numbers. Variations are related to the time of life, the patient's environment and sexual activity, and, in premenopausal patients, even the time of the month (3). The desirable effects of preoperative cleansing by douching and scrubbing with antibacterial soaps, such as those containing povidone-iodine (Betadine) or chlorhexidine gluconate (Hibiclens), will assure a significant reduction in bacterial quantity, but this procedure in itself does not "sterilize" the vagina.

There seems to be a significant risk of postoperative infection when an operative procedure combines surgical manipulation and dissection of the vagina with a large opening of the peritoneal cavity and, at its conclusion, leaves areas of surgically traumatized and devascularized tissue crushed by forceps and tied into pedicles. This clinical risk can be reduced considerably if an appropriate broad-spectrum antibiotic is present at the time of surgery in the tissue being operated upon as suggested by Burke (2). Such protection is especially desirable when the surgical procedure carries an appreciable risk of clinical infection. Ledger et al. (12) and others (7, 14, 18, 24) have found this to be especially likely in premenopausal patients subjected to vaginal hysterectomy and have formulated a useful set of guidelines for antibiotic prophylaxis in gynecology, which include Burke's recommendation that the "antibiotic must be circulating in the patient's tissue before the operation begins and should be promptly discontinued if there is no specific reason for continuing it after the patient recovers normal physiology.'' Burke emphasized, however, that: ''Preoperative preventive antibiotics will not eliminate all postoperative septic complications. There will be situations in which the level of bacterial resistance, extent of trauma, size of inoculum of bacteria, or combination will be such that antibiotics will be of little use. Antibiotics are but an adjunct to the natural resistance to bacterial invasion. They by no means replace it.'' We are in accord with this thinking, and in addition, firmly believe that there is no substitute for meticulous precision and efficiency in technique and hemostasis to minimize tissue trauma.

Preventive antibiotics are thus particularly useful in curbing morbidity when major vaginal surgery is performed and especially when local hemostasis has been augmented by preliminary infiltration of tissue with a vasoconstrictor. An initial intramuscular injection of an antibiotic 1 hour before the start of surgery ''on call to the operating room'' seems to provide an effective tissue level when needed; but because there is often an unpredictable time variable of 1/2 to 3 hours between ''on call to the operating room'' and the actual initial incision, it appears that a proper level of antibiotic can be delivered to the tissues for surgery if it is given intravenously in the operating room immediately before the onset of anesthesia. Initial intravenous administration of prophylactic antibiotics *during anesthesia* is not recommended (20). The antibiotic probably will reach an effective tissue level within 20 to 30 minutes of the time of intravenous administration. If the operation is to be of less than 2 hours total duration, a single dose of antibiotic is desirable. If the operative time is longer than 2 hours duration, the intravenous dose should be repeated 2 hours from the beginning of the operation. Our first choice of antibiotic is 2 gm of a first generation cephalosporin such as cefazolin (Ancef or Kefzol), which has a half life of eighty minutes; and if a second dose is given 2 hours after the first, the half life totals 120 minutes.

The decreased febrile morbidity has been impressive and noteworthy and, by shortening the patient's hospital stay, cost effective. Although, in general, cephalosporins are contraindicated for the patient with a history of ''penicillin allergy,'' a single preoperative dose may occasionally be used if the surgeon feels that the indication is warranted and the risk:benefit ratio is favorable and if the allergic manifestation after penicillin injection was of the nature of a mild skin rash. If, on the other hand, the patient had a previous anaphylactic reaction to penicillin, this must be thoroughly respected and an alternate such as minicycline, metronidazole (9), or clindamycin and gentamycin chosen. There has been much speculation as to why reduced postoperative morbidity has been demonstrated using antibiotics to which anaerobic organisms are not sensitive. Perhaps the antibiotics suppress the aerobic flora, permitting the body to concentrate its defensive energy on the surviving anaerobes even though the latter were not sensitive to the antibiotic. Another possibility relates to possible interdependence of an anaerobic infection on a coincident aerobic colonization. The reverse of this situation might explain the similar effectiveness of preoperative metronidazol (Flagyl) (5, 9).

## POSTOPERATIVE CARE

Antibiotics or antibacterials to ''cover'' the bacteria often associated with the use of an indwelling bladder catheter need not be started until the day the catheter is to be removed. This sequence seems to avoid or retard the development of an antibiotic-resistant type of urinary tract infection such as often intrudes when antibacterial "coverage" is instituted immediately postoperatively and continued through the patient's postoperative course. (The exception will be after urinary fistula repair, in which one would wish to "sterilize" the urine during the early healing phase.) A urine culture and sensitivity study should, of course, be obtained the day the catheter is removed; when a positive culture is reported, the most appropriate antibiotic should be used until the culture becomes negative. Gentle percussion of the costovertebral angles should be accomplished postoperatively the evening after surgery and for the next several days. Unexpected or pronounced unilateral tenderness should be promptly investigated by infusion intravenous pyelography to exclude ureteral obstruction. Postoperative intravenous fluids should be continued until one is assured the patient will take and retain by mouth sufficient fluids, at which point the intravenous route should be discontinued. Liquids by mouth are usually permitted as soon as the patient has recovered from anesthesia, but in sips rather than by glassfuls, and preferably tea or tap water. Carbonated beverages, milk products, and fruit juices should be avoided initially to decrease the production of intestinal gas (18). When frequently repeated, this regime will usually assure the ingestion of an adequate 2 quarts of liquid per day. Solid foods can be offered as soon as the patient is interested; but, other than an occasional nibble, a significant intake is unlikely until the patient's appetite returns, usually on the second or third postoperative day. There are exceptions, of course, particularly after the repair of rectovaginal fistula or an old fourth-degree laceration, in which instance the patient is best maintained on an initial clear liquid nonresidue diet, followed during the second week after surgery by a low-residue diet.

The cessation of smoking in a postoperative patient may inhibit intestinal peristalsis due to the withdrawal of nicotine, so some problems with bowel function should be anticipated.

Stool softeners and laxatives should be considered if there has been a posterior colporrhaphy or perineorrhaphy, and it is desirable for bowel movements to be resumed by the third postoperative day. If not, a laxative suppository (Dulcolax) or low enema at this time, repeated if necessary, will lessen the chance of unexpected and unwanted fecal impaction. Under no circumstances should the patient recovering from gynecologic surgery be permitted to sit up to strain on a bedpan in an effort to accomplish a bowel movement without resorting to an enema. Surgery in the female pelvis is not infrequently followed by thrombosis in relatively large veins communicating with the internal iliacs and vena cava. The possibility exists that, under such circumstances, the suddenly increased intra-abdominal pressure as a result of a patient's efforts to accomplish a bowel movement is associated with an increased incidence of embolism of a large, soft, bland thrombus via the iliacs and vena cava, occasionally, with disastrous results. This risk should be reduced significantly by (a) early ambulation of the patient, (b) the prohibition of any major postoperative straining efforts of the patient to accomplish a bowel movement, and (c) the use of stool softeners and enema to assure postoperative bowel movement without exertion or strain on the patient's part.

Pain relief should be offered as necessary, preferably by the use of small doses of medication repeated at frequent intervals in order to avoid an accumulative effect and a systemic or respiratory depression. Little seems to be gained by having a patient dangle her legs over the edge of the bed the evening following surgery, and it seems this might even increase venous stasis. We do believe, however, that the patient should be encouraged to flex her legs, bend her ankles, and gently move from side to side and change position in bed, beginning soon after awakening from surgery and continuing throughout her entire postoperative period. Beginning the day after surgery, she should be helped to a bedside chair for a few minutes three or four times daily. This may also improve the transit time of intestinal gas (19). Sitting upon a rubber doughnut may strain new sutures and is not recommended. Warm sitz baths or showers can be started on the second or third postoperative day if the patient is willing. Any pre-existing medical conditions under treatment (i.e., hypertension) should be frequently re-evaluated, the postoperative routine modified, or appropriate therapy reinstituted as necessary.

Prolonged visiting with the patient should be discouraged, particularly during the first few postoperative days, when the patient needs ample opportunity to rest. These periods of rest should, however, be carefully interspersed with periods of ambulation and physical activity, and to assure the latter it is important that oversedation be avoided. Regular periods of deliberately deepened breathing should be encouraged as soon as the patient becomes conscious, and frequent repetition of forced inspiration or incentive spirometry has proven effective in reducing postoperative pulmonary problems.

The patient should be seen at least once daily by her surgeon during hospitalization and should receive an additional daily visit at a different time of day by a house officer, and more frequently when necessary.

Appropriate blood studies should usually be obtained before a postoperative patient is discharged from the hospital, but often this need be only a postoperative hemoglobin and hematocrit on the third or fourth postoperative day if, by that time, the patient's condition seems satisfactory. A postoperative hemoglobin of 9 gm/ml or greater and a hematocrit of at least 27 in a patient without cardiovascular disease will respond to oral therapy, and transfusion is unnecessary.

When elastic stockings have been applied preoperatively and the patient is resuming physical activity in a satisfactory manner, the stockings can be removed, usually by the third or fourth postoperative day.

If the patient is postmenopausal and sexually active, oral ingestion of an estrogen can be started as soon as the patient is taking fluids by mouth. This can be supplemented by nightly and later weekly instillations of an intravaginal estrogen that will aid wound epitheliazation, help preserve vaginal blood supply and elasticity, and avoid the vaginal atrophy that would otherwise become even more evident with postoperative contraction of the vaginal incision.

During her postoperative course, it is well to review on several occasions the patient's ingestion of all medications, for conflicting or unnecessary orders may be recognized for which timely correction can be made.

The probable date of discharge from the hospital should be discussed with the patient a day or 2 ahead of time, to allow the patient and her family adequate time to make arrangements and preparations. The patient should be given very specific instructions before discharge as to what she may and may not do during her convalescence. Written or printed postoperative instructions can be given to the patient, of which the following might be useful:

### Instructions on Going Home

1. "Go directly home and rest for the remainder of the day.
2. During the first week at home increase activity gradually. Expect unanticipated tiredness, and let no days' activities become an endurance contest.
3. Beginning the third week you may go out of doors and if able drive at the end of the month. Rest several times daily during the first week.
4. Please call the office within the first week to arrange for a postoperative appointment.
5. Do not hesitate to call for further advice if you have any questions.

### Activities

Gradually increase activity for the first 2 weeks. Do NOT engage in heavy lifting, scrubbing, douching, or intercourse until you have checked at the office.

### Diet

You may return to your usual diet. For constipation, drink some prune juice, extra water, or take 1 ounce of milk of magnesia, as necessary. Bran with breakfast is often helpful.

### Baths

You may shower, take tub baths, and wash your hair at any time.''

The patient should also be instructed as to the circumstances (fever, excessive bleeding, etc.) for which she should call for help postoperatively. Many patients will appreciate a summary and an interpretation of the laboratory studies recorded while in the hospital, and every patient should be given specific directions as to when to return to the surgeon's office for postoperative examination.

Measures designed to avoid as well as to recognize specific postoperative complications are discussed in Chapter 22, where indicated treatment will also be considered.

## Getting the Postoperative Patient to Void

The bladder has a triple nerve supply—somatic, sympathetic, and parasympathetic—and the perception and balance between these sometimes opposing influences vary from patient to patient and from time to time. Because this harmony is easily disturbed, it is not surprising that postoperative resumption of voiding is a rather common problem, but not often predictable with any degree of certainty. Difficulty in this area may occur after any surgical procedure, but especially after those involving the abdomen and pelvis. Noteworthy are episiotomy, colporrhaphy, hysterectomy, herniorrhaphy, hemorrhoidectomy, and laparotomy.

### Prevention of the Difficulty

Although the balance of complex physiologic and psychologic events associated with the act of voiding is often taken for granted by the patient, minor alterations in the facility of these habit patterns can produce major disturbances in resumption of function. Prevention of any difficulty is of prime importance. The circumstances under which one's patient is expected to void must be as private and comfortable as possible, and there is no substitute for promptness and calm on the part of the patient's attendants. Von Peham and Amreich (16) wrote years ago of the difficulty some encounter of voiding in the recumbent position. It at all possible, the patient should be permitted to void in a natural sitting position, using a nearby toilet if feasible, a portable commode if not, or sitting on a bedpan if confined to bed. Careless overdistention of the bladder is to be avoided at all costs, as it is not only painful but, as Lapides (11) has pointed out, appears to interfere temporarily with the blood supply of the bladder sufficient to lower local resistance to infection. Overdistention may effectively induce a temporary paralysis of detrusor activity that can require days to overcome.

The use of synthetic absorbable sutures, such as polyglycolic acid-type (Dexon, Vicryl) instead of catgut, appears to be associated with a considerable reduction in postoperative intravaginal adhesions as well as swelling and edema of the pelvic tissues. This is particularly noteworthy following colporrhaphy that includes any reconstructive plication or support of the vesical neck, where we now use longer lasting monofilament absorbable synthetic sutures of polydiaxanone (PDS, Ethicon Co.) or polygluconate (Maxon, Davis and Geck Co.). When transurethral drainage has been used, a silicone-coated Foley catheter is undoubtedly less irritating to the urethral mucosa than the uncoated rubber of the standard catheter, and it is thus associated with reduced mucosal edema and lessened consequent partial urethral obstruction. If the patient has a history of long-standing bladder decompensation, as may be associated with the aging large or massive cystocele, some intrinsic detrusor hypotonia can be predicted and bladder tone increased by judicious use of bethanechol chloride (Urecholine) befpre removal of the catheter and for several days thereafter until comfortable voiding has been re-established. In obviously anxious patients, preliminary sedation with barbiturates and judicious use of analgesics will be rewarding, employing a dose tailored to the needs of the individual patient.

Recall that the bladder neck is well supplied with alpha-adrenergic receptors that, when stimulated, tend to cause smooth muscle contraction in this area, in contrast to stimulation of beta-receptors that tend to produce relaxation of the bladder neck and trigone in the presence of low amounts of noradrenaline (21). Alpha-adrenergic blocking agents such as phenoxybenzamine or prazocin will thus selectively block spasm resultant from alpha-adrenergic receptor stimulation in this area. Success has been reported (13, 15) from the use of the alpha-adrenergic blocking agent phenoxybenzamine (Dibenzyline) in a dose of 10 mg by mouth 4 to 5 hours after surgery and repeated, if necessary, once or twice during the first 24 hours. Our experience with this drug for this circumstance has been favorable. Remember that any beta blockers such as propranolol hydrochloride (Inderal) may not only stimulate detrusor tone inducing a hypertonia but, by selective blocking, may induce some spasm of the bladder neck.

## Etiology of Inability to Void

*Anxiety*. When postoperative voiding difficulty has developed, it can be considered the result of one or more etiologic factors, some of which were characterized by Jeffcoate (10). Powerful among these factors is anxiety on the part of the patient or her attendant staff that gives rise to strong psychologic influences on her voiding patterns. Sometimes this is preconditioned by fear, conversation with other patients, hearsay, or observation of other patients. Treatment, of course, includes appropriate counseling, gentle calmness, cheerful confidence and empathy on the part of the attendant staff, and appropriate sedation and pain relief. The administration of tea or beer has been recommended, the former to induce some detrusor hyperactivity and the latter some general body sedation.

*Mechanical Interference*. Local physical factors may interfere with the physiology of voiding. Among these are the presence of vaginal packing, local edema, rectal fullness, or any obstruction of urethra or ureters. Any mechanical factors that interfere with the opening of the internal urethral sphincter may play a role, especially those causing failure of physiologic obliteration of the posterior urethrovesical angle during attempts at voiding. For example, very few women can void while a tight vaginal packing is in place (Fig. 6.1) and treatment of this etiologic circumstance is the removal of any mechanical obstruction of the vagina or urethra. It is important that overhydration be avoided at the time an indwelling catheter is to be removed, as this, although frequently urged by some nursing staff, exaggerates any difficulties that may be present and produces rapid and unnecessary overdistention of the bladder.

*Reflex Interferences*. A major etiologic factor can be related to neurologic

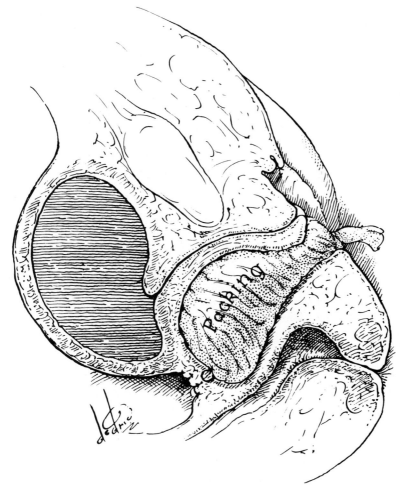

**Figure 6.1.** Spontaneous voiding after surgery may be inhibited if the vagina is so tightly packed with gauze that physiologic descent of the vesicourethral junction is precluded. (From Nichols DH: Getting the postoperative patient to void. *Contemp Obstet Gynecol* 12:41–45, 1978; reproduced with permission of Contemporary Ob/Gyn, Medical Economics Co.)

relfex interference with the normal physiology of voiding. This may be coincident with levator spasm, as is so often seen after parturition, episiotomy, and hemorrhoidectomy, which may give rise to reflex spastic contraction of both the internal and external urethral sphincters. This is, of course, accentuated by nervousness and patient embarrassment. Sitz baths, analgesia, and time are of the greatest help, because when painful but temporary levator spasm has finally been overcome, the bladder and urethral sphincters will once again begin to relax. Similarly, pain in the rectus abdominus muscles, from laparotomy incision, will often reflexly induce levator spasm, interfering with the physiologic descent of the vesical neck during the voiding process. Again, patience and analgesia will help. Temporary use of an alpha-adrenergic blocker, such as phenoxybenzamine, will often relieve urethral spasm, as mentioned above. Undiagnosed or unsuspected overdistention of the bladder will introduce a temporary detrusor paralysis and is, therefore, to be avoided at all costs. It can develop insidiously in the patient who has been oversedated and overhydrated and has failed to perceive or respond to bladder fullness. Once pathologic overdistention has developed, the treatment is primarily expectant, awaiting the return of bladder tone 1 or 2 days after continuous decompression by indwelling catheter and prevention of additional or future episodes of overdistention.

*Neurological Abnormality.* Another etiologic circumstance may be that of primary neurologic defect. Neuropathy giving rise to chronic bladder hypotonia may be associated with diabetes, central nervous system lues, or multiple sclerosis. Sometimes this correlation can be suspected from the patient's medical history. Neuropathy coincident with herniated intervertebral disc may be evident; there is coincident constipation and usually a history of sudden onset. Low discs that involve the cauda equina but are too far caudal to be evident on myelography may be present. Skillful neurologic evaluation is required for appropriate diagnosis. Hypotonia can often be suspected preoperatively, and subtle detrusor stimulation by postoperative bethanechol (Urecholine) may be advisable. Dosages may start as low as 10 mg three times a day but rapidly increase to the point of clinical effectiveness, sometimes to as much as 50 to 75 mg three times daily.

*Drug-induced Detrusor Hypotonia.* Last, one must consider drug-induced hypotonia, as coincident and often long-term consumption of the common tranquilizing agents may be associated with unexpected and sometimes chronic detrusor hypotonia. This effect should be suspected among patients accustomed to daily doses of diazepam (Valium), chlordiazepoxide hydrochloride (Librium), thioridazine hydrochloride (Mellaril), chlorpromazine (Thorazine), prochlorperazine (Compazine), and meprobamate (Miltown). In many instances, these drugs may have been supplied by other physicians, and the patient may have become so accustomed to taking them that she has forgotten to include her consumption of them in her medical history. Discontinuation of the drug, when it is a factor producing detrusor hypotonia, may result in a rather prompt reappearance of normal bladder tone.

### Treatment

Generally speaking, the most comfortable and successful treatments at present are those outlined above. Detrusor hyperactivity induced by deliberate production of a chemical cystitis such as the instillation of intravesical Mercurochrome or ether is neither popular nor recommended, as the results are not only unpredictable, but the method may unexpectedly give rise to a long-standing, chronic cystitis, sometimes of massive degree. Some postoperative patients will find they can at first void more comfortably from a semistanding position, probably one that reduces levator spasm, and others may find comfort from aiding voiding once it has begun by manual suprapubic compression over the bladder, more effective when the patient is leaning somewhat forward during the voiding process.

Patients recovering from suprapubic sling procedures who have been accustomed to emptying their bladders by tightening the rectus muscles to increase intra-abdominal pressure must be instructed not to do so in the future, as voluntary rectus muscle contraction may tighten the sling sufficiently to occlude the urethra.

Any significant urethral stricture obstructing normal flow can be relieved by gentle urethral dilation.

### Protocol for Removal of the Catheter

Special attention is needed concerning removal of the catheter in someone recovering from reparative surgery.

Make sure the patient's bowel function has been established by the third postoperative day. This is aided by having placed the patient on a house diet the first or second postoperative day, and at the same time starting the administration of stool softeners with a gentle laxative (Pericolace). If no movement has occurred by the evening of the third postoperative day, milk of magnesia 30 ml and 4 ml of cascara are given and, if ineffective, an irritant suppository such as bisacodyl (Dulcolax) or a saline enema ordered. If this has not brought about a bowel movement, the patient should be given a gentle rectal examination to rule out a fecal impaction. If one is found, it is gently broken up digitally, and an oil retention enema followed by a saline enema are given.

A useful protocol concerning patient management after removal of a transurethral catheter is as follows: Between 7:00 and 8:00 am a urine culture is obtained, and the patient is started on an antibacterial such as nitrofurantoin (50 mg of Macrodantin three times daily), methenamine (23) (1 gm three times daily), or trimethoprim sulfa. An alpha-adrenergic blocker (such as 10 mg of phenoxybenzamine) is given by mouth.

After removal of a transurethral Foley catheter, the nursing staff should be instructed to catheterize as necessary if the patient is unable to void. An alternate is to catheterize two or three times daily immediately after voiding until a postvoiding residual of no more than 100 ml have been recorded on two consecutive occasions. The amount that the patient voids is usually of prognostic significance, even when the initial urinary residual volume may have been undesirably high. It is of greater significance and much more encouraging if a patient is voiding 100 to 200 ml with a residual of 200 to 250 ml than if the patient is voiding only 10 to 20 ml at a time with a residual volume of 200 to 250 ml. In the first situation, one would expect the amount voided to increase in relative amounts as the quantity of residual urine decreases.

The attitude of the nursing staff is of utmost importance in the management of patients unable to void after surgery. Knowledgeable and friendly confidence, smiles, and infinite gentleness in catheterizing these individuals, already apprehensive with understandably tender tissues, is most likely when personnel are experienced in postoperative urinary tract care.

If, after removal of the catheter, the patient is still unable to void in adequate amounts, she may be taught the technique of self-catheterization using the soft plastic Mentor female catheter, or she may be discharged with a Foley catheter in place and clamped. The clamp is to be opened and the bladder drained periodically as necessary. It should be explained that the temporary inability to void is by no means rare or unusual and will probably not lengthen or change her convalescence one bit. A handout sheet is provided for the patient to refer to jconcerning the care of the catheter, and it is often quite helpful. One we have found useful is reproduced herewith:

### Care of the Catheter

The bladder must be given time to rest and heal, during which the swelling and irritation from surgery must be given time to subside. This involves a variable length of recovery time from person to person lasting anywhere from a few days to several weeks. The more extensive the need for repair, the greater the scope of the repair, and the longer the period of recovery of comfortable bladder function.

During this recovery period, a person's kidney system continues to work, of course, and it is necessary to drain the urine from the bladder until functional recovery of the bladder has been completed. This outlet is provided by an indwelling catheter inserted in the bladder as at the time of surgery.

When the catheter is inserted through the urethra, the usual external canal between vulva and bladder, the urethral catheter can be clamped, to stop its flow, until there is sufficient fluid in the bladder to produce urgency and the sense of wanting to void at which time the clamp can be removed and the bladder emptied, then the clamp reapplied. After about 2 weeks of bladder rest the catheter is removed by cutting it across with clean scissors sometime during the midmorning hours, and the patient is requested to call the office that weekday afternoon to inform us how the bladder is working. If adequate amounts of urine are being passed and at intervals greater than 2 hours between voidings, it is good evidence that comfortable bladder function has returned. There will often be a mild sense of burning or irritation during voiding until the swelling in the urethra from the catheter has subsided, usually within 1 or 2 days. Should urinary burning and frequency increase beyond this point, instead of getting progressively better, be sure to call the office.

## Suprapubic Catheter

We have used the suprapubic catheter in two particular instances: one, after repair of a fistula at the vesical neck as a means of keeping the catheter away from the site of the fistula repair or another, after the creation of a neovagina in a patient requiring the postoperative use of a vaginal obturator (Chapter 21). Should the surgeon be an advocate of suprapubic catheterization, a handout concerning care of the suprapubic catheter may be of advantage to the patient. This is as follows:

### Care of the Suprapubic Catheter

Under many circumstances, the doctor may wish to put the recently repaired tissues around the urethra, bladder, and vagina at complete rest while they recover from surgery, and a catheter will be placed into the bladder through a tiny incision in the skin of the lower abdomen. This is a temporary way of diverting the urine until the patient's own bladder system is able to function again and does save a patient the nuisance, discomfort, and irritation from repeated catheterization during the healing process.

By the time preliminary healing is underway, usually after the fourth postoperative day, this catheter may be fitted with a screw type clamp that, when tightened, will stop the flow of urine through the catheter and permit the bladder to fill. When the patient feels bladder fullness and the desire to void, she is encouraged to do so, and following voiding, or if unable to pass water through the urethra at that time, the screw clamp is opened and the bladder drained through the suprapubic catheter. This procedure is continued on a regular basis as long as necessary until most of the urine is being passed naturally through the urethra, and less than 2 ounces or two is drained from the suprapubic catheter after each voiding. For this reason, it is important to keep a running account of the amount of urine voided each time and the amount obtained from the catheter after each voiding.

When the amount left behind has remained less than 2 ounces in volume, the suprapubic catheter clamp should be left firmly applied for a full 1 or 2 days to see whether regular urinary voiding remains well established. If so, and at the end of 2 days, the catheter is removed by simply cutting across its midpoint. The opening left by the catheter will usually close within a day or 2, but a small amount of urine will often drip at first from this opening, requiring a small dressing until the opening has closed.

A word of caution regarding estrogen supplementation in postmenopausal women: If a postmenopausal patient has not been taking estrogen preoperatively, its introduction during the immediate postoperative phase may be associated with some hyperemia and edema of the vesical neck. This swelling may produce some degree of temporary partial obstruction of the urethra.

There must be additional factors present that we cannot yet predictably or accurately underestand or measure that influence the process of voiding. Not the least of these is the degree of strong motivation on the part of the patient. There are some whose confidence in their own bladders is sufficient to overcome almost any disturbance of reflex activity, and such people are a joy to behold as their resumption of normal physiology occurs unexpectedly. But for those who are experiencing difficulty, there is no substitute for calm, optimistic, and peaceful understanding on the part of the patient's attendants through that brief time that, for the patient, may become a temporarily disquieting and disabling crisis.

## References

1. Alexander JW, Fischer JE, Boyajian M, et al: The influence of hair removal methods on wound infections. *Arch Surg* 118: 347–352, 1983.
2. Burke JF. Use of preventive antibiotics in clinical surgery. *Am Surg* 39:6–11, 1973.
3. Galask RP, Larsen B, Ohm MJ: Vaginal flora and its role in disease entities. *Clin Obstet Gynecol* 19:61–81, 1976.
4. Clarke-Pearson DL, LeLong ER, Synan IS, et al: Complications of low-dose heparin prophylaxis in gynecologic oncology surgery. *Obstet Gynecol* 64:689–694, 1984.
5. Hamod KA, Spence MR, Rosenshein NB, et al: Single-dose and multidose prophylaxis in vaginal hysterectomy. *Am J Obstet Gynecol* 136:976–979, 1980.
6. Harwood A: The hot-cold theory of disease. *JAMA* 216:1153–1158, 1971.
7. Hemsell DL, Cunningham FG, Kappus S, et al: Cefoxitin for prophylaxis in premenopausal women undergoing vaginal hysterectomy. *Obstet Gynecol* 56:629–634, 1980.
8. Hunt TK, Ehrlich HP, Garcia JA, et al: Effect of vitamin A on reversing the inhibitory effect of cortisone on healing of open wounds in animals and man. *Ann Surg* 170: 633–640, 1969.
9. Jackson P, Ridley WJ: Simplified antibiotic prophylaxis for vaginal hysterectomy. *Aust NZ J Obstet Gynaecol* 19:225–227, 1979.
10. Jeffcoate, TNA: *Principles of Gynecology.* New York, Appleton-Century-Crofts, 1967.
11. Lapides J: Neurogenic bladder: Principles of treatment. *Urol Clin North Am* 1:81–97, 1974.
12. Ledger WL, Gee C, Lewis WF: Guidelines for antibiotic prophylaxis in gynecology. *Am J Obstet Gynecol* 121:1038–1045, 1975.
13. Leventhal A, Pfau A: Pharmacologic management of postoperative overdistention of the bladder. *Surg Gynecol Obstet* 146: 347–348, 1978.
14. Mickal A, Curole D, Lewis C: Cefoxitin sodium: Double-blind vaginal hysterectomy prophylaxis in premenopausal patients. *Obstet Gynecol* 56:222–225, 1980.
15. Nichols DH: Getting the postoperative patient to void. *Contemp Obstet Gynecol* 12:41–45, 1978.
16. von Peham H, Amreich J: *Operative Gynecology.* Philadelphia, JB Lippincott, 1934.
17. Polivy J: Psychological reactions to hysterectomy: A critical review. *Am J Obstet Gynecol* 118:417–426, 1974.
18. Polk BF, Shapiro M, Goldstein P, et al: Randomised clinical trial of perioperative cefazolin in preventing infection after hysterectomy. *Lancet* 1:437–440, 1980.
19. Sawyers JL: Questions and answers. *JAMA 253:705, 1985.*
20. Spruill FG, Minette LJ, Sturner WQ: Two surgical deaths in association with cephalothin. *JAMA* 229:440–441, 1974.
21. Stanton SL: *Female Urinary Incontinence.* London, Lloyd-Luke (Medical Books), 1977.
22. Turner GM, Cole SE, Brooks JH: The efficacy of graduated compression stockings in the prevention of deep vein thrombosis after major gynecological surgery. *Br Obstet Gynecol* 91:588–591, 1984.
23. Tyreman NO, Anderson PO, Kroon L, et al: Urinary tract infection after vaginal surgery. Effect of prophylactic treatment with methenamine hippurate. *Acta Obstet Gynecol Scand* 65:731–733, 1986.
24. Whelton A, Blanco LJ, Carter GG, et al: Therapeutic implications of doxycycline and cephalothin concentrations in the female genital tract. *Obstet Gynecol* 55: 28-32, 1980.

# CHAPTER 7

# Vaginal Surgery for the Older Woman

The increase in the number of older women coming to the gynecologist may be due partly to the larger numbers of older women in the community. It may also be due to the individual woman's expectation of a longer life and her unwillingness to accept discomfort or disability if she believes it can be relieved.

Biologic age is of greater importance than chronologic age (12). There is no unequivocal association between age, per se, and surgical risk (1, 12, 20) and no significant increase in postoperative complication rate because of age alone (16). Surgery should not be denied the elderly on the basis of age alone (8).

The surgeon being consulted by an elderly patient concerning possible reconstructive pelvic surgery must always bear in mind the goals of reconstructive surgery: (a) relieve the symptoms, (b) restore the anatomy to normal, (c) restore the function to normal. Each goal must be studied objectively in relation to the surgical benefits that will aid in restoring or enhancing the quality of life of the older woman.

"The safest operative procedures are considered those that are elective, away from the diaphragm, not involving suppurative disease, allowing early mobilization, and minimal postoperative sedation and analgesia" (9). To the patient's advantage, this spectrum of reduced risk clearly embraces the discipline of vaginal reconstructive surgery designed to improve the quality of a patient's life with the characteristics of the older woman that merit special attention when gynecologic surgery is being contemplated.

By common usage, the individual becomes an "older woman" after her 65th birthday. In 1954 Studdiford and Douglas (22) reported that during the years 1941-1953, 139 women 65 years of age or older had major gynecologic surgery in Bellevue Hospital. That number represented only 3.1% of the 4450 women operated on the gynecologic service during that period. In 1975, McKeithen (15) stated that 33.4% of the women admitted to the Bayfront Medical Center (St. Petersburg, FL) in 1973 had been 65 years old or older.

Elective gynecologic surgery is being done increasingly often on women over 65, over 70, and often for women over 80, but this does not indicate that such surgery on older women involves less risk in 1980 than was recognized in 1950. Anesthesia now involves techniques that reduce the risks of postoperative pulmonary and circulatory complications.

## PREOPERATIVE EVALUATION

It is the surgeon's obligation to have made a careful and thorough preoperative appraisal of the older woman's mental and emotional, as well as her physical and functional, status. It is important to learn whether she wants to recover quickly and be able to engage in increased activity. A desire to recover is probably as important as the older woman's blood count and nutritional status. Certainly neither should be ignored when major surgery is being considered. The gynecologist should have the following considerations in mind during a preoperative assessment of the older woman's readiness for surgery:

Many older women do not take in enough fluid to maintain adequate stores of body water. If dehydration is increased during surgery and during the first few postoperative days, the thermal buffer effect of body water will not be adequate to help keep the body temperature within a nearly normal range. An appreciable degree of dehydration will also result in a higher tissue concentration of whatever drug dosage has been calculated on the expectation of a body weight.

There are increasing numbers of the aging population in the United States who are relatively affluent. These individuals want and are expecting to continue living active lives that are a source of satisfaction to themselves, their families, and their friends.

McKeithen in Florida and Eton (8) in England, have emphasized the importance of recognizing the attitudes and expectations of the more well-to-do older women. Both have stated that good results can be expected when elective gynecologic surgery is done on older women living in comfortable circumstances who are well informed and who expect, as a result of the surgery, to live in better health for a longer time. When a woman's living conditions have been depressing, however, and there are no reasons to expect improvement in her activities and home life, she is not likely to feel much better or to enjoy a better life after "successful" repair of the procidentia she believed had for years been the cause of discomfort and fatigue.

Obviously the gynecologist should not assume that the patient's state of mind, her outlook, and her expectations are determined solely by economic factors. The affluent can also be depressed. Agitation can be as depressing as anxiety. The elderly matron exasperated by the behavior of a child or distraught by the misfortunes of her children may be on tranquilizers or other drugs. There is, therefore, no substitute for a carefully taken history, which must include knowledge of drugs taken in the past as well as recently. The patient may need to be impressed with the importance to her of revealing all such relevant information.

One must not, however, merely conclude that the prognosis for a good result will be dependent upon the patient's state of mind. The rapidity with which she regains strength and resumes activities will also be dependent upon her general health. The all-important parameters to be considered in a preoperative assessment of the older woman's readiness for surgery include her state of nutrition and the possibly related degree of anemia. It is equally important to look for evidence of chronic infection, particularly in the respiratory or urinary tract.

Among women in the United States, personal dietary habits are largely responsible for nutritional deficiencies. The older woman who lives alone is particularly likely to have been on an inadequate diet. Economic status does not assure the individual of an adequate intake of essential foods. Depression often serves to aggravate chronic fatigue, which makes the preparation of meals "not worth the effort." Either alcohol or smoking a cigarette or both are too often substituted for a meal. Too often there has been a conviction that to stay thin is healthy. The result is likely to be a nutritional state that does not respond to the tissue-building needs on which the rate of recovery after surgery will depend. Not infrequently, elective surgery might better be postponed until a period of "building up" demonstrates that the patient appreciates her dietary needs and is likely to continue a more adequate diet, at least during several months of convalescence.

No responsibility of the gynecologic surgeon is greater than that involved in the obligation to weigh the risks of somewhat elective vaginal surgery for an older woman against a realistic appraisal of what the patient has to gain, even if the result of a repair is altogether satisfactory.

The questions that should be considered by both the patient and her gynecologist can for the most part be answered if they are both willing to face up to the probabilities. However, not all individuals can be expected to approach such questions in an objective manner. One woman will want to know all her doctor can tell her about the risks of surgery and the complications that may develop as well as what she can expect in the way of discomforts and disabilities after the operation. Another will prefer that the doctor only tell her that he recommends an operation; she would rather not know the details or hear about the possible complications. The current medicolegal climate does obligate the surgeon to explain to the patient more about the operative procedure and the probabilities of how she will be afterward than some patients want to hear. The informed consent process will assure that patients will at least know what to expect.

The individual woman who is in generally good health at age 65 is likely to live longer than the age of average life expectancy, which in the early 1980's approximates 77 years of age for women in the United States. Kent (11) has called attention to the significant difference of two "ages." The term familiar to most Americans is "life expectancy," which we know as the average age attained by a man or woman born in the United States during this century. Kent has emphasized, however, the importance of also being familiar with and giving consideration to the current figure for the "maximum life span." The latter we should recognize as the age at which the aging process currently can be expected to terminate the lives of humans who have reached "old age."

The current figures for life expectancy have increased from 30 years in the era of the Roman empire to 50 years in the 1900's and, in the United States, to 77 years in the 1970's. We are aware also that the elimination of large numbers of infant and childhood deaths (which had largely accounted for the earlier figures for average life expectancy) has in fact largely accounted for what we have erroneously regarded as a progressive lengthening of human life. Few of us have recognized what Cutler (3–5) has emphasized: that the maximum human life-span has remained practically unchanged during the past 100,000 years. Cutler's studies indicate that the life expectancy of an adult in good health at age 65 is little if any higher than it was in 1900.

The gynecologist should be mindful of Cutler's concepts and the data that suggest that a woman 75 years of age who is in good health in the United States can be expected to live at least another 25 years. Actually Cutler has stated that the maximum life span of the individual "over 65 and in good health" should approximate 100 years.

We should consider that the woman 75 years old and in good health is not likely to be disabled soon or to die within a short time simply because she is approaching the current age of life expectancy. If chronic disease does not contraindicate gynecologic surgery, the capable gynecologic surgeon should expect to rid a 75-year-old woman of her prolapse and in good conscience assure her of a postoperative return to comfort, unrestricted activities, and probably years of continuing good health.

Although such optimism is justified under the favorable circumstances increasing numbers of older women now enjoy, the gynecologic surgeon must remember that the risks of elective surgery are appreciable and ever present. The competent and conscientious gynecologist will not be satisfied to play the percentages and assure the older woman with whom he is considering an elective gynecologic repair that she will get along fine and realize an excellent result. Not until the older woman's attitude, habits, and health have been carefully appraised can her family doctor or her gynecologist appreciate how well or how poorly she will bear the brunt of major surgery.

In most instances a close friend or favorite relative will accompany the older woman when she is considering surgery. It is highly desirable that the gynecologist make certain that a responsible member of the family as well as the patient understand what is proposed, what the risks are, what convalescence will involve, and what results can be expected. The most desirable relative or close friend to whom such information can be given is someone who will be in a position to be of help to the patient during her recovery after leaving the hospital. Should the patient indicate that she does not want the doctor to discuss her condition or the contemplated operation with anyone, the gynecologist must exercise great care and tact in discussion of the patient's expressed preference. Unless there is reason to believe the patient will be quite able to arrange for all of the care she may need, the doctor should be unwilling to accept the dual responsibility of doing the surgery and making certain of the adequacy of the patient's care after she leaves the hospital. For a number of reasons, the doctor should want to make certain that someone of the patient's choice is fully informed of the indications for surgery and the possible problems during the patient's convalescence.

Any iron deficiency anemia may best be treated by infusions of packed red cells. It is not only important to recognize anemia preoperatively, it is equally important to determine its significance, for transfusions alone will, of course, provide only temporary improvement.

Chronic infection is most likely to be identified preoperatively in the vaginal flora or in the urinary or respiratory tract. Significant vaginal infection is likely to be recognized clinically when there are grossly ulcerated areas of prolapsing vaginal membrane, particularly when atrophic or senile vaginitis has preceded secondary infection or when a patient's diabetes has been poorly controlled.

When major vaginal surgery is being considered for a woman over 65, prophylactic preoperative estrogen may be advisable several weeks before surgery, especially when a clinically evident secondarily infected vaginitis is present. Eton (8) has advised discontinuing preoperative estrogen "a week or two before surgery to allow dissipation of any effects on blood coagulation." Continuing estrogen until the day of surgery also seems to appreciably increase the vascularity within perivaginal connective tissues. There is, of course, no objection to resuming estrogen postoperatively as soon as ambulation, pelvic mobility, and leg exercises can be advised.

The older woman may not have engaged for years in physical exercise or exertion to a degree that causes deep inspiration and accelerated respiration. Her lungs may not have been fully expanded for so long that her respiratory capacity may be reduced by passive congestion and edema. If she has a chronic cough, she may have made a habit of quiet respiration or she may have developed a significant degree of bronchiectasis and be harboring a chronic bronchitis. Her pulmonary function should, therefore, be evaluated by an internist who may institute a course of appropriate antibiotics combined with a bronchial dilator, postural drainage, and incentive spirometry therapy before clearing her for general anesthesia and a period of postoperative inactivity.

If the contemplated surgery is to be an extensive vaginal repair and the patient has a chronic cough, it is particularly desirable to schedule the surgery at a time of the year when respiratory infections are at a minimum and to plan a postoperative regimen designed to maintain adequate respiratory excursion while minimizing the likelihood of coughing.

Mayer (14) has emphasized the frequency of chronic urinary tract infection among women over 65 years of age. Considering the probability of repeated catheterization or an indwelling catheter after extensive vaginal surgery, the urinary tract must be considered a potential source of postoperative morbidity and a prolonged convalescence. A history of recurring urinary tract infections suggests the possibility of upper urinary tract involvement, in which case diagnostic studies, including intravenous pyelography, urinalysis, and cultures, may indicate adequate antibiotic therapy preceding any elective surgery. A lower urinary tract infection in an ambulatory patient can usually be effectively treated without cultures, but an upper tract infection or a postoperative urinary tract infection should be managed on the basis of cultures and sensitization determinations. Whenever treatment is indicated, it should be specific, adequate, and, if necessary, repeated rather than prolonged.

The decrease in glomerular filtration rate is the most important renal change associated with advanced aging, which is of special importance in calculating the reduced dosages of medication excreted primarily in the urine (10, 19). Interference with tubular resorption diminishes the ability of the kidneys to concentrate urine. These factors combined with decreased renal blood flow inhibit prompt restoration of fluid and electrolyte balance.

Most preoperative study and testing can be performed on an ambulatory basis before admission. When the patient and all of the data have been studied, a risk:benefit ratio is developed and a decision made to offer surgical treatment when the likely benefit of surgery clearly exceeds the risk (19). The length of postoperative stay is not prolonged over that of the younger patient when preparations have been made for convalescence at home.

Comprehensive preoperative medical assessment is required, to include drug and nutritional history. Laboratory evaluation should include a hemogram, urinalysis, blood chemistry, chest X-ray, and electrocardiogram. Pulmonary function assessment is advisable when obstructive disease is suspected, and creatinine and creatinine clearance are good measures of degree of suspected impairment of renal function (21). Hypertension (160/95 or greater) is frequent among the elderly (10). Because drug elimination may be slower in the elderly, the surgeon should order with caution low doses of drugs postoperatively and limit carefully the number that are used, to minimize adverse drug reactions.

## SPECIAL FEATURES OF POSTOPERATIVE CARE

It appears that length of postoperative hospitalization is not prolonged for the elderly (6, 15, 17). Surgical morbidity and mortality apparently are not related to the length of an operation (13), provided competence in anesthesiology is exercised, but the duration of spinal anesthesia suggests it is most effective when the planned surgery is of 2 hours duration or less. Epidural anesthesia is a suitable alternate when an operation of longer duration is planned or cardiovascular instability is likely. Competent general anesthesia is also a legitimate choice for the elderly, as it provides excellent control of patient oxygenation, and preoperative evaluation and discussion between patient and anesthesiologist is of inestimable value.

Pulmonary wedge pressure appears to be a more dependable means of interpreting blood pressure changes than is central venous pressure monitoring during surgery of the patient at risk. Higher pulmonary capillary wedge pressure may be necessary in the elderly to maintain preload and cardiac output (19).

Both anesthesiologist and surgeon must be mindful that tachycardia and tachypnea are often unreliable as signs of hypoxia in the elderly, and the patient must be assured of adequate operative and postoperative supplemental oxygen therapy when indicated and as measured by any significant change in arterial blood gases and adequate circulatory hemoglobin.

It is advisable preoperatively to apply elastic stockings onto both legs from the ankle to the upper thigh to avoid a rapid postoperative pooling of blood in the lower extremities. If the legs are not so wrapped, the rapid return of blood to the lower extremities will be likely to lower the blood pressure alarmingly a short time after the legs are lowered.

Postoperative care of the elderly patient should emphasize pulmonary recovery including deep breathing, incentive spirometry, and early ambulation. Lack of the pain of an abdominal incision promotes effective patient cooperation, but she must be reminded to participate.

Fluid intake and urinary output must be carefully measured and balanced. Oral fluids up to 2 liters per day provide some latitude in quantity. Because the sense of thirst is blunted with aging, there must be continuous surveillance as to the quantity consumed.

Postoperatively the older patient may require up to 5 days to recover full mental function after anesthesia (2). A subtle change in mental status may be the first sign of hypoxemia, acidosis, myocardial infarction, acute infection, or impending septic shock (10, 18). Careful personal observation of the patient's breath and breathing will alert the disciplined and astute observer and help to clarify the patient's status. Pain is less a symptom of acute illness than in the younger patient, so careful observation of progressive recovery is made through daily and unhurried rounds.

## SUMMARY

It is not enough for the gynecologic surgeon to have mastered the techniques of vaginal repair. Before the older woman can be assured of a good result if one operates, the gynecologist must have made certain of the patient's readiness for surgery. Measures must have been undertaken to correct any factor likely to delay either her recovery from the operation or her resumption of desired activities. Successful gynecologic surgery for older women will depend as much upon the adequacy of the preoperative appraisal and preparation of the patient as on the technical skill and clinical judgments of the gynecologist.

### References

1. Blake R, Lynn J: Emergency abdominal surgery in the aged. *Br J Surg* 63:956–960, 1976.
2. Blundell E: A psychological study of the effects of surgery on 86 elderly patients. *Br Soc Clin Psychol* 6:297, 1967.
3. Cutler RG: Evolution of human longevity and the genetic complexity governing aging rate. *Proc Natl Acad Sci USA* 72:4664–4668, 1975.
4. Cutler RG: Nature of aging and life maintenance processes. *Interdisciplin Top Gerontol* 9:83–133, 1976.
5. Cutler RG: Evolution of longevity in primates. *J Hum Evolution* 5:169–202, 1976.
6. Ellenbogen A, Agranat A, Grunstein S: The role of vaginal hysterectomy in the aged woman. *J Am Geriatr Soc* 29:426–428, 1981.
7. Eton B: Gynecologic surgery in elderly women. *Geriatrics* 28:119–123, 1973.
8. Glenn F: Pre- and postoperative management of elderly surgical patients. *J Am Geriatr Soc* 21:385–393, 1973.
9. Hooyman N, Cohen HJ: Problems associated with aging. *Clin Obstet Gynec* 29:353–373, 1976.
10. Johnson JC: Surgery in the elderly. In Goldman DR, Brown FH, Levy WK, Slap GB, Sussman EJ (eds): *Medical Care of the Surgical Patient.* Philadelphia, JB Lippincott, pp 578–590, 1982.
11. Kent S: The evolution of longevity. *Geriatrics* 35(1):98–104, 1980.
12. Lewin I, Lerner A, Green S, et al: Physical class and psysiologic status in the prediction of operative mortality. *Ann Surg* 174:217, 1971.
13. Marshall WH, Fahey PJ: Operative complications and mortality in patients over 80 years of age. *Arch Surg* 88:896–904, 1964.
14. Mayer TR: UTI in the elderly: how to select treatment. *Geriatr Med* 35(3):67–77, 1980.

15. McKeithen WS Jr: Major gynecologic surgery in the elderly female, 65 years and older. *Am J Obstet Gynecol* 123:59–65, 1975.

16. Panayiotis G, Ellenbogen A, Grunstein S: Major gynecologic surgical procedures in the aged. *J Am Geriatr Soc* 26:459–462, 1978.

17. Pierson RL, Figge PK, Buchsbaum HJ: Surgery for gynecologic malignancy in the aged. *Obstet Gynecol* 46:523–527, 1975.

18. Polacek DJ: Monitoring high-risk and critically ill Patients. In Buchsbaum JH, Walton LA (eds): *Strategies in Gynecologic Surgery.* New York, Springer-Verlag, p 127, 1986.

19. Polacek DJ, Buchsbaum HJ: Surgery in the aged. In Buchsbaum HJ, Walton LA (eds): *Strategies in Gynecologic Surgery.* New York, Springer-Verlag, pp 181–194, 1986.

20. Robbins RE, Budden MK: Major abdominal surgery in patients over 70 years of age: results during 1962 to 1966 compared with those during 1950 to 1959. *Can J Surg* 15:73–78, 1972.

21. Rowe JW, Andres R, Tobin JD, et al: The effect of age on creatinine clearance in men: a cross-sectional and longitudinal study. *J Gerontol* 31:155–163, 1976.

22. Studdiford WE Jr, Douglas GW: Major gynecological surgery in the aged patient. *Am J Obstet Gynecol* 68:456–465, 1954.

# CHAPTER 8

# Instruments and Sutures

Effective and successful surgery is more dependent upon the surgeon's judgment and technical competence than upon the design or the quality of the instruments used. No set of instruments will consistently be associated with a satisfactory surgical result without the skills of the surgeon. The carpenter is more important than his or her tools, but fine tools may help the good carpenter to make one's good work even better. There are significant choices available in the surgeon's armamentarium, and the right choices will enable the operator to accomplish with greater ease and efficiency the best of which he or she is capable.

Quality standard instruments available for vaginal surgery in standard operating room set-ups might well include sharpened curved Mayo scissors, narrow Deaver retractors, curved and straight Kocher's forceps, Allis clamps, Rochester or curved Kelly hemostats, Crile hemostats, Lahey thyroid or Gordon uterine vulsella, and double-toothed Jacobs-type tenacula. For vaginal hysterectomy, the set-up should include several Heaney-type hysterectomy forceps as well as the Heaney-type needle holder.

The operating room should be of an adequate and comfortable size, in a quiet location, with elbow room and moving space around the table for the surgeon and assistants, the anesthesiologist and his or her equipment, and the nursing staff and instrument tables (Fig. 8.1). Continuous suction equipment is desirable, including one weighted speculum equipped with a suction tip. A separate suction with a hand-held tube should be provided. The trap for each suction device provides a quick and accurate estimate of surgical blood loss.

Adequate modern anesthesia equipment provides for continuous monitoring of the patient's pulmonary and cardiac status. Adequate amounts of appropriate suture material and sterile supplies, including any packing that might be called for, should be at hand, where they can be provided on short notice without the necessity of sending out a hurried call for additional supplies. Efficiency in surgery is developed not through rushing, but in the effective use of each minute of operative time and avoidance of waiting for special instruments or sutures that are needed but were not requested ahead of time. Blood loss during surgery is the product of ml per minute X the number of minutes. Fearing AIDS and hepatitis, most patients are frightened by blood transfusion. When operative blood loss is minimized, so is the need for transfusion.

## SUTURE MATERIAL

Basic requirements concerning the suture materials to be used in the closing of surgical wounds are indicated in the following quotation (1):

"The purpose of a surgical suture is to maintain approximation of tissues until the healing process has progressed to the point where artificial support is no longer

**Figure 8.1.** The arrangement of personnel within the operating room is depicted. The surgeon is in the central position at the foot of the operating table with the second assistant to the right and the first assistant to the left. There is a spotlight over a right-handed surgeon's shoulder illuminating the perineum, and the instrument table is to his back and somewhat to the right. The instrument nurse is behind the instrument table, facing the back of the surgeon. This enables her to share in a full view of the operative field and to follow visually the progress of the surgical procedure. The positions of the spotlight, the nurse, and the instrument table are reversed if the surgeon is left-handed.

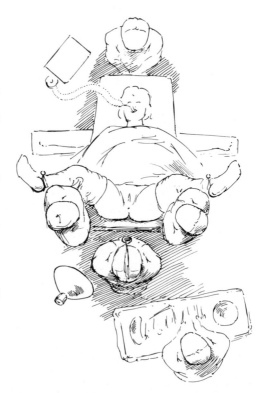

necessary for the wound to resist normal stresses. Beyond this point, the sutures serve no useful purpose, and may, in fact, be the source of irritation or serve as a nidus for persistent infection. Thus, the ideal suture should persist and maintain tensile strength until the tissue has healed sufficiently, and then disappear.''

## RELATIONSHIP OF SUTURES TO WOUND HEALING

The strength of a closed surgical wound is the sum of the scar plus the suture material. Immediately after the wound has been closed and for the next 3 or 4 days the suture material provides all the strength of the wound. This strength has been estimated at about 40% of the original strength of the tissues before surgery. As healing develops and scar tissue is formed, the strength increases. In the absence of infection, it has been estimated that the wound is about one-third healed on the sixth postoperative day and two-thirds by the tenth. The remaining one-third may require several months. Variances from these generalizations may be caused by many factors, including the tension applied to the margins of the wound, the biochemistry and physical condition of the particular patient and of the suture material, and the presence of infection. The suture material has become superfluous once wound healing has finished and a strong scar is produced. In the presence of infection, sutures may be absorbed with unusual speed and fail to supply adequate support during the initial and critical healing. When nonabsorbable suture has been used in the presence of infection, a sinus may form postoperatively. The suture behaves as an infected foreign body. The sinus will close only after the sutures or foreign body is extruded or surgically removed.

Tissue reaction to suture material does not determine wound strength, although it is proportional to the bulk of the suture material present in the wound. Knot pull strength (Fig. 8.2) is important. Time should not be taken in

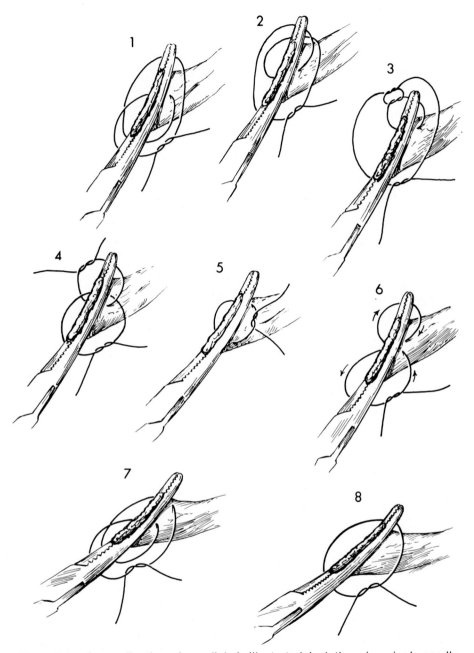

**Figure 8.8.**  Suture ligation of a pedicle is illustrated. In *1*, there is a single needle penetration of the pedicle, but the base is doubly ligated. In *2*, the toe is doubly ligated. After a small loop over the toe of the hemostat has been tied, a second loop goes around the entire pedicle, as shown in *3*. Interlocking loops in *4* provide security but require a double penetration of the pedicle by the needle. The double penetration in *5* leaves a small portion unligated. *6* provides security, but also requires a double penetration. *7* fixes the suture at two points. *8* is a single free tie, which is most likely to slip under certain circumstances. *2* is recommended for the infundibulopelvic ligament, reinforced by a free tie. *7* represents the Heaney stitch, especially useful for the cardinal or uterosacral ligament. It is unlikely to slip, but does require a double penetration of the pedicle. (Reproduced with permission of the American College of Surgeons from Nichols DH: A technique for vaginal oophorectomy. *Surg Gynecol Obstet* 147:765, 1978.)

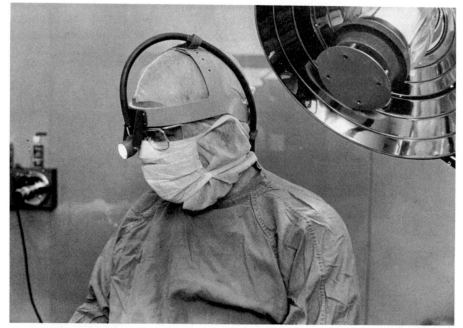

**Figure 8.9.** The fiberoptic headlight is shown, which will provide literally shadow-free bright illumination to the depths of a body cavity, even in a horizontal plane.

line drawn between the two stirrups will intersect each acetabulum or hip socket. The operating table should also be equipped to assure rapid adjustment into varying degrees of Trendelenburg and reverse Trendelenburg positions, as individual and, occasionally, emergency circumstances may require. The table height should be sufficiently adjustable to permit the operator either to stand during the operative procedure or to be seated should that be his or her preference.

A lithotomy sheet should have ample casings for the feet, so that it can be placed in position readily even though the patient's legs are placed somewhat vertically in the extended leg holders or stirrups.

Elastic stockings for the patient are advisable and they should be in place before the start of the anesthesia. Whether their use will result in a significant reduction in postoperative pulmonary embolism may be debatable; but they do provide venous compression. When the patient's legs are taken out of the stirrups and are lowered into the horizontal recumbent position at the conclusion of the operative procedure, the resultant rapid pooling of blood into the large venous beds of the legs has been reduced. Lowering the legs without compression as they come down out of the stirrups may result in a precipitous and significant drop in blood pressure as a result of what, in effect, has been a sudden increase in the size of the venous pool into which a fixed volume of blood is circulating.

## SPECIAL INSTRUMENTS

Vaginal surgeons usually develop preferences for a few special instruments that are well designed for vaginal work. Although it is desirable that the surgeon have two assistants for vaginal operations, this is not always possible. When one must occasionally work with a single assistant, the large Rigby retractor (Fig. 8.10*h*) is of considerable help, freeing the assistant's hands for

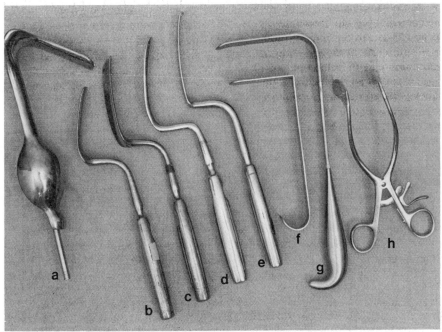

**Figure 8.10.** Various retractors are depicted. The Remine weighted suction speculum is shown in *a*. Some of the various shapes and sizes of the Briesky-Navratil vaginal retractors are shown in *b*, *c*, *d*, and *e*. The small Heaney retractor is shown at *f*, along with the long-handled Heaney retractor at *g*. A large-sized Rigby self-retaining retractor is shown in *h*.

knot cutting, sponging, and holding the movable retractors. A weighted speculum usually will be found quite helpful for the frequent situation in which virtually all of the surgical dissection must be accomplished within the vagina. A modification of the standard weighted speculum, which provides for built-in continuous suction (Fig. 8.10*a*), has been our preference for many years. The suction tubing may be built into the retractor blade, further increasing operative exposure (Fig. 8.11). Examination of the wall-mounted trap of the suction apparatus aids at a glance in keeping track of estimated blood loss during surgery.

The instruments attributed to N. Sproat Heaney were especially designed for use within the vagina. The Heaney needle holder is particularly valuable, as it provides for considerable range of the angles at which the needle can be grasped (Fig. 8.12*c*). This variability facilitates placement of curved needles and sutures at almost any conceivable angle with relative ease when placing sutures deep within the pelvis (Fig. 8.13). The Heaney hemostats have a desirable "pelvic curve," which assures placement and a grip on tissues that provides security with minimal risk of slippage. For use in the hysterectomy in which there might not be much prolapse at the start of the operation, the Heaney-Glenner hysterectomy forceps (Fig. 8.12*b*) are valuable. They have both an upward curve and a lateral curve adapted to both the right and left sides of the patient as is stamped on the forceps. The Heaney-Ballantine hysterectomy forceps (Fig. 8.12*a*) are useful, as are the Masterson forceps and the Maingot. The Merz hysterectomy forceps (Fig. 8.14) has the standard Heaney curve and utilizes the principle of the Glassman noncrushing jaws, invoking minimum trauma to the tissue to which it has been applied. It is useful for

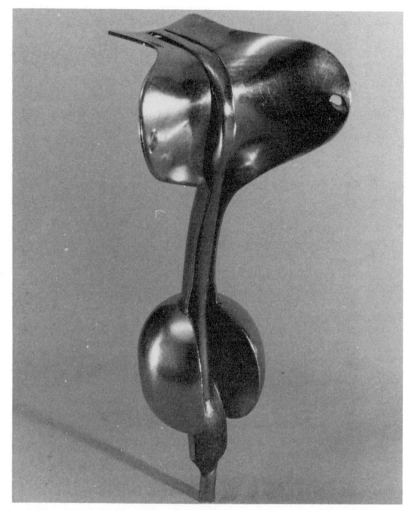

**Figure 8.11.** A weighted suction speculum for the posterior wall of the vagina is shown. The suction tubing has been buried in the posterior blade of the retractor, improving the exposure in the operative field. It is available from the custom order department of Codman-Shurtleff, New Bedford, MA, 02745.

clamping the mesovarian during oophorectomy because it neither slips nor tears tissue even when traction is necessary.

During performance of vaginectomy or the Schauta radical vaginal hysterectomy, the long mouse-toothed forceps of Krobach (Fig. 8.12*d*) provide an effective means of temporarily occluding the vagina. When the operator is familiar with their use, one or two of these can be of considerable help during a usual type of perineorrhaphy and posterior colporrhaphy.

Bonney forceps (Fig. 8.15*b*) are highly recommended, as they combine a rat tooth for holding the tissues, with occlusive serrated edges for grasping of the needle deeply placed in tissues. Long Singley forceps (Fig. 8.15*c*) are particularly desirable for handling peritoneum and intra-abdominal organs with minimal trauma. So-called Russian forceps (Fig. 8.15*a*) are comfortable to use on the vaginal surface of the bladder during anterior colporrhaphy, as they distribute the compression given the tissue within their grasp equally over a wide area.

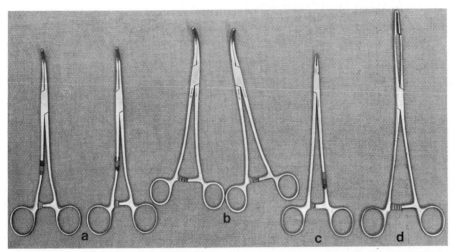

**Figure 8.12.**  Clamps and needle holders are shown. A pair of Heaney-Ballantine hysterectomy forceps, with right and left curve are shown in *b*. The Heaney needle holder is shown in *c*, and the Krobach mouse-toothed clamps is shown in *d*.

Heaney retractors (Fig. 8.10*f*) are easier to hold than the narrow Deaver. The short-handled Heaney retractor is lightweight, the handle is unobtrusive, and it can be very helpful during colporrhaphy. The long-handled Heaney retractor (Fig. 8.10*g*) is particularly helpful during vaginal hysterectomy as a means of holding the bladder safely out of the way after the anterior vesicouterine peritoneal fold has been identified and opened.

Breisky-Navratil retractors (Fig. 8.10*b*) come in an almost limitless assortment of sizes. They are widely used in vaginal surgery on the European continent, but are not very well known in America. An assortment in the varying widths and depths available will provide useful retraction in an infinite variety of clinical circumstances.

The handle of the retractor, being parallel to the blade, may be grasped easily and securely, much like a dagger. Thus, it can be held comfortably with less tendency toward slippage or wandering and without obstructing the surgical team's view of the operative field. Even greater exposure may be provided in

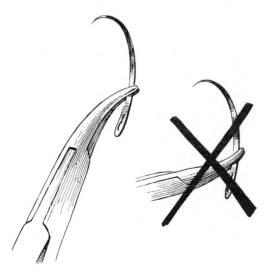

**Figure 8.13.**  The correct (*left*) and incorrect (*right*) ways to grasp the needle with a Heaney needle holder.

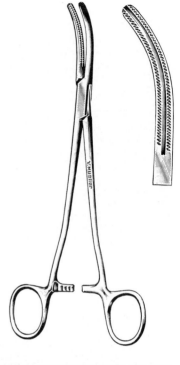

**Figure 8.14.** The Merz hysterectomy forceps is shown, and the Glassman type jaws and the Heaney curve are noted.

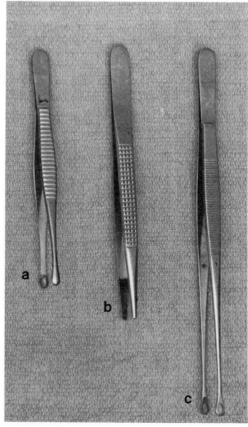

**Figure 8.15.** Tissue forceps are shown. The Russian forceps is shown in *a*, the Bonney is in *b*, and the Singley is in *c*.

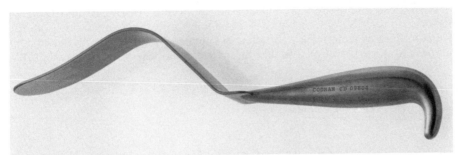

**Figure 8.16.** FLat blade vaginal retractor CD 1106 or 09804, available in various sizes from special order department, Codman-Shurtleff Inc, New Bedford, MA, 02745, or from Mr. William Merz, American V. Mueller, Chicago, IL, 60648.

the depths of the wound by the flat blade retractor (Fig. 8.16), which should be held as shown in Figure 8.17.

The 28-cm Deschamps ligature carrier for the right hand is particularly useful during a sacrospinous fixation procedure, but it is also useful during oophorectomy, because the blunt point tends to push adjacent blood vessels to one side, thus avoiding the lacerations that would be more likely to occur with a sharp-pointed needle. Some various modifications of the Deschamps carriers are shown in Chapter 16. A long hook to grasp the suture after it has penetrated the tissue is a desirable accessory.

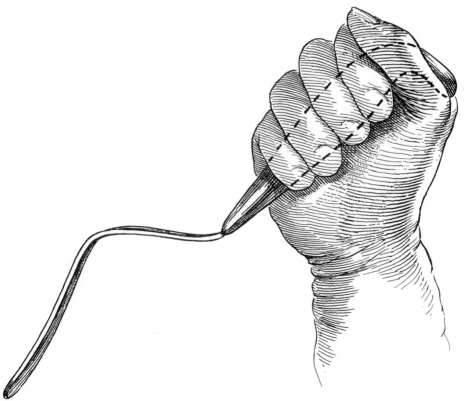

**Figure 8.17.** The preferred method of holding a flat-bladed retractor is shown, which keeps the assistant's hand out of the operator's field of view.

All of these instruments are available from various American and European makers and distributors, and may be obtained, for instance, on order from Mr. William Merz of American V. Mueller of Chicago, Illinois, or from the custom instrument department of Codman-Shurtleff in New Bedford, Massachusetts.

## Reference

1. Hermann JB: Changes in tensile strength and knot security of surgical sutures in vivo. *Arch Surg* 106:707–710, 1973.

# CHAPTER 9

# Minor and Ambulatory Surgery

Some minor gynecologic surgery is regularly performed in an office setting, whereas that requiring more surgical dissection may be performed in an operating room of an ambulatory care center or hospital.

The simplest maneuvers, such as endometrial biopsy, may often be performed without anesthesia, but effective anesthesia should be provided, often by local infiltration, if the discomfort is likely to be severe or more than momentary.

## BIOPSY OF THE VULVA

Biopsy of a suspicious lesion of the vulva should be accomplished under local anesthesia. A sample of the full-thickness of the vulvar skin can be obtained using the Keyes skin biopsy drill (Fig. 9.1). Alternatively, a sharp biopsy punch can be used to obtain one or more specimens. The base of the donor site should be coagulated to minimize bleeding.

## SURGERY OF BARTHOLIN'S GLAND

A Bartholin's cyst is a cyst of the duct and not of the gland, the latter usually compressed around the deep periphery of the cyst and not necessarily visible to the naked eye. After surgical excision of a cyst, often a formidable procedure associated with an unexpectedly high blood loss due to the vascularity of the tissues in this area, the future secretions of the remaining and buried but functional glandular tissue can reaccumulate and, without an opening to the external skin, may re-create a new and often symptomatic cyst requiring re-excision.

Acute initial Bartholin's abscess can be treated by aspiration through a no. 19 needle and syringe. The aspirate should be sent for bacteriologic identification, culture, and sensitivity. The patient, meanwhile should be started on 400 mg of metronidazole twice daily and 250 mg of penicillin four times daily, both for 7 days. If it is later determined that the offending organism is of gonorrhea, the patient should be given 1 gm of Probenecid and 3.5 gm of Ampicillin. When tissue edema subsides, the patency and function of the duct will return in about 80% of cases (6).

Incision and drainage of a Bartholin's abscess can be performed in the vestibular area close to the hymen through an area of fluctuation. The incision should be between 1 and 2 cm in length, and a drain or wick inserted for 24 hours. Because the skin heals and seals itself rapidly, reoccurence is not uncommon particularly if the duct has been damaged by the infection.

An alternative method of great simplicity is offered by the placement and inflation of a Word catheter through a stab wound into the cyst cavity (Fig. 9.2), where it will remain for 3 to 4 weeks until the track of the wound has become epithelialized forming a new duct (16). Inflation of the bulb should

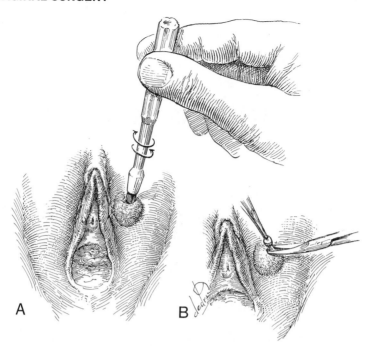

**Figure 9.1.** Biopsy of vulvar skin using a Keyes punch. The site has been infiltrated with a local anesthetic and the cutting end of the punch applied to the site selected for biopsy. Pressure is applied lightly and the punch rotated back and forth (see *arrows*) drilling a hole through the full-thickness of the skin. The specimen disk is elevated with fine pointed forceps and cut away from the subcutaneous tissue. The wound is cauterized for hemostasis. (With permission from Nichols DH, Evrard JR (eds): *Ambulatory Gynecology.* Philadelphia, Harper & Row, 1985, p 432.)

always be performed using saline rather than air, as the latter may permit premature deflation. During this 3- to 4-week period, the protruding proximal end of the small catheter can be tucked out of the way into the vagina. At the end of 3 to 4 weeks, the bulb on the catheter is deflated and the catheter removed. This procedure is particularly useful in the presence of infection. A small Foley catheter can be used instead of the Word. The bulb is inflated and the entire catheter tightly ligated about 3 inches from where it enters the skin. It may be transected just distal to the point of ligation, which has occluded both the central and side lumens, and the free end should be tucked into the vagina.

A Bartholin's cyst may also be marsupialized when large and uninfected. A window may be cut from the vestibular skin including the cyst wall. The edge of the residual cyst lining may be sewn to the vestibular skin by a series of interrupted through-and-through stitches. When healing has been completed, a permanent fistula will have been created between the cyst cavity and the skin essentially becoming a new "duct," the size of the ostium gradually contracts over a period of months, and in time, is scarcely visible though functional.

A solid lesion within Bartholin's gland should be sampled by needle biopsy or surgical excision (1) to exclude the presence or absence of malignancy that can be either adenocarcinoma if the tumor is of the gland, or transitional or squamous cell carcinoma if it is a malignancy of the duct. Bartholin's carcinoma is serious and is generally treated by radical vulvectomy and bilateral groin dissection.

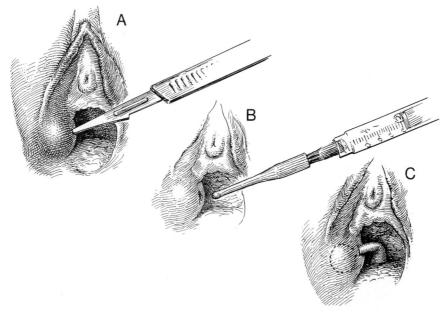

**Figure 9.2.**   Marsupialization of a Bartholin's cyst using a Word catheter. In *A*, a stab wound is made through the full-thickness of the right Bartholin's cyst at the site chosen for the new duct. In *B*, a Word catheter has been attached to a syringe containing 2 ml of sterile saline and the tip of the catheter is quickly introduced into the cyst cavity. In *C* the catheter bulb is inflated with saline, the syringe removed, and the free end of the catheter tucked back into the vagina. The catheter should remain in place for several weeks, until the new duct has become epithelialized. Then the bulb is deflated and the catheter removed. (With permission from Nichols DH, Evrard JR (eds):*Ambulatory Gynecology.* Philadelphia, Harper & Row, 1985, p 433.)

## LESIONS OF THE PROXIMAL URETHRA

Prolapse of the urethra is not uncommon, particularly in postmenopausal women but occasionally in newborns. If asymptomatic, it need not be treated. It rarely causes bleeding. But if it is a source of annoyance to the patient, it may be treated by excision of the circular area, and the wall of the urethra sewn to the skin of the circumferential tissue by a series of interrupted sutures. When a lesion of the distal urethra is associated with bleeding, differentiation must be made between the benign and relatively harmless urethral caruncle, and the more ominous invasive carcinoma of the urethra. The carcinoma tends to be harder when palpated and somewhat more friable, but the distinction is made by histologic examination of biopsy material. The treatment of caruncle is by simple excision, but the treatment of carcinoma varies between interstitial radiation and radical surgery depending upon the circumstances of the particular case.

## SURGERY OF THE HYMEN

Incision and hymenectomy is the treatment of coice and will be curative for an imperforate hymen. A small but rigid hymen producing obstruction to the vagina may be treated by hymenotomy at the four- and eight-o'clock positions, kept open during the healing phase by digital stretching performed by the patient. A rigid inelastic perineum may be overcome by midline perineotomy, sufficient to admit three finger breadths into the vagina. The edges of the incision should be sewn to the perineal skin transversely, at right angles to the original incision.

When recurrent postcoital cystitis occurs, examination should be made for the presence of a congenital anomaly of thick lateral bands connecting the urethral meatus to the hymenal margin. Urethrolysis at this site is curative (Fig. 9.3).

Introital stenosis, usually postmenopausal and too inelastic to permit relief by perineotomy, will respond effectively to Z-plasty (Fig. 9.4).

## VULVAR VESTIBULAR SYNDROME (FOCAL VULVITIS)

This condition may be suspected from an abrupt onset of severe dyspareunia, usually in a young Caucasian patient with no visible outlet obstruction or palpable endopelvic pathology. The patient may have one or more areas of exquisite tenderness that have been identified in the vestibule, most commonly in the posterior portion between the hymen and the vulvar skin. Gently touching this area with the end of a cotton-tipped applicator will produce instant discomfort, and the site can be sharply demarcated. The condition has been identified from time to time for over 100 years (22), and the most recent interest has been initiated since 1981 (9, 10, 18, 28, to 30). The vestibule is of endodermal origin from the urogenital sinus, making it embryologically quite distinctive from the other tissues of this area. Four percent aqueous Xylocaine on a cotton ball applied to this area some 15 minutes before coitus will often

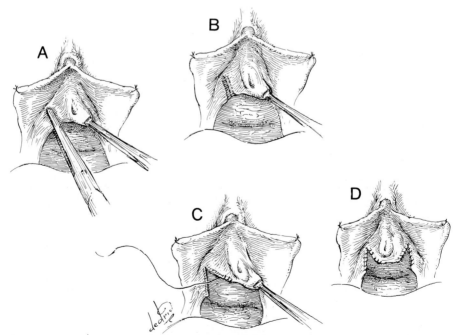

**Figure 9.3.** Urethrolysis is shown. The site of the hymenal attachment to the urethra is being crushed in a forceps *(A)*, first on one side and then the other. An incision to be made through the crushed tissue is shown by the *broken line (B)*. The cut edge of the incision is overcast by a running locked suture *(C)*, and the end result demonstrated *(D)*. (After C. Wood, the Mason Clinic, Seattle, WA.)

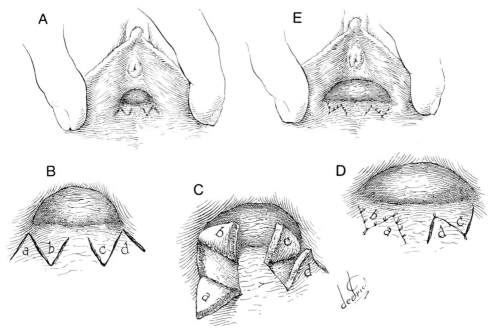

**Figure 9.4.** The Z-plasty is depicted. Preoperative introital stenosis is seen *(A)*. The lines of incision are shown. Note the introital enlargement at the conclusion of the procedure *(E)* after the full-thickness flaps have been undermined, rotated, and sewn in place *(B, C,* and *D)*.

provide sufficient temporary anesthesia for consumation of the marriage. Xylocaine ointment may be applied to the area during the day to obtain temporary relief. Because the taking of oral contraceptives may exacerbate the condition, for reasons unknown, they should be stopped for at least 6 months. Remission will occur in about one-half of the cases.

If the syndrome is persistent after 6 months of observation and treatment as described above, including the suggestion of alternative or noncoital means of sexual gratification for the couple, a surgical approach of vestibulectomy and perinealplasty may be expected to provide relief in most cases. Diagnosis is reconfirmed preoperatively by examination of the vestibule with a magnifying glass or low power colposcope, and often a cluster of raised pinkish or yellowish papules will be present in the area of pain. This specific site of pain may be carefully mapped out with a marking pen immediately preoperatively and before anesthesia so that the affected area may be totally excised (Fig. 9.5). The full epithelial thickness including the adjacent hymen of this sensitive area within the vestibule should be excised. The full-thickness of the posterior vaginal wall should be mobilized for 2 or 3 cm so that it can be brought down to cover this raw area at the conclusion of the operation, where it is attached to the skin of the perineum by two layers of interrupted sutures (28). Because postoperative oozing at this site is common, the patient may be kept in the hospital for a day or two postoperatively.

## TREATMENT OF AN OBSTRUCTED HEMIVAGINA

A hemivagina associated with a didelphic uterus, bicornuate or septate vagina may be completely or partially obstructed. When completely obstructed, there will be dysmenorrhea from the accumulated monthly blood and

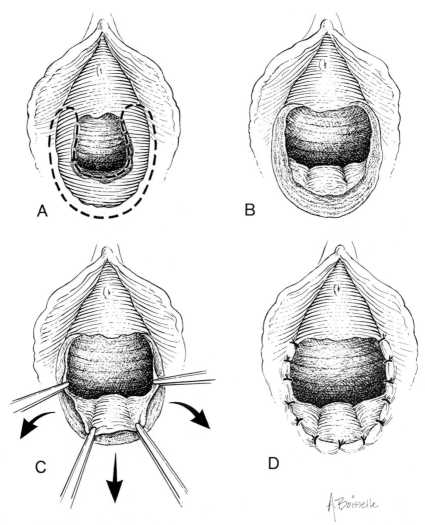

**Figure 9.5.** Vestibulectomy is illustrated. The painful area of vestibular skin is carefully demarcated preoperatively and an incision made lateral to this line of demarcation as noted by the *dotted line* in *A*. The full-thickness of the skin including the adjacent hymen has been removed, *B,* and any bleeding vessels clamped and ligated or electrocoagulated. In *C,* the posterior vaginal wall has been mobilized and pulled down as indicated by the *arrows* to cover the raw area. The full-thickness of the vagina is sewn to the skin of the vulva by two layers of interrupted synthetic absorbable sutures a shown in *D*. Raw areas anterior or lateral to the urethra are left open to granulate and avoid stricture.

a mass will be palpated in the lateral wall of the vagina (27). Congenital urinary abnormalities may co-exist. Diagnosis is confirmed by aspiration of old blood from the mass, and treatment is by prompt marsupialization, creating a large vaginal window connecting the cavities of the two vaginas.

## EXCISION OF THE VAGINAL APEX

A precancerous lesion of the posthysterectomy vaginal apex may be treated by full-thickness excisional biopsy as shown in Figure 9.6. It may represent

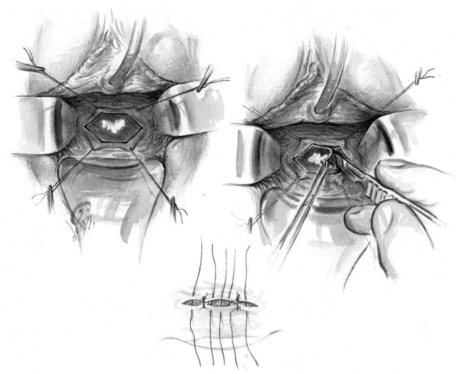

**Figure 9.6.** Excision of the vagina apex is shown. The lesion is carefully demarcated as by Schiller's stain and four guide sutures are inserted as shown. The subepithelial tissue may be infiltrated by 0.5% lidocaine in 1:200,000 epinephrine solution for hemostasis, and the tissue to be excised indicated by incision through the full-thickness of the vaginal wall as shown. This is excised by sharp dissection and the vaginal edges are brought together by a series of interrupted polyglycolic acid sutures placed as shown. If there is concern about preserving vaginal depth, a closure may be made in a vertical direction rather than a horizontal direction.

vaginal intraepithelial neoplasia in a patient with previous surgical intraepithelial neoplasia treated previously by hysterectomy, but the tissue must be studied in the laboratory to exclude unexpected invasion of the subepithelial tissues.

## CULDOCENTESIS

This procedure, usually performed at a site in the midline of the upper posterior vaginal wall between the uterosacral ligaments, is useful in identifying the nature and character of fluid distending the cul-de-sac of Douglas (Fig. 9.7). When abscess is suspected the culdocentesis should take place in an operating room and the procedure performed at the site of fluctuation as determined by the bimanual abdominal-rectal-vaginal palpation. The nature and character of fluid distending the cul-de-sac of Douglas is identified and, if purulent, the needle is left in place, the entry into the cavity enlarged by surgical colpotomy, and drainage promptly instituted. The abscess contents are sent for prompt bacterial identification, culture, and sensitivity. Other aspirates are treated appropriately.

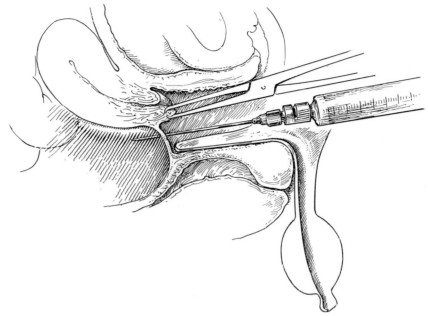

**Figure 9.7.** Culdocentesis is illustrated. The cervix has been steadied with a tenaculum, and a sharp pointed no. 18 needle attached to a syringe inserted directly into the bulging cul-de-sac. The fluid is then aspirated and examined. (With permission from Nichols DH,Evrard JR (eds): *Ambulatory Gynecology*. Philadelphia, Harper & Row, 1985, p 443.)

## EXCISION OF ENDOMETRIAL OR ENDOCERVICAL POLYP

A polyp protruding through the external cervix should be excised in its entirety and sent for prompt laboratory study. The base of a small polyp can be grasped within the jaws of a small hemostat and twisted off. Larger polyps are better removed by excision of their entire stalk and, because its site of origin and attachment to the endocervix or endometrium is usually nonvisible, the polyp can be fed through the loop of a tonsil snare (Fig. 9.8). The loop is advanced within the endocervical or endometrial cavity until its progress stops, at which point the snare is slowly tightened, crushing and transecting the pedicle of the polyp. The polyp is sent for laboratory examination. The patient should be re-examined after a month to determine whether or not other polyps might be present that should also be removed and studied.

## TREATMENT OF A WOLFFIAN DUCT CYST

Large Wolffian duct cysts are occasionally found along the side walls or beneath the lateral surface of the vaginal apex. They are anatomically separate from the urethra and bladder and are filled with clear mucus (20). If enlarging, or if they are a source of dyspareunia, they should be treated preferably by marsupialization instead of excision. This is because excision is occasionally accompanied by unexpectedly profuse bleeding and risks ureteral ligation when hemostatic deep sutures are placed at the base of the cyst cavity at the time of controlling bleeding.

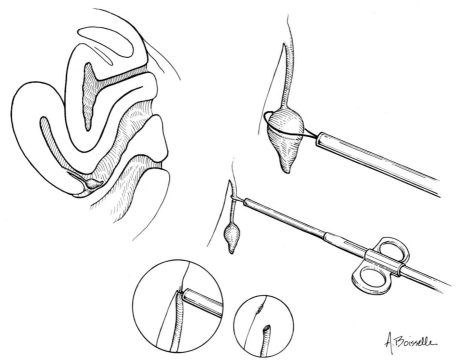

**Figure 9.8.** Removal of an endocervical or endometrial polyp is shown. The polyp protruding through the cervix is seen in sagittal section through the pelvis. It is threaded through the eye of the wire of a tonsil snare, as shown, which is advanced along the stalk as far as it will go. The snare is tightened slowly *(insert)* first crushing then transecting the stalk and the polyp removed for laboratory examination.

## TREATMENT OF CERVICAL INTRAEPITHELIAL NEOPLASIA

When a patient with cervical intraepithelial neoplasia wishes to preserve her uterus and its reproductive function, treatment other than hysterectomy can be chosen from:

1. cryosurgery;
2. laser surgery;
3. electrocoagulation.

These require that the:

1. abnormal epithelium be visualized completely;
2. endocervical curettage is negative;
3. there is agreement between the findings of cytology and colposcopy;
4. the patient is willing to participate in long-term and adequate follow-up activity.

### Cryosurgery and Laser Therapy

Coincident with careful cytologic interpretation of the screening Papanicolaou (Pap) smear, experienced colposcopy added to the usual armamentarium of gynecologists has made it possible to locate with specificity the site of epithelial abnormalities of the cervix, vagina, and vulva, and to biopsy these suspicious areas under colposcopic guidance for histologic study to rule out invasive cancer. Obviously invasive malignancy should be confirmed by the examination of tissue obtained by punch biopsy. When a premalignant condition has been identified and the entire lesion visualized colposcopically, a spectrum of definitive treatment can be offered to the patient. When the endocervical extent of a lesion cannot be estimated with certainty and the endocervical curettage is inconclusive, conization will provide adequate material for study. Although laser conization is popular with some gynecologists, our experience has found the so-called "cold-knife" conization to be entirely effective.

Premalignant lesions can be treated by cryosurgery (17, 23, 25) or laser vaporization (2–5, 15, 19, 21, 24, 25, 31) as alternatives to surgical excision.

When a colposcopically directed biopsy is reported as showing microinvasion of a malignancy, or possible microinvasion, conization becomes necessary for study of the entire lesion. When this is discovered during pregnancy, when the squamocolumnar junction everts, a shallow "coin biopsy-type" of conization avoids the potentially dangerous excision of the endocervix (8). Eversion of the squamocolumnar junction and excessive blood loss is reduced by the introduction of a purse-string of six hemostatic sutures placed close to the vaginal reflection(8).

## Conization of the Cervix

In recent years, gynecologists have discontinued the practice of the routine preoperative shaving of vulvar and suprapubic hair before a conization or dilatation and curettage (D&C) (or any other vaginal surgery). Clipping of long hair is sometimes helpful in keeping it out of the way (26).

Although diagnostic conization has been largely replaced by colposcopically directed biopsy, it is of value in the investigation of patients with a malignant noninvasive lesion or an abnormal Pap smear in whom the squamocolumnar unction is too high to be visualized and biopsied. Although the procedure is primarily diagnostic, it may be therapeutic under certain circumstances, such as when an entire noninvasive lesion of the cervix may be visualized and included within the surgical specimen. (Because intraepithelial neoplasia is commonly multicentric, this does not preclude the future development of other areas of dysplasia or carcinoma in situ.

## Technique

A simple technique that provides acceptable hemostasis consists of infiltration of the cervical stroma with not more than 50 ml of 0.5% lidocaine (Xylocaine) in 1:200,000 epinephrine (Adrenalin) solution. This produces marked spasm of cervical blood vessels, confirmed by a visible blanching of the cervix. With a No. 11 pointed scalpel for the incision, a cone of tissue of the proper size is removed, up to but not including the internal cervical os.

It is absolutely essential that the axis of the cone parallel the axis of the vagina and cervix; perforation of the uterus at the apex of the cone can damage the neighboring organs and tissues. The twelve-o'clock position on the operative specimen may be marked for orientation by a suture. Bleeding or oozing points should be coagulated with the electrosurgical unit. An alternative procedure for preliminary hemostasis requires the insertion of deep hemostatic sutures of absorbable material placed in the three- and nine-o'clock positions. The cone of cervix is obtained, numerous bleeding points coagulated, and the cervix packed for 24 to 48 hours with 1/4-inch iodoform gauze. If significant oozing is immediate, which is rare, a more hemostatic "hot" electroconization may follow. The difficulty with this as a routine procedure is that if the initial cone has not removed the entire lesion, there is no more fresh adjacent tissue to study by immediate biopsy. Because of tissue destruction, postoperative cervical scarring will be great. When a D&C and conization are to be performed on the same patient at the same time, the D&C is done immediately after the conization, never before.

## Complications

Hemorrhage may be seen either at surgery or within the first postoperative weeks after conization. Visible bleeding points should be electrocoagulated, and if there is a general ooze, the area should be suture-ligated. Mild bleeding may be stopped by application of the tip of a silver nitrate stick, or a cotton applicator soaked in Negatan or Monsell's solution. If this is not successful, packing the affected area with microfibrillar collagen (Avitene) is generally effective. (Avitene exerts its hemostatic effect by attracting functioning blood platelets, which adhere to the microfibrils, triggering the formation of thrombi in the adjacent tissue. Although more expensive, it is more effective than Gel-Foam or Surgicel.) A "pulsating" ooze should be treated by a carefully placed suture. If bleeding recurs, bilateral transvaginal ligation of the uterine artery may be required. Rarely, hysterectomy or internal iliac ligation may be indicated to control excessive recurrent postoperative bleeding, particularly if the conization has transected a major branch of the uterine artery that has subsequently retracted into the substance of the cervix or lower uterine segment.

Cervical stenosis is the principal long-range complication after unintended resection or trauma to the internal cervical os. Because cervical conization heals by scar formation, contraction will cause the diameter of the canal to become smaller, inducing a stenosis or stricture in some patients. The gynecologist who does a conization of the cervix must assume a responsibility to make certain that the patient's cervical canal does not become stenotic a few weeks or several months after the operation. The patient must be advised to return for postoperative examinations at regular intervals for at least 6 months, during which period, at each visit, the gynecologist should test the patency of the cervical canal by carefully passing a small dilator or sound through the canal and inner os. To let stenosis develop and progress to occlusion will lead to amenorrhea, hematometria, possibly endometriosis, and certainly to a rightfully dissatisfied patient. The cervix tending to stenosis cannot always be dilated sufficiently without anesthesia to alter the progressive tightening of scar tissue. If the os cannot be dilated in the office without intolerable discomfort, the use of a laminaria tent for 24 hours has been recommended (12). The operator must be careful not to let the laminaria tent slip into the uterine cavity, however, for it will become swollen, stuck, and difficult to remove without reinsertion of a second laminaria tent to dilate the cervix. If a stenosis does develop, dilatation of the canal under anesthesia and suturing an old-fashioned stem pessary in the canal to be worn for several months (or until it falls out) maybe preferable to occasional, but usually futile, sounding or dilation in the office or clinic. A stenosis may require long-term treatment by periodic endocervical dilatation until the surface of the cervix has been re-epithelialized and scar formation and healing have stabilized.

There is little place for "hot" conization in the treatment of chronic cervicitis. The procedure is not cost-effective and it carries additional risks, including the cicatrix of scar tissue formation and its troublesome sequelae. When endocervicitis causes a chronic leukorrhea that has become sufficiently troublesome to the patient to require treatment, strip cauterization or electrocoagulation of the affected area of the cervix may be the procedure of choice. Because infection often involves the depths of the endocervical glands, superficial cauterization of the cervix by local applications of a caustic or of silver nitrate is not indicated.

## CONIZATION AND CURETTAGE: PREFERRED SEQUENCE

Better results will usually be assured if the conization is done after the cervix and uterus have been "sounded" but before the curette is used in the canal or uterine cavity. The indications for conization and fractional curettage do not often coexist, but the procedures are not mutually exclusive. An external mucocutaneous junction around the margin of an"erosion" can, of course, be removed with a large biopsy loop without coagulating the endocervix. Even when a usual conization includes excision of 1 or 2 cm of the endocervix, the small, sharp curette can still be used to determine if malignancy is suggested by friable tissue of a softened area in the lower uterine segment adjacent to the inner os. When such curettage of the endocervix does not suggest carcinoma, it will probably be necessary to dilate the inner os in order to admit a larger curette and polyp forceps to the uterine cavity. If careful conization precedes curettage, a satisfactory fractional curettage can still be accomplished (14).

## DILATATION AND CURETTAGE (D&C)

The most frequently performed surgical procedure in gynecology is cervical dilatation and uterine curettage. Referred to universally as a D&C, this operation is often the first surgical procedure to be undertaken by the doctor preparing to be a specialist in obstetrics and/or gynecology. It is generally recognized that the technique of D&C is not difficult or tricky to learn. Few surgical procedures are as straightforward or more suitable for unvaried routine performance (11).

Conventional D&C of the uterus is indicated under the following circumstances.

1. D&C is used to evaluate abnormal uterine bleeding in persons in whom the cervical os is so tight that an endometrial biopsy cannot be performed.
2. D&C is used to evaluate and diagnose the cause of postmenopausal uterine bleeding when a diagnosis has not been made clear by endometrial biopsy. Knowledge of the presence of an endometrial polyp or malignant tumor is essential to the patient's treatment.
3. Immediately preceding hysterectomy in a patient with abnormal uterine bleeding, D&C is used because positive or suspicious endometrial findings may influence the operative decision.
4. D&C is used to empty the uterus of its contents when unwanted products of conception remain, as after an incomplete abortion.
5. For the patient with intractable menorrhagia and an enlarged uterus, D&C will clearly distinguish between adenomyosis interna and uterine leiomyomata, particularly submucous leiomyomata, clarifying a recommendation for treatment.
6. D&C is part of the workup of an infertility patient with leiomyomata when a hysterogram has not resolved the issues of location and types of leiomyomata present (e.g., submucous).
7. In the evaluation of a patient with an abnormal Pap smear, D&C is used when there is no gross or colposcopically visible lesion of the cervix.
8. D&C is used to treat known or suspected intrauterine synechiae (Asher-

21. Stafl A, Wilkinson EJ, Mattingly RF: Laser treatment of cervical and vaginal neoplasia. *Am J Obstet Gynecol* 128:128,1977.

22. Thomas TG: Hyperaesthesia of the vulva. In: *The Diseases of Women*. Philadelphia, Henry C Lea, 1880, pp 145–146.

23. Townsend DE: Cryosurgery for CIN. *Obstet Gynecol Surv* 34:828, 1979.

24. Townsend DE, Levine RU, Crum DP, et al: Treatment of vaginal carcinoma-in-situ with the CO2 laser. *Am J Obstet Gynecol* 143:565, 1982.

25. Townsend DE, Richart RM: Cryotherapy and the carbon dioxide laser management of cervical intra-epithelial neoplasia: A control comparison. *Obstet Gynecol* 61:75, 1983.

26. Walton LA, Baker VV: Mechanical and Chemical Preparation of the Abdomen and Vagina. In Buchsbaum HJ, Walton LA (eds): *Strategies in Gynecologic Surgery*. New York, Springer-Verlag, 1986, pp 46–47.

27. Wiser WL: Mass in the Lateral Wall of the Vagina. In Nichols DH (ed): *Clinical Problems, Injuries and Complications of Gynecologic Surgery,* 2nd ed. Baltimore, Williams & Wilkins, 1988, pp 139–143.

28. Woodruff JD, Genadry R, Poliakoff S: Treatment of dyspareunia and vaginal outlet distrotions by perineoplasty. *Obstet Gynecol* 57:750–754, 1981.

29. Woodruff JD, Parmley THG: Infection of the minor vestibular gland. *Obstet Gynecol* 62:609, 1983.

30. Woodruff JD, Friedrich EG: The vestibule. *Clin Obstet Gynecol* 28:134–141, 1985.

31. Wright CV, Cavies E, Riopelle MA: Laser surgery for cervical intra-epithelial neoplasia: Principles and results. *Am J Obstet Gynecol* 145:181, 1983.

# CHAPTER 10

# Vaginal Hysterectomy

In the selection and recommendation of an operative procedure for hysterectomy, there is no place for surgical histrionics or dogmatic pronouncements.

It should be the intention of the gynecologist to gain by personal experience equal confidence in his or her abilities and the results that can be expected by both the transabdominal and transvaginal operations. In this course of evaluating each patient's problem, he or she may choose the approach that seems clearly in the best interests of that individual.

As the operator's experience grows and confidence in his technique is gained, he or she will probably realize that indications for abdominal hysterectomy may evolve ultimately as the contraindications to the vaginal approach. As the operator's experience in transvaginal surgery increases, it becomes apparent that in general the patient's convalescence is more comfortable after a vaginal than after an abdominal hysterectomy. Moreover, the vaginal operation provides optimal opportunity for the correction of frequently coexistent problems of pelvic relaxation during the same operative procedure.

The gynecoid pelvis provides the most room for successful transvaginal hysterectomy, while the android type may compromise exposure. The type of pelvis can often be appreciated by the slant the vulva makes with the body axis (Fig. 10.1). The width of an adequate vaginal outlet can be judged by the distance between the ischial tuberosities measured during the pelvic examination by inserting the operator's closed fist between them (Fig. 10.2).

The most important single observation in evaluating the feasibility of vaginal rather than abdominal hysterectomy might well be the demonstrable "mobility" of the uterus. Usually a movable uterus can readily be removed from below. Conversely, the uterus that is not movable should rarely be approached transvaginally even when the vaginal operation seems otherwise indicated, as might be the case in an extremely obese patient or one for whom there is evident need for a vaginal or perineal repair.

A desirable degree of mobility may be demonstrable by the phenomenon of pseudoprolapse, whereby, with the pelvic musculature effectively relaxed under anesthesia, moderate traction will bring an ordinarily well-supported cervix of the nonfixed uterus nearly to the introitus. Under such circumstances a vaginal hysterectomy can be readily accomplished even when removal of the uterus is the primary and perhaps the only objective of the operation.

## VAGINAL HYSTERECTOMY FOR THE PATIENT
## WITHOUT PROLAPSE

The vagina is often indicated as the route for hysterectomy when the uterus is movable. It is the easiest of vaginal hysterectomies to perform, as the anatomy of the supports of the uterus is constant and unaltered by disease. Hospitalization can be shortened and the patient often may be home by the second or third postoperative day. Vaginal hysterectomy can be performed easily on the nulligravida patient.

Provided the uterus is movable, the less the prolapse, the easier the

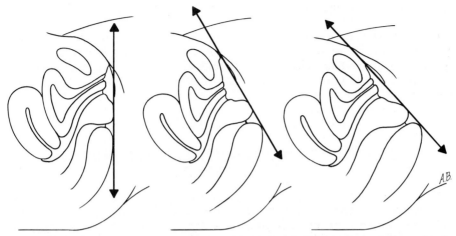

**Figure 10.1.**   With a narrow android pelvis the soft tissue slant of the vulva is perpendicular to the long axis of the body as shown in the drawing to the *left*. A more favorable vulvar slant is noted in the roomy gynecoid pelvis depicted in the *center* drawing, while the axis of the platypelloid pelvis is depicted in the drawing to the *right*.

hysterectomy. The greater the prolapse, the more difficult the hysterectomy. This is because the anatomic differences between cases are less in the former and greater and less predictable in the latter. Massive vaginal eversion with procidentia can be among the most challenging of all gynecologic surgical cases, demanding precise surgical judgment with each progressive step and creative resourcefulness with its resolution. One may perform a hundred such

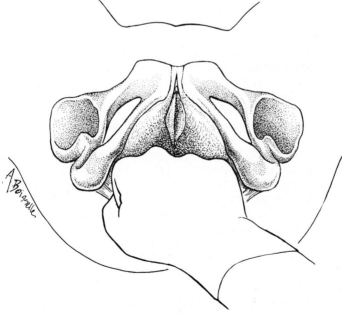

**Figure 10.2.**   The operator's fist can be inserted comfortably between the ischial tuberosities in the gynecoid pelvis, indicating adequacy of the bony pelvis for transvaginal surgical exposure.

operations and the anatomic challenges, findings, and solutions of no two will be identical.

When the anus itself seems to be the most dependent portion of the patient's perineum and she literally sits on her anus, this uncommon finding usually correlates with a major defect in the integrity of the levator ani. The latter may be associated with postmenopausal estrogen deficiency and loss of tissue tone, but it is more likely to be a consequence of major trauma to the levator ani and pelvic diaphragm or to be due to an acquired or congenital deficiency of innervation or to degenerative neurologic disease (see Chapter 13).

## CONSERVATION OR PROPHYLACTIC REMOVAL
## OF THE OVARIES

From a theoretical standpoint, the desirability of ovarian removal at the time of hysterectomy should be considered by the vaginal surgeon by the same criteria as would be observed during an abdominal operation (5). Because the ovaries are not technically as readily accessible during a vaginal hysterectomy as during abdominal laparotomy, there is a significantly decreased frequency of ovarian removal on a prophylactic basis when hysterectomy is accomplished by the vaginal approach.

When evaluating the indications for castration, the surgeon should consider seriously and critically whether the effects of removing the ovaries justify the relatively small chance that the individual may in the future develop a neoplasm of the ovary if the ovaries are preserved (27). Because estrogen replacement is readily available after castration, many will argue that the usual replacement therapy relieves only the subjective vasomotor symptoms of the menopause and, unless long continued, does not prevent the degenerative changes that may progress in diverse forms after castration. It is essential to remember that estrogen replacement therapy, to be effective, must be given prophylactically. Although the particularly undesirable bony changes are preventable, once developed they apparently are not reversible. Moreover, Robinson et al. (30) pointed out that the standard postmenopausal daily dose of 1.25 mg of conjugated estrogen will be only partially successful in altering postmenopausal blood serum lipid levels, that a dose of 2.5 mg per day is somewhat more effective, but that the optimal effect may require 5 mg per day or more, a dose likely to produce such distressing secondary effects as breast tenderness, fluid retention, and weight gain.

Randall (28) notes that patients for whom estrogen supplementation or replacement had been prescribed after a surgical menopause tended to discontinue the medication after 1 or 2 years. He suggested the reason might be the fact that the more significant of the degenerative effects that may follow estrogen withdrawal may not become symptomatic until long after estrogen effects are no longer demonstrable, and as a result the patient does not associate immediate cause and effect. Mattingly and Huang (21), describing their studies of steroidogenesis in the postmenopausal ovary, have demonstrated that although estrogen production fails precipitously after cessation of menstruation, stromal steroid production persists for a long time after the menopause, for which reason they have emphasized that the postmenopausal ovary continues to have a significant metabolic function. The same authors report a survey of published reports of patients in whom ovaries had been conserved at the .time of hysterectomy. In reports totaling 7765 patients followed for varying intervals after hysterectomies, only 12 individuals were known to have developed cancer in the preserved ovaries, an incidence of only 0.15%. However, the overall incidence of ovarian malignancy suggests that the eventual frequency of ovarian cancer is likely to approximate one per 100 patients. We believe, therefore, that castration should not be routine at any arbitrarily designated age, but we would agree that so-called prophylactic oophorectomy should be considered after the age of true ovarian senescence, whether that be demonstrable at 40 or 70 years of age. If there are indications for intraperitoneal surgery in a postclimacteric patient with nonfunctioning ovaries, one should certainly consider prophylactic oophorectomy, because the tendency of the ovaries to neoplasia does not disappear when steroidogenesis ceases. The postmenopausal ovary should not be considered too old to develop malignancy, but if the ovaries are still functioning at the time of hysterectomy, the operator should consider the advantages as well as the risks of ovarian preservation. Because there seems no arbitrary age at which all ovaries should be removed, we believe the view of the surgeon who elects not to perform routine oophorectomy is defensible, and that one's philosophy concerning ovarian preservation should determine the procedure recommended, whether surgery involves the transabdominal or the transvaginal route.

## PROPHYLACTIC OOPHORECTOMY IN THE PREMENOPAUSAL PATIENT

If the patient has a family history positive for ovarian cancer, she might be considered a candidate for prophylactic oophorectomy at the time of vaginal hysterectomy. She should be told this would reduce her chances of developing carcinoma of the ovary, although not be offered a guarantee that this possibility would be eliminated, as the disease seems to have certain potential general coelomic manifestations. Elective oophorectomy in the premenopausal patient is a preoperative decision in which the patient should be a participant.

Transvaginal removal of the grossly normal ovary might be encouraged in the patient over 55, discouraged in the patient less than 35, and the operator's advice somewhat flexible in between (3), depending more upon the present degree of ovarian activity than upon the chronologic age of the patient. Castration of the younger patient will accelerate the onset of osteoporosis and other degenerative changes.

### Manner of Operating

One contemplates the evolution of his or her own technique as a result of personal experience and comparison with the procedures described by other operators. It usually becomes apparent that a surgeon learns to identify and embrace a large group of basic fundamental principles and has not merely memorized a sequence of operative steps. Step four need not follow step three; for example, it may even follow step six or seven, or be skipped altogether, depending upon the characteristics of a particular patient's tissues and the operator's development of tissue relationships. The "whys" of doing something are every bit as important as the "whats." Illustrations enhanced by sagittal drawings have helped us visualize important operative details. By adding a third dimensional or spatial geometric concept to the reader's way of surgical thinking it can be shown that only in cases of advanced prolapse does the surgery start in tissues that actually come out of the pelvis.

The techniques to be described have not been used in all cases but have been used in the cases reported in which we consistently have achieved the best results. Obstetrician-gynecologists who prefer to stand doing episiotomy repairs will find advantages to standing during vaginal hysterectomy and repair (Fig. 8.1). This position seems to provide desirable mobility with minimal muscle tension on the part of both operator and assistants. When standing it will be necessary to elevate the operating table almost to its maximal height. Regardless of operative technique, some operators will prefer to be seated.

Horizontal light sources are very desirable while working within the pelvis. Because operating room spotlights tend to wander during the course of the procedure, some operators find that a fiberoptic forehead lamp (Fig. 8.9) provides a readily directed shadowless illumination in the very depths of the wound and into the hollow of the sacrum. It is important that the operator and all assistants keep their visual attention on the operative field; no one but the anesthesiologist need watch the patient, and no one needs to watch the nurse, clock, technician, or one another. A retractor held by a disinterested assistant can become a source of injury if allowed to wander, or it may obscure the telltale spurt of a small unsecured artery. When tension upon a pedicle or adjacent structure is relaxed, bleeding from a momentarily exposed vessel may remain undetected because the visual attention of the operator and his assistants has not been concentrated upon the operative field.

## Initial Procedures

The rectum should have been carefully cleansed by an enema given approximately 8 hours before and not just shortly before surgery. The patient should have been instructed to void just before coming to the operating room. Only if it is palpably distended must the bladder be catheterized at the beginning of surgery. It is our opinion that the bladder with a little urine in it is easier to identify than one that is empty. If desired, 30 ml of dilute indigo carmine, methylene blue solution, or sterile evaporated milk can be instilled into the bladder preoperatively as a means of assuring recognition of an unanticipated bladder opening that will occasionally occur during the course of a gynecologic operative procedure. We recommend this routinely for every patient who has experienced a previous cesarean section.

A careful preoperative bimanual pelvic re-examination under anesthesia should then be performed, for this helps the operator to conclude whether to proceed with the hysterectomy vaginally or abdominally (Fig. 10.3). The size, position, shape, and especially the mobility of the uterus should be carefully determined. The freedom and position of the cul-de-sac should be noted and the thickness and length of the uterosacral ligaments evaluated. Elongation of the cervix should be noted, as this will help identify the point at which incision through the vagina should begin. The direction and depth of the vaginal axis at rest should be noted.

A preliminary D&C should be performed, particularly if there has been any history of abnormal bleeding, and this will usually suggest the cause of the bleeding.

The preliminary curettage gives additional information in regard to the size, mobility, consistency, position, and "internal architecture" of the uterus. The position of the uterus is also important. A prolapsed uterus will rarely be found in anteversion, unless there has been a previous suspension or fixation procedure. A retroverted uterus is usually accompanied by pathologic elongation of the infundibulopelvic ligaments, with the ovaries in the cul-de-sac, making them much more accessible to surgical removal through the vaginal incision if the decision is to do so during the course of the operation.

One alternative is to discontinue the vaginal approach to hysterectomy if during the course of the procedure unexpected difficulties are encountered. An interrupted vaginal operation can be completed through a transabdominal approach, but in most instances this sequence should be regarded as evidence of an initial error in surgical judgment.

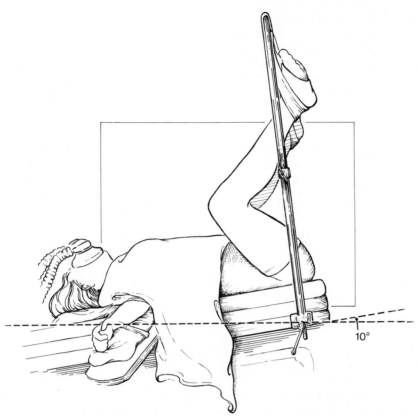

10°

**Figure 10.3.** A thorough bimanual re-examination of the genitalia under anesthesia should immediately precede any type of vaginal surgery. The size, position, shape, and mobility of the uterus should again be carefully determined. The side and freedom of the cul-de-sac should be noted, and any thickening of the uterosacral ligaments should be evaluated. The direction and depth of the vaginal axis should be carefully noted. The operating table is then tilted and locked in a 5 to 10° Trendelenburg position.

Following examination under anesthesia and preliminary curettage of the uterus, traction is made by a double-toothed tenaculum applied to the anterior lip of the cervix, and the integrity of the urogenital diaphragm and the anterior vaginal wall in relation to the pubis is identified. This gives the operator considerable insight as to whether coexistent suspension or support of the urethra and lower vagina should accompany the repair and the extent to which restoration of the normal vaginal axis and depth is likely to be achieved by his planned reconstruction. Another tenaculum applied to the posterior lip of the cervix makes it easier to also evaluate the location and size of the cul-de-sac of Douglas as well as the strength and size of the uterosacral ligaments that become more readily demonstrable as they are placed on a stretch (Fig. 10.4). The attachment of the cul-de-sac to the cervix then usually becomes more obvious, helping to indicate the site for the operator's placement of the initial incision to circumscribe the cervix.

If the labia minora are large enough to interfere with adequate exposure of the vagina, they should be temporarily fixed to the skin lateral to the labia majora by one or two sutures on each side.

**Figure 10.4.**   Traction is made to a tenaculum applied to the posterior lip of the cervix and the site of the cul-de-sac of Douglas palpated as shown. The length and strength of the uterosacral ligaments are noted.

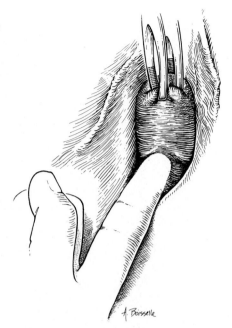

The cervix, having been grasped anteriorly and posteriorly with two double-toothed tenacula, is drawn downward as the cervix and upper vagina are adequately exposed by suitable vaginal retractors.

We are convinced that blood loss during surgery, particularly in premenopausal nonhypertensive women, can be lessened considerable by selective paracervical infiltration of not more than 50 ml of 0.5% lidocaine (Xylocaine) in 1:200,000 epinephrine (Adrenalin) solution (11), the so-called "liquid tourniquet." Use of this agent has been beneficial to us in three ways: First, it has markedly decreased operative blood loss and the consideration for transfusion. Second, it has seemed to lessen anesthesia and the need for postoperative analgesia; and third, it has allowed much greater ease of identification in the development and separation of cleavage planes. We inform the anesthetist before the injection. Because of the temporary ischemia produced, the immediate resistance to infection could be reduced (9). However, if prophylactic antibiotics have been started preoperatively, a therapeutic concentration should already be disseminated within the pelvic tissues (see Chapter 6). In our hands there has been no demonstrable increase in morbidity. We usually do employ this vasoconstrictive solution. When a patient is receiving halothane or cyclopropane anesthesia, or has been taking a beta blocker such as Propranolol, when unstable, or severe hypertension or coronary heart disease are recognized, we may in such patients substitute infiltration by normal saline solution.

The actual infiltration is most easily accomplished by use of a pressure syringe and a 22-gauge spinal needle (Fig. 10.5). The areas of the bladder pillars are injected, along with the lower cardinal ligaments and the insertions of the uterosacral ligaments. Before injecting the solution, traction is made on the plunger of the syringe to make certain that no blood is obtained, thus avoiding intravenous or intra-arterial injection of the solution. If a bloody aspirate is obtained, the needle is repositioned. The emphasis is placed on injecting the tissues around the cervix into the tissues to which the cervix is attached, rather than injecting the cervical tissue itself. While employment of the "liquid tourniquet" may reduce blood loss considerably, it is not a substitute for

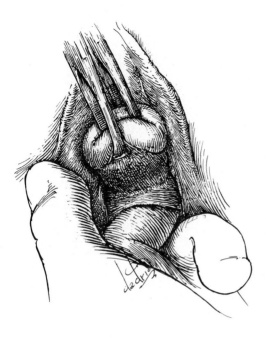

**Figure 10.9.** So as to reduce unnecessary bleeding, the opening in the peritoneum is made no larger than to admit one or two examining fingers. The nature of any intraperitoneal fluid is noted. The uterosacral ligaments should not be detached by this incision, but their thickness and possible elongation and site of attachment to the cervix are noted. The interior of the cul-de-sac should now be explored, and any enterocele or potential enterocele recognized so that it may be excised later in the operation. Any pathologic adhesion or cul-de-sac nodularity should be identified. The operator's exploring index finger sweeps superiorly, identifying the freedom of the posterior surface of the uterus, confirming the size of the uterus, and noting the position of any fibroids or other pathology that will be encountered later in the operation.

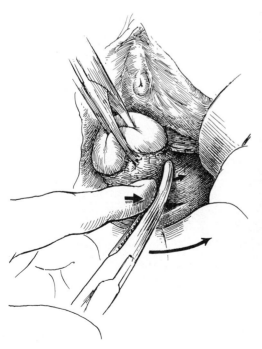

**Figure 10.10.** The uterosacral ligaments are identified and clamped, and if these appear elongated and seem strong, the clamps may be so placed as to assure some shortening of the ligaments as they are cut from the uterus. The tip of this clamp usually includes the lower portion of the cardinal ligament. Necessary shortening is accomplished by placement of the *unlocked* clamp across the uncut uterosacral ligament. The operator's finger presses the clamp as shown; the heel is moved a further distance than the tip. A lateral retractor, shown, displaces the vaginal wall, previously stripped from the surface of the ligament.

**Figure 10.11.** When the desired amount of shortening has been achieved, the jaws of the clamp are locked in the lateral portion of the ligament as shown.

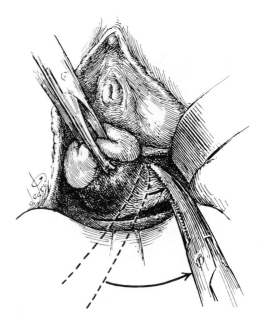

when oozing persists, because such sutures so frequently result in an increased risk of future enterocele if later in the operation the operator fails to resect any excess of peritoneum in the cul-de-sac before placing the purse-string closure of peritoneum cranial to these sutures. Any excess of peritoneum should always be excised before the cul-de-sac is closed.

The uterosacral ligaments are clamped and, if elongated and strong, should at this time be shortened (Figs. 10.10–10.12), after which they are cut from the uterus. (We believe that double clamping "for safety" is purely elective, according to the surgeon's preference.) The tip of the clamp should include the uterosacrals and the lower portion of the cardinal ligaments.

When placing a suture around this pedicle, it is important that the flexibility

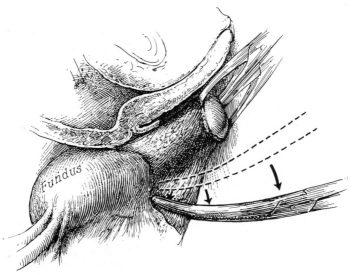

**Figure 10.12.** Shortening of the uterosacral ligament, when desirable, before cutting it, is shown in sagittal section.

of the operator's wrist provide impetus that follows the needle's curve. The needle should be pushed through the tissues only along the course of its curved direction, and pulled through along the axis of the needle's curve, to avoid the laceration of tissue more likely to occur when the needle is pushed through in a straight line. As the follow-through of the player's golf swing or tennis stroke affects the accuracy of the ball's flight, the swing and flexibility of the surgeon's wrist minimize the size of the opening and the trauma to tissues that can result from each placement of a hemostatic suture around the pedicles.

The uterosacral ligaments are secured by transfixation ligature to the posterolateral surface of the vagina at about the four and eight-o'clock positions. This suture should include the full thickness of the vaginal wall so that the ligaments will be firmly and permanently reattached to the vagina at this point (Fig. 10.13). These uterosacral sutures should be held without cutting to facilitate later identification and possible inclusion in the repair.

The operator's attention may now be directed anteriorly where the full thickness of the cut edge of the vagina may be identified between forceps at either side of the twelve-o'clock position. The cervix should be steadied in position by the tenacula, but excess traction is to be avoided for excess traction at this stage may pull the "knee" of the ureter into the operative field and appreciably increase its vulnerability. Using Mayo scissors, with the points directed away from the bladder, a 1-cm snip is made in the midline and the vesicovaginal space is now entered. The opening may be enlarged by spreading the tips of the Mayo scissors, which are then withdrawn without closing them (Fig. 10.14).

The midline incision (Fig. 10.15) is then extended through the full thickness of the upper anterior vaginal wall, which has previously been separated from the bladder by dissection within the vesicovaginal space. The full thickness of the vaginal wall is now separated from the bladder (Fig. 10.16). If the position of the cervix at this point suggests that there is not as much prolapse as the operator suspected, this inverted T incision becomes especially advantageous. If, however, there is as much or more prolapse than the operator expected (increased somewhat because the uterosacral ligaments have been released

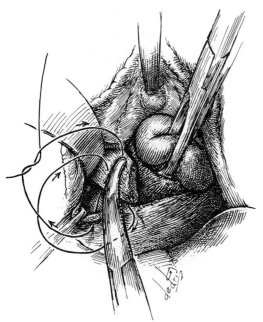

**Figure 10.13.** The cut ends of the ligaments are secured to the posterolateral surface of the vagina by a transfixion ligature at about the four- and eight-o'clock positions. These sutures include the full thickness of the vaginal wall, and by this means the ligaments should be firmly and permanently reattached to the vagina at this point. The ends of these uterosacral sutures are left long, however, to facilitate later identification and probable involvement of the ligaments in closure of the repair.

**Figure 10.14.** An incision of upper vagina into vesicovaginal space is shown. The operator's attention may now be directed anteriorly where the full thickness of the cut of the vagina is picked up between Kocher hemostats at the twelve-o'clock position. Using Mayo scissors with the points now directed upward and away from the bladder, a 1-cm snip is made in the midline of the anterior vaginal wall, the vesicovaginal space is entered, and the opening is enlarged by spreading the tips of the Mayo scissors.

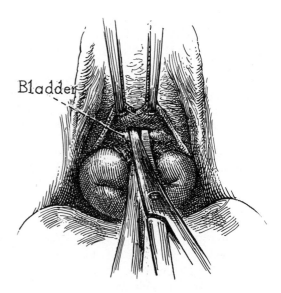

from their hold upon the uterus), then only a horizontal vaginal incision may be necessary, because in the latter situation the vesicouterine peritoneal fold becomes noticeably closer to the surgeon's hand and vision.

The bladder, readily identified by its looseness, may be picked up in the midline with forceps and placed on some tension. The supravaginal septum is incised and entered in the midline with the points of the curved Mayo scissors pointing downward or posteriorly (Fig. 10.17). The plane of separation follows the line of fusion between the posterior layer of the connective tissue of the anterior vaginal wall as it fuses with the encapsulation of the cervix (Fig. 1.25). The handles of the Mayo scissors should be elevated during this maneuver to assure directing the tips of the scissors away from the undersurface of the bladder (Fig. 10.18). Sharp dissection of the bladder from the cervix is

**Figure 10.15.** A midline incision is often made in the upper 2 inches of the vagina, again through the full thickness of the anterior vaginal wall that has been separated from the bladder by the preceding dissection.

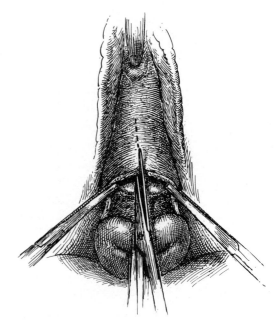

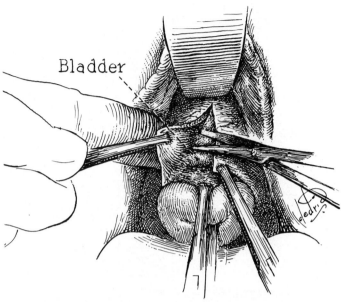

Bladder

**Figure 10.16.** Mobilization of the vaginal membrane is accomplished by extension laterally within this opening in the vesicovaginal space, while the full thickness of the vaginal wall is separated or reflected upward and away from the bladder.

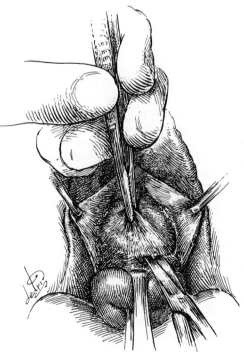

**Figure 10.17.** The bladder is identified by its looseness and picked up in the midline by lightly applied forceps. The bladder wall is then placed on slight tension, and the supravaginal septum is identified in the midline and incised with a curved Mayo scissors, the curve and the scissor points directed downward along the anterior cervix, opening through the tissue normally fusing the posterior wall of the bladder to the cervix.

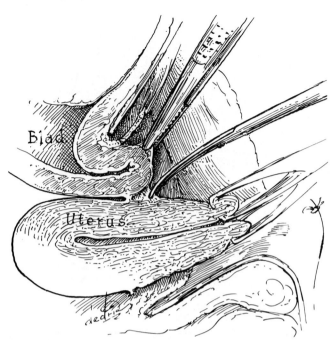

**Figure 10.18.** A sagittal drawing shows how the handles of the Mayo scissors should be consciously elevated during this maneuver to aid in pointing the scissor tips away from the undersurface of the bladder. As the scissors approach the vesicouterine peritoneal fold, the tissue can be safely rendered more visible by the following maneuver: Firm pressure is made with the closed but curved tips of the Mayo scissors pointed toward the cervix. While elevating the handles of the scissors above the horizontal, the tips of the scissors are spread apart and withdrawn, all the while maintaining pressure by the tips against the cervix. In this way the correct cleavage plane may be kept bloodless while this tissue plane is safely entered and the opening enlarged.

accomplished by meticulously snipping the fine fibers that bind the connective tissue capsule of the bladder to that of the cervix. This is much safer than bluntly stripping the bladder away from the cervix with either the finger or with a sponge. Laceration of the bladder from blunt stripping commonly occurs in the lowest section of the bladder fundus at some distance from the ureteric orifice (15). As the scissors approach the vesicouterine peritoneal fold, the tissues will usually become readily distinguished, but recognition of the peritoneum can usually be assured by the following maneuver: Making firm pressure with the closed, curved tips of the Mayo scissors pointing toward the cervix, and while elevating the handles of the scissors above the horizontal, the tips of the scissors are spread apart and withdrawn while maintaining pressure of the scissor tips against the cervix. In this way, the proper cleavage plane will be entered bloodlessly and safely, after which the opening may be readily enlarged. This dissection is carried upward until the freedom of the anterior vesicouterine peritoneal fold is recognized by its almost frictionless smoothness to palpation, or it may be visualized as the white line of a double fold of peritoneum. Having established the desired opening along the proper cleavage plane, a retractor is then placed beneath the bladder to hold it away from the cervix. The anterior vesicouterine peritoneal fold may be opened at this time (Figs. 10.19 and 10.20) and a long-handled retractor inserted. Either immediately before or after this retraction of the bladder superiorly, the "bladder

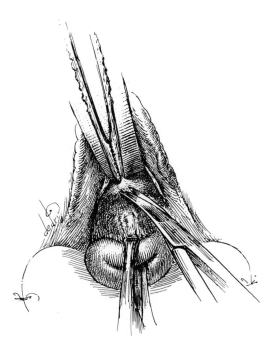

**Figure 10.19.** If not opened earlier or adequately, the anterior peritoneal fold, which is readily picked up by a Bonney forceps, may be confidently opened at this time.

pillars''may be clamped, cut, and ligated near their attachments to the cervix.

The so-called "bladder pillars" are never as strong as they may appear to be. Figure 10.21 indicates how portions of the cervical capsule will usually be included in this tissue. Surgical utilization of this maneuver provides an appreciable degree of protection to the ureters by assuring that dissection will be closer to the cervix and relatively away from the ureteral knee.

Although the gauze-covered thumb may readily strip the bladder capsule along a cleavage plane indistinguishable from the supravaginal septum up to the

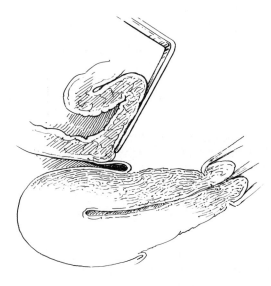

**Figure 10.20.** Exposure of the anterior peritoneum is facilitated at this time by displacing the bladder anteriorly and holding it out of harm's way with a retractor. The anterior vesicouterine peritoneal fold is at this time much easier to observe, and it may be brought closer to the operator after detachment of the cardinal ligaments. Usually it may be identified by the somewhat frictionless sensation that is imparted to the operator's examining finger, or it may appear as a whitish fold of tissue because of the doubled thickness of peritoneum where it folds back upon itself to extend beneath the bladder, the latter held out of harms way by a retraction, as shown.

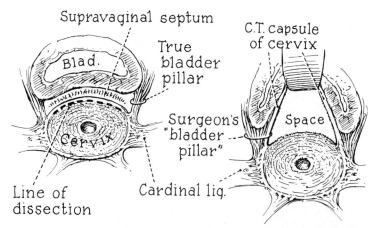

**Figure 10.21.** When the dissection between the cervix and bladder is carried out beneath the connective tissue capsule of the cervix, as indicated by the *dotted line,* there is an apparent increment in the thickness of the "bladder pillar," as indicated in the drawing to the *right.*

anterior peritoneal fold, there is a risk of tearing the bladder if the correct plane has not been entered. This plane may be obscured by adhesions and fibrosis following previous low cervical cesarean section, and careful sharp dissection will lessen the risk of unwanted bladder penetration. Occasionally the operator's readiness to dissect and desire to stay as far away from the bladder as possible, will cause him or her to incise within the connective tissue capsule of the cervix. This is particularly likely to occur if the initial incision around the cervix is too close to the external cervical os. As the operator continues by sharp dissection he or she may, by not entering the anatomic plane between bladder and cervix, dissect further and beneath the peritoneum covering the anterior uterine segment. The smooth undersurface of the peritoneum may be recognized by palpation but is not readily visualized, and it should not be opened blindly, as it is difficult to be assured of the actual site of its reflection from the superior surface of bladder unless it is accessible under direct vision. Failure to proceed with caution at this stage is one of the most common reasons for unintentional bladder penetration. Fortunately, if bladder injury does occur at this point, it will be well above the bladder trigone and relatively easy to repair after the uterus has been removed. Recognition of bladder injury is usually assured by the escape of a sudden gush of urine. The indication for and technique of immediate repair will be considered in the discussion of operative complications in Chapter 22.

A proper time to open the peritoneum during the course of extending the mobilization and identification of the bladder is soon after the smooth thin layer of peritoneum has been visualized, usually as a fold or double reflection appearing after the cardinal and uterosacral ligaments and the surgeon's "bladder pillars" have all been separated from the uterus. Cutting all pedicles close to the cervix results in further descent of the uterus, and this descent brings the peritoneum down with it. After the anterior peritoneal fold has been recognized by palpation and visualized but not yet opened, the portion of the bladder pillars closest to the cervix may be included in the clamp (Fig. 10.22) across the adjacent portion of the cardinal ligament. However, a small, rather superficial artery in the bladder pillar will often bleed as the vaginal membrane is reflected from the midline over the cervix. When such bleeding occurs it is advisable to separately clamp and ligate the vessel and adjacent bladder pillar on each side close to the cervix. Similarly, one should identify the cardinal

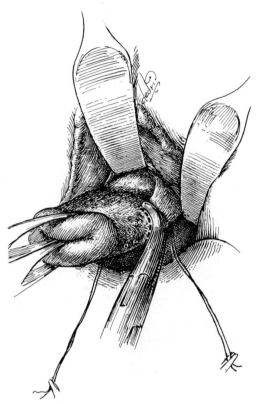

**Figure 10.22.** Separation of the lower cervical portion of the cardinal ligaments of the uterus is depicted. The anterior peritoneum has been palpated or visualized but not yet opened. That portion of the bladder pillars closest to the cervix may be included in the clamp across the remaining lower portion of the cardinal ligament, which should be clamped near the cervix. The cardinal is then cut from the cervix, and the hemostat is replaced with a transfixion Heaney type of ligature, which some operators will prefer to cut rather than leave long as a means of later identification of the cardinal ligaments. Preferably the clamp on the cardinal ligament will not include the uterine artery and adjacent veins. The fascia of the cardinal ligament is cut from its continuation anterior and posterior to the cervix. During this time, the uterine vessels, as they are released from the fascia encircling and attaching to the cervix, will often stand out conspicuously. Under such circumstances, the suture securing the cut ends of the cardinal ligaments may be tied and left long to facilitate later identification of the ligaments. However, if the uterine vessels have been included in the suture transfixing the cut ends of the cardinal ligament, the suture should be cut promptly in order to avoid later traction on the ligature of the uterine vessels.

ligament tissue to each side of the cervix, at which point we believe it advisable to make an effort to clamp, cut, and ligate that structure without picking up the uterine vessels separately.

With vaginal hysterectomy one good clamp at a time is used on the cardinal ligament. With this approach traction to the cervix brings with it the uterine artery that pulls the ureter down, and a second clamp decreases the distance from the clamp to the ureter putting the latter at some degree of risk. With a total adbominal hysterectomy, on the other hand, one may use two clamps at a time on each portion of the cardinal ligament detached from the uterus, as upward traction on the uterus pulls the uterine artery *away* from the ureter.

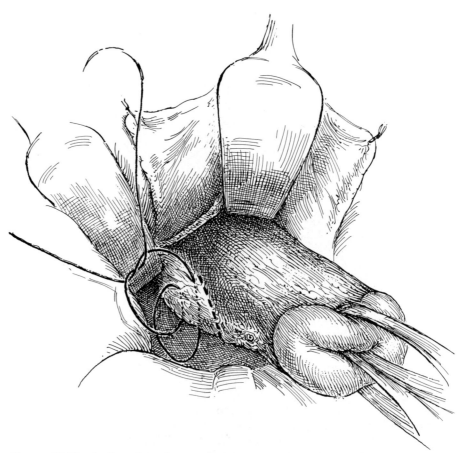

**Figure 10.23.** In the clampless technique, the suture is placed as in a Heaney stitch and the first cast of the knot tied. Then the pedicle is cut from the uterus and the Heaney stitch is tightened and a second and third cast placed to make it secure.

Occasionally when one encounters an intermediate or advanced degree of uterine prolapse, a clampless technique may be employed, in which uterine pedicles are ligated by primary passage of the needle, without preliminary clamping (Fig. 10.23). If using this technique, one should be careful *not* to cut the pedicle until the first cast of the stitch has been placed and tightened. Then the pedicle of the ligated tissue should be cut, the first cast of the knot tightened *again*, and the second cast placed and tightened.

If separately identified, the uterine vessels should be safely clamped and ligated with a tie that is cut short so it will not be used for subsequent traction. When there is a large uterus or when an irregular or intraligamentous fibroid has distorted the usual anatomic relationships, it is particularly useful to make such a deliberate attempt to exclude the uterine artery and adjacent veins in the initial clamping across the cardinal ligaments. At this point a cautious push or pull on the clamped tissues should be made in the axis of the ascending branch of the uterine artery (which may tear a small vein that can be readily clamped along with the uterine artery). This cautious but deliberate pull or push on the cardinal ligament tissue caught in the initial clamp will invariably result in enough separation of the anterior and posterior layers of ligament attaching to the lower uterine segment to disclose an underlying segment of the uterine vessels, which usually promptly and literally bulge into the operator's view. The uterines can then be clamped (extraperitoneally, without including the peritoneum either anteriorly or posteriorly), cut, and ligated with a minimal amount of ligamentous tissue. After ligation of the vessels, the remaining superior portions of the broad ligament, including adjacent peritoneum both anteriorly and posteriorly, may be clamped and caught in a transfixing ligature without risk of disturbing or jeopardizing the ligation of the uterine vessels.

Safe entry into the peritoneal cavity through the anterior vesicouterine peritoneal fold can be accomplished by a variety of techniques, each best chosen according to plan and correlated with the specific degree and type of prolapse involved. The presence or absence of coexistent cystocele that the operator intends to repair, the size of that cystocele, the extent of cervical descent, the degree of mobility by which the cervix can be brought closer to the operator by traction on the tenaculum, and the length of the cervix are all factors that must be taken into consideration. Often the site of the anterior vesicouterine peritoneal reflection is at the same level as the reflection of the posterior peritoneal reflection (within the cul-de-sac of Douglas) to the uterus.

The anterior peritoneal fold should be opened only under direct vision, never blindly, because the latter procedure could easily unnecessarily damage the bladder. Grasped with forceps, the peritoneum is tented as a vertical fold and may be readily opened with the scissors. The operator's index finger explores the anterior cul-de-sac, noting any pathology or adhesions, while making certain the incision has properly entered the peritoneal cavity anteriorly. Both index fingers may then be inserted into this anterior peritoneal opening, enlarging it by spreading the fingers laterally. A long-handled Heaney or Deaver retractor may then be inserted (Fig. 10.24) as a means of keeping the bladder up and out of the operative field. The relationship of the uterer to the uterine artery during hysterectomy is shown in Figure 10.25.

Had the operator been unable to identify the anterior peritoneal plication with certainty, further attempts at an anterior opening into the peritoneal cavity should have been delayed until a point of safe opening could be positively identified by either longitudinal section of the cervix or by inserting the operator's first and second left fingertips through the posterior peritoneal opening over the fundus of the uterus (17) and spreading them beneath the vesicouterine peritoneal fold, making it both palpable and visible (Figs. 10.26 and 10.27). To facilitate later identification of the edges of the peritoneum, it is permissible to tag the midline of both the anterior and the posterior edges with a suture left long so as to be readily retrievable when the operator is ready to close the peritoneum.

With the peritoneum opened both posterior and anterior to the uterine fundus, the upper cardinal and lower broad ligaments are then clamped, cut, and ligated. During application of these clamps, from the cornual angles downward, the tips of the hemostats should be so placed that each is within the peritoneal cavity, both anteriorly and posteriorly. This placement serves to seal off the broad ligament by compressing both anterior and posterior peritoneal leaves of the broad ligament between the jaws of the hemostat (Fig. 10.28). This step effectively prevents extension of any laceration into the very vascular venous plexus located within layers of the broad ligaments. These hemostats should be immediately replaced by transfixing ligatures.

During the course of the procedure after the cardinal and uterosacral ligament complex has been ligated and both anterior and posterior cul-de-sac opened, it may become apparent that traction applied to the cervix fails to move the uterus any further in a downward direction. One or more of several factors may be interfering with the delivery of the uterus, for under normal

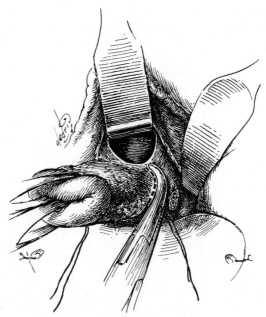

**Figure 10.24.** Clamping, cutting, and ligating the upper cardinal and lower broad ligaments are shown. Maintaining somewhat lessened traction on the cervix and uterus, the upper portions of the cardinal and lower broad ligaments are now clamped, cut, and ligated. With each application of these clamps, the tips of the hemostats should be so placed as to be visible within the peritoneal cavity, both anteriorly and posteriorly, thus assuring that the broad ligaments will be sealed off by bringing together the anterior and posterior peritoneal leaves of the broad ligament between the jaws of the hemostats. This step should effectively prevent extension of any tendency toward laceration of the tissues thinly supporting the very vascular venous plexuses usually located within the layers of the broad ligament. As soon as the uterus is removed, the hemostats on the ligaments should be replaced by transfixion ligatures. A single correctly placed ligature securely tied and promptly cut (leaving ends not less than 3 nor more than 5 mm long) will assure reliable ligation of the uterine vessels. A second ligation suture "to make sure" doubles the risk of the suture-placing needle entering a uterine vessel, doubles the risk of the needle puncturing or fixing a ureter, and, unless the second tie is squarely and simply atop the first one, the two ties per side technique appreciably increase the amount of tissue devitalized by the ligatures, which must be absorbed during convalescence. Considering all of the possible consequences, we have long believed that one properly placed ligature is the better technique.

circumstances the broad ligament and its contents, including both round and ovarian ligaments, offer little resistance to downward traction. At this point, one should suspect and determine with certainty whether the patient has had a previous ventral fixation or Gilliam-type uterine suspension or whether there are adhesions binding the uterus to other intra-abdominal organs. Any one or more of the following conditions also could be arresting descent of the uterus: (a) parametrial and broad ligament fibrosis from previous or chronic infection, (b) pelvic endometriosis, (c) undiagnosed pelvic carcinoma, extending from either the uterus or an extrauterine site.

Another possibility that should not be overlooked in one's preoperative assessment is a mechanical obstruction to further descent of the uterus by a

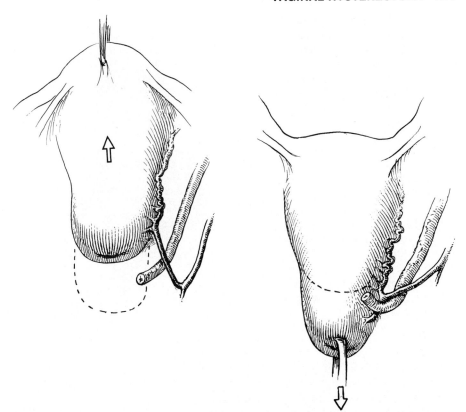

**Figure 10.25.** The relationship of the ureter to the uterine artery during hysterectomy is depicted. The *dotted line* represents a usual position of the uterus. In the drawing on the *left,* the relationship between the uterine artery and the ureter is shown when upward traction is applied to the uterine fundus as in abdominal hysterectomy. The drawing on the *right* demonstrates the change in this relationship when downward traction is applied as during vaginal hysterectomy. The risk of ureteral injury is greater during a vaginal hysterectomy.

large fibroid uterus with leiomyomata so situated as to interfere with delivery of the uterus. The operator is then faced with a choice among several alternate procedures. The first is to abandon the vaginal approach to hysterectomy at this point and finish the operation through a transabdominal incision. Allen's caution (1), with which we concur, was as follows:

"I do not believe that large tumors should be attacked through the vagina. How large a tumor one should attack depends on one's experience and skill, but also on the location of the tumor in the uterus. Relatively small tumors immediately beneath the bladder or extending out into the broad ligament, where the uterine blood supply is reached with difficulty, are much more important as contraindications than large tumors if they are in the fundus. Once the lower blood supply is secured, these upper tumors can be reached and morcellated with, shall I say, impunity."

The alternative would be to consider the possibility of amputation of the cervix and morcellation of any fibroid tumors of the uterus (Figs. 10.29 and 10.30), providing they could be grasped safely through the vagina. Werner and Sederl (33) and others have recommended bisection of the noncancerous uterus with sequential removal of one side of the hysterectomy specimen and then the

**Figure 10.26.** The first and second fingers of the operator's left hand have been inserted through the opening the posterior cul-de-sac and flexed above the uterine fundus. The anterior vesicouterine peritoneal fold, now identified and distended by the tips of the operator's fingers as shown, may be opened safely under direct vision. At this point the midpoint in the anterior peritoneum may be tagged by a single suture and left long to facilitate identification of the edge of the peritoneal opening. A long-handled Heaney or Deaver retractor may then be inserted to hold the bladder anteriorly while the uterus is removed.

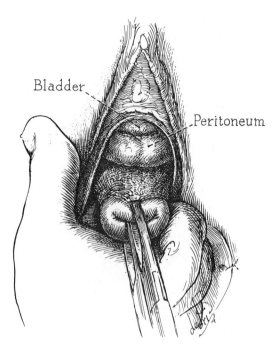

other (Fig. 10.31). The option chosen by the operator should be one that reflects both the patient's own best interests at that time and the confidence, experience, and technical ability of the operator.

Traction is continued on the cervix, drawing it closer to the operator. The middle portion of the broad ligament may then need to be separately clamped, cut, and ligated, with care again being taken to make certain that both anterior and posterior leaves of the broad ligament peritoneum are included within the grasp of the hemostat on either side. Transfixion ligatures should by now have

**Figure 10.27.** Flexing of the operator's fingers over the fundus of the uterus to visualize the anterior vesicouterine peritoneal fold is shown in the sagittal section.

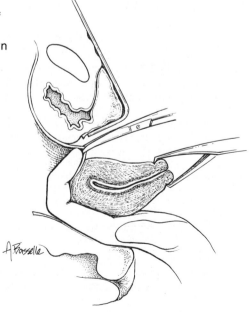

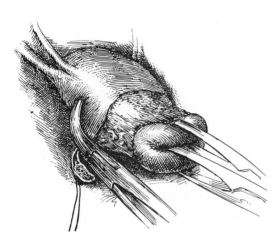

**Figure 10.28.** Clamping, cutting, and ligation of the middle broad ligament are shown. Traction is continued on the cervix, drawing it closer to the operator. This maneuver also makes apparent any tissues to which the remainder of the uterus may still be attached. Any remaining portions of the middle broad ligaments are clamped, cut, and ligated, again taking care to make certain both anterior and posterior leaves of the broad ligament and covering peritoneum are compressed within the grasp of the forceps.

secured the blood supply to the uterus (including both the ascending and descending branches of the uterine artery), and the operator has determined that the uterus is not held by any previously unsuspected adhesions.

When it is low in the pelvis, the fundus of the uterus may be delivered through either anterior or posterior peritoneal opening (Fig. 10.32); but when the fundus is freely movable and can be readily visualized, it can be delivered without flipping it (Fig. 10.33). Hemostats are applied to the cornual angle of the uterus on either side, and the uterus is removed.

The latter technique decreases the potential risk of contaminating peritoneal surfaces as a result of contact with a bacteriologically dirty cervix. Recognizing that the frequency with which retroperitoneal infection in the cellular tissues as compared to the infrequency of peritonitis accounts for posthysterectomy morbidity, prophylactic amputation of the external cervix may be indicated whenever uterine size or relative immobility of the uterus seems likely to result in more than the usual manipulation of the uterus as the fundus is being freed up and removed.

If at this point it is determined that the body of the uterus is movable but too large to permit comfortable delivery by ''flipping'' the fundus through either the anterior or posterior peritoneal opening and morcellation is not desired, the myometrium can be incised circumferentially (Fig. 10.34). Incision for this purpose should be placed parallel to the axis of the uterine cavity and parallel with the serosal covering of the uterus (Figs. 10.35 and 10.36). It frees the uterus much as a banana is peeled by turning the skin inside out, bringing the cervix still closer to the operator, but without violating the integrity of the endometrial cavity (Fig. 10.36). The incision is carried symmetrically around the full circumference of the uterus through the myometrium just beneath the serosa (Fig. 10.37). Incision of the lateral portions of myometrium medial to the remaining attachment of the broad ligament results in considerable additional descent of the uterus and greatly increases the mobility of the as yet unremoved fundus (Fig. 10.38).

The cornual angle hemostats are, in turn, replaced by transfixion ligatures (Fig. 10.39). After these are tied, an additional bite is taken through the round ligament on each side, and the suture is tied again (Fig. 10.40). This will permit traction on the adnexal pedicles to be born principally by the round ligament (which has been ligated higher than the infundibulopelvic ligament by virtue of

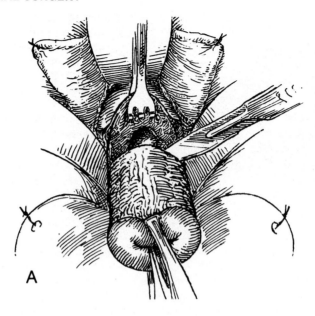

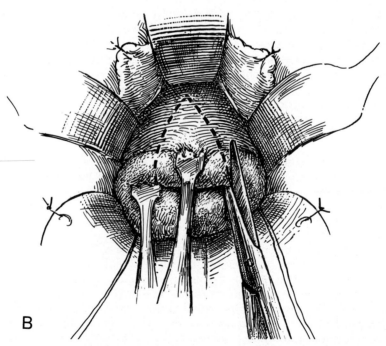

**Figure 10.29.** Morcellation is depicted. The uterosacral and cardinal ligaments have been cut and ligated and the cervix amputated as shown in *A*. The myometrium is firmly grasped by Leahy clamps, and the first of several wedges of anterior or posterior uterine wall may be excised in the midline as shown in *B*, gradually reducing the size of the uterus.

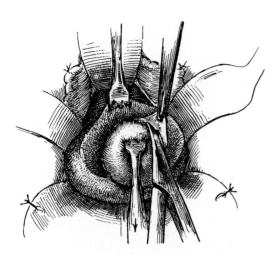

**Figure 10.30.** This piecemeal excision is continued in the direction of the closest fibroid until its pseudocapsule is reached and opened. The fibroid is grasped with a Leahy clamp, traction is applied, and almost bloodless dissection continues in the plane of the pseudocapsule as shown until the fibroid can be removed either intact or piecemeal, depending upon its size.

the extra bite). It is important not to pull the ligature off the pedicle of an ovarian artery within the ovarian ligament.

At this time the adnexa should be carefully inspected on each side, and, if removal is desired, it should be accomplished with particular care to assure ligation of the ovarian vessels (5, 25) (Figs. 10.41 and 10.42).

When vaginal oophorectomy of an obviously benign ovarian tumor is to be performed, one should first clamp and cut the mesovarium and then remove the ovary, using the clamp on the mesovarium as a handle so as to not fill the vagina with the ovarian tumor obstructing the operator's vision of its pedicle.

If the operator has decided upon castration and the uterus is being removed, one may remove the ovaries alone, sparing the tube and mesosalpinx, which may aid appreciably in subsequent peritonealization by covering the intraperitoneal mesovarium stump. Should the operator prefer to preserve the tube, care must be taken when ligating the ovarian pedicle to preserve the mesosalpinx and tubal blood supply. When the tube also is to be removed, the slanted Deschamps ligature carrier with its blunt point is good for ligation of the infundibulopelvic ligament. After the cornual angle stitches have been tied, the uncut ends of the sutures can be secured in a clamp and held long for use later

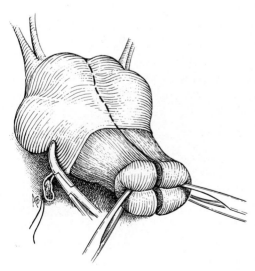

**Figure 10.31.** Bisection of the uterus when it is enlarged or fixed in position. It can be bisected and removed one-half at a time. The cardinal ligament and uterine artery are clamped, cut, and ligated, and a clamp has been placed on the lower portion of the broad ligament. The cervix may be split in the midline, as shown, and the hemisection of the uterine corpus made along the path indicated by the *dotted line*.

**Figure 10.32.** The fundus of the uterus may be delivered by way of either anterior or posterior peritoneal opening, and hemostats may be applied to the cornual angles as shown. After both sides have been clamped, the uterus is cut away.

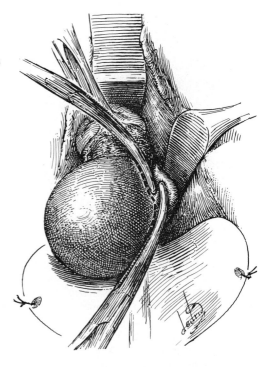

in the procedure. If adhesions are great, the leaves of the broad ligament may be spread by funneling with the scissor tips for mobilization of the components ligated separately (4).

An enterocele, enterocele sac, or potential enterocele may be identified at this time by exploration of the cul-de-sac with the operator's finger (Fig. 10.43). At times it will be helpful to pack the interior of the sac with a moistened gauze sponge to facilitate identification and to aid dissection. Because the patient should already be in a 5 or 10° Trendelenburg position (Fig. 10.3), the contents of the abdomen can usually be readily packed away from the operative field by

**Figure 10.33.** When the fundus is freely movable and descends without undue traction, the uterus may be freed and delivered without "flipping" the fundus either anteriorly or posteriorly. Hemostats are applied to the cornual angles of the uterus on either side, after which the uterus is cut away from these hemostats and the cut ends are securely ligated.

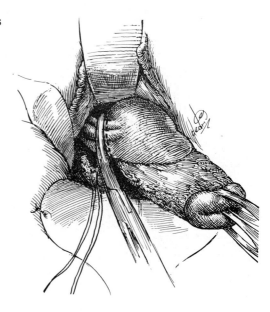

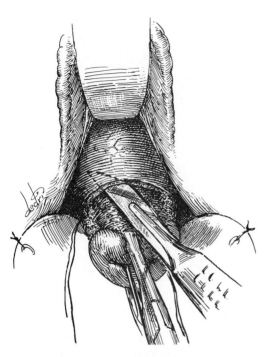

**Figure 10.34.** A Lash incision into the myometrium is shown. The operator has already secured by transfixion ligature the inferior and major blood supply of the uterus (the ascending and descending branches of the uterine artery) and has determined that the uterus is not being deviated or fixed by any previously unsuspected adhesions. If it is now determined that the body of the uterus is too big to permit delivery, the outer superficial myometrium can be incised circumferentially.

relatively little gauze packing. An enterocele sac can be easily separated from the surrounding connective tissue by alternating sharp and blunt dissection as far down as the anterior surface of the rectum, which is identified by the small condensations of fat adherent to the peritoneum and by the noticeably longitudinal muscle layer of the outer rectal wall. As the anterior or vesicouterine peritoneum is inspected, any excess of redundant peritoneum left after the opening and dissection of the anterior peritoneal cul-de-sac should be excised at this time to lessen the possibility of an anterior postoperative enterocele. The bladder, if at all distended, should now be emptied of urine by catheter, as this will often seem to facilitate reperitonealization by making the anterior cut edge of the peritoneum more readily visible and accessible. Should difficulty be encountered in locating the anterior peritoneum, tissues inferior to the anterior peritoneum may be lightly grasped with successive gentle bites of

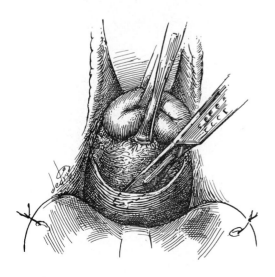

**Figure 10.35.** Both anterior and posterior myometrial incisions should be kept parallel to the axis of the uterine cavity and should completely traverse the outer myometrial layer of the uterus.

**Figure 10.36.**  If the circumferential incision has been properly placed, this will permit enucleation of the bulk of the uterus without transgressing the endocervical or endometrial cavity, much in the manner of peeling a banana as its skin turns inside out. The large bulky uterus is thereby increased in length and decreased in width, which in essence "makes the cork smaller than the neck of the bottle."

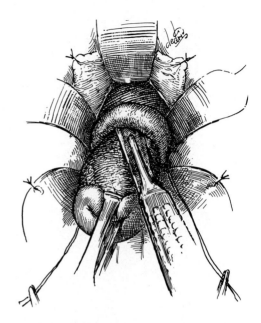

an unlocked hemostat in such fashion as to "walk up" or roll these tissues toward the operator until the anterior peritoneal edge is identified. When unmistakably visible, the peritoneal edge is grasped by a hemostat while sutures are being placed to close the peritoneal opening.

Traction is made on the previously clamped and held transfixion ligature of the uterosacral ligament (Fig. 10.44). By pulling on this suture, the ligament on tension is readily identified. Peritoneal closure is begun using a full length of

**Figure 10.37.** The large but movable uterine corpus is shown by the *dotted line* in relationship to the myometrial incision.

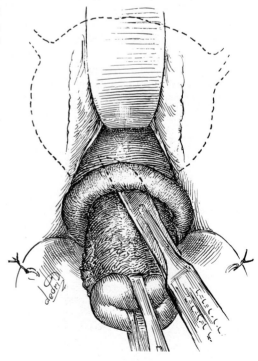

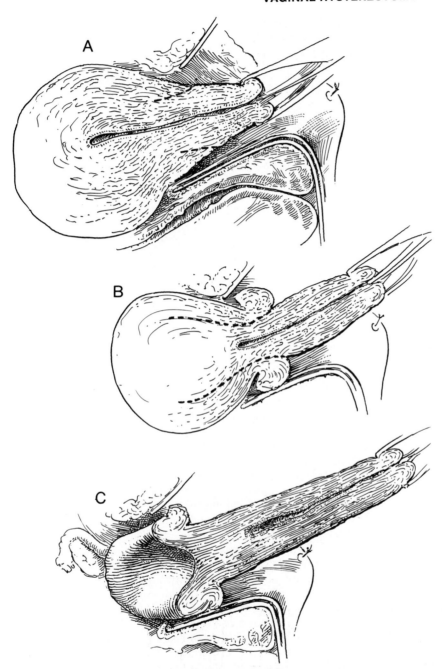

**Figure 10.38.**   A sagittal drawing of a large bulky uterus is noted in *A*. The cardinal and uterosacral ligaments have been separated from the sides of the uterus, but delivery of the body is difficult because of its size. The pathway for incision into the myometrium parallel to the axis of the uterus is identified by the *broken line*. In *B*, the incision has been deepened, as traction further exteriorizes the cervix. The myometrial incision will be extended further as indicated by the *broken line*. In *C*, the uterus can now be delivered outside the pelvis. The length has increased as the diameter has been decreased, as shown. The cornual angle can now be clamped under direct visualization and the uterus cut free.

**Figure 10.39.** Ligation of the adnexal pedicle. Each hemostat is then replaced by transfixion ligature as shown.

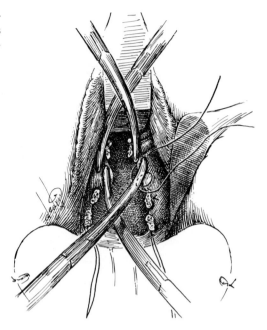

absorbable 0 suture, a single strand of polyglycolic or polydiaxonone suture, and a doubled strand of chromic catgut is used. Beginning with a stitch through the peritoneal surface and into the left uterosacral ligament, the posterior peritoneum is then reefed in a linear fashion by a series of bites until the same level on the opposite uterosacral ligament location is reached (Fig. 10.45). This posterior peritoneal reefing should be along the level of the reflection of peritoneum from the anterior wall of the rectum. The operator should not place reefing sutures higher than this level, for to do so would displace an undesirably excessive amount of rectum into vaginal space.

The purse-string sutures to close the peritoneum and any suture placed for the purpose of bringing the uterosacral and/or the infundibulopelvic and round ligaments together should be carefully placed above or proximal to the ligature on the pedicles. The purpose of the suture that brings the ligamentous structures together is 2-fold: to promote a firm tissue union, and to assure that all ligated pedicles will be extraperitonealized. The ligatures on the uterine vessels will not be caught up on an approximating suture. Although the vessels will retract into the parametria, their ligated pedicles also remain extraperitonealized.

After the peritoneal closure stitch has been passed through the uterosacral ligament and adjacent peritoneum, first on the patient's left and later similarly on the right side, traction on the previously held uterosacral transfixing ligatures is relaxed. The homolateral adnexal pedicle suture on the patient's right side is then grasped, and gentle traction is again made in order to bring the round ligament into view. The peritoneal closure stitch is passed through the round ligament proximal and medial to the previously placed pedicle ligation. The round ligaments do not support the vagina, they are incorporated in the purse-string stitch only to better peritonealize the pelvis. The anterior peritoneum is then identified, and any excess is excised and reefed by a series of bites that continue to and through the left round ligament, at which point the stitch has been continued in clockwise fashion entirely around the peritoneal opening and through the round and uterosacral ligaments on each side. Peritoneal

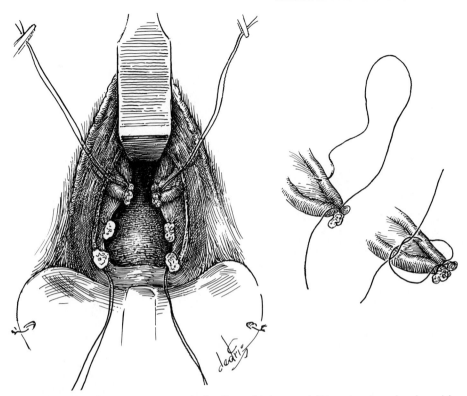

**Figure 10.40.** The sutures are tied, after which an additional suture is placed in the round ligament on either side, to which the pedicle is again tied as shown on the *right*. This maneuver assures that later traction on the adnexal or the cornual angle pedicle will, in fact, be exerted on the round ligament that has been ligated more proximal than the infundibulopelvic ligament by virtue of the extra ligature. This technique reduces the risk that a tie that has secured the ovarian artery within the pedicle of the ovarian ligament may be pulled off the pedicle during only moderate traction. Because of this risk, the ovarian pedicles as well as the adnexa should be carefully reinspected on each side just before the peritoneum is closed. When the cornual angle stitches have been secured, the ends of these sutures should be tagged long enough to be readily identified when the adnexa and ovarian pedicles are to be reinspected later in the procedure.

closure following vaginal hysterectomy is done primarily to incorporate the strength of the subperitoneal connective tissue retinaculum into a firm scar at the bottom of the pelvis that will resist increases in intra-abdominal pressure. The mesothelial lining of the peritoneal cavity per se has little supportive value.

Care must be taken to remove all intra-abdominal intraperitoneal packing, after which all slack in this purse-string type of peritoneal suture is taken up by reefing the tissues fairly snugly along the suture both anteriorly and posteriorly. Only after such reefing should the purse-string suture closing the peritoneum be tied. To be effective all reefing should be accomplished before, not as, this stitch is tied. This plication of tissues at the bases of the uterosacral ligaments actually draws the pubococcygei and their fasciae together (19, 20), narrowing the genital hiatus. After the purse-string peritoneal closure stitch has been tied, both ends of the stitch should be left long without cutting and held for later use.

Because the uterosacral ligaments are relatively fixed in position, the

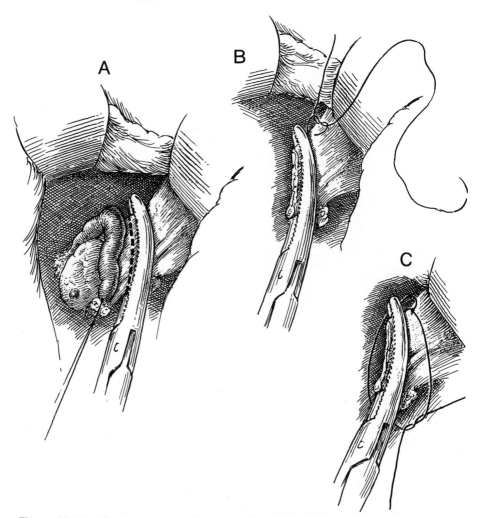

**Figure 10.41.** If adnexal removal or resection is desirable, it should be performed at this time. Vaginal salpingo-oophorectomy may be accomplished as follows: Downward traction is applied to the round ligament suture. The ovary may be grasped in a spongeholder and a forceps applied across the infundibulopelvic ligament as shown in *A*. The ovary and tube are excised, and a transfixion suture of medium thickness is placed, as illustrated in *B*. The tie is completed, as shown in *C*, as the forceps is removed.

movable round ligaments that are also included in the purse-string suture will be brought to the semifixed uterosacral ligaments, rather than the opposite, fixing the peritonealization in a posterolateral direction over the levator plate, tending to re-establish the horizontal axis of the upper vagina and appreciably lessening the chances of the postoperative development of an enterocele.

The round ligament pedicle stitches may be tied together beneath the base of the bladder, providing for additional safety as auxilliary support to the intra-abdominal contents should the peritoneal sutures be broken or become untied. The retracting sutures in the labia minora may now be cut and the vagina prepared for closure. If no colporrhaphy is to be done and to preserve maximal vaginal depth, the inverted T-shaped incision in the anterior vaginal

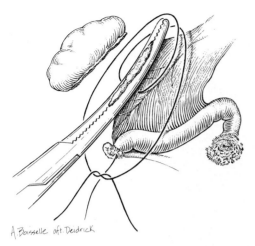

**Figure 10.42.** When the infundibulopelvic ligament is short, transvaginal oophorectomy may be accomplished as shown. The mesovarium has been clamped and the ovary removed. There is a single penetration of the mesovarium at its midpoint, and each end of the suture is passed around the distal tip of the hemostat and tied beneath the heel of the clamp.

A. Boisselle aft. Deidrick

wall is trimmed to an inverted V (Fig. 10.46) and the vagina closed in a sagittal direction.

After completion of the anterior colporrhaphy, as closure of the anterior vaginal wall begins, the needle on one end of the preserved peritoneal closure stitch is passed through each side of the uppermost portion of the anterior vaginal wall, from the inside out on one side and outside in on the other, at

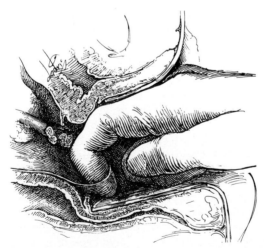

**Figure 10.43.** The importance of recognizing evidence of a potential enterocele or the demonstration of an existing enterocele sac always warrants careful exploration of the cul-de-sac by the operator's fingers as shown in this sagittal section. For demonstration or identification purposes, a suspected sac can be packed with a gauze sponge to facilitate demonstration of excess peritoneal connective tissue by both sharp and blunt dissection down to a point where the excision of excess peritoneum will extend across the anterior surface of the rectum. Any fat that is present belongs on the rectal side of the dissection. Rectum should be recognized promptly during this dissection either by the characteristic condensations of fat or by the longitudinal muscle fibers of the outer layer of rectal wall. In the same manner, the anterior peritoneum should be inspected. If there is excessive redundant peritoneum anteriorly, it should be excised at this time, lessening the postoperative possibility of an anterior enterocele.

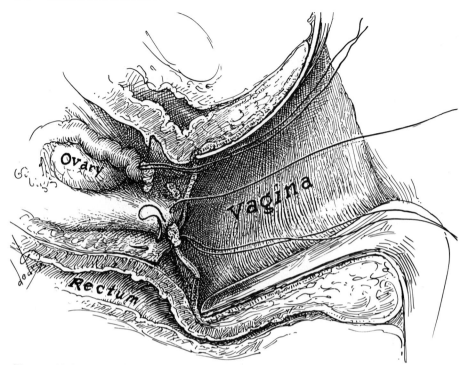

**Figure 10.44.** The beginning of the high peritoneal closure stitch through the peritoneal surface of the uterosacral ligament, then the posterior peritoneum just above its cut edge, is shown.

precisely the level at the vault that will correspond to the previous attachments in the cardinal ligaments and held for tying later. The end of the peritoneal closure stitch sewn beneath the anterior vaginal wall at its apex as noted above is then tied to its other held end (of the previously tied peritoneal purse-string suture), taking care, as when previously preparing to tie the peritoneal purse-string suture, to reef the tissues to be tied rather snugly together before seating and tying the knot (Fig. 10.47). This suture fixes the anterior vault to the edge and level of the peritoneal purse-string, effectively lengthening the anterior vaginal wall and aiding in the support of the vaginal vault.

Tying the held end of the peritoneal closure stitch to an uppermost stitch in the anterior vaginal wall with a bite or two to either side of the midline also effectively unites the anterior connective tissue capsule of the vagina to the area in which the uterosacral ligaments have been brought together as a result of the placement of the peritoneal stitch. Because each uterosacral ligament has in effect been united to the posterolateral surface of the vaginal wall, this has the effect of uniting the tissue capsule of the anterior vaginal wall to that of the posterior vaginal wall (16).

The anterior vaginal wall is closed by either running or interrupted subcuticular sutures. A subcuticular closure assures a more exact and smooth approximation of the epithelial layers. This alignment effectively reduces the development of postoperative foci of granulation tissue in the suture line, and in virtually doing so, the opportunity for future development of an enterocele is reduced and the vault is appreciably strengthened (4, 26).

By having closed the vagina from side to side in a longitudinal direction (Figs. 10.48 and 10.49) rather than front to back, an additional 2 or 3 cm of vaginal length will have been developed, which at times may mean the

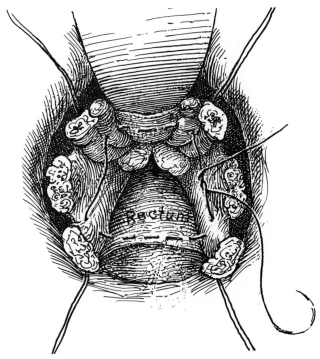

**Figure 10.45.** If a marking suture has not been placed and difficulty is experienced in locating the anterior peritoneum, the tissue caudal to the anterior peritoneum is lightly grasped with successive gentle bites of an unlocked hemostat, in such fashion as to "walk up" this area until the anterior peritoneum is recognized and grasped in a forceps. Peritonealization is accomplished using a full length of absorbable 0 or 2/0 suture, held in a light hemostat for identification later. We prefer to begin this stitch on the peritoneal side of the left uterosacral ligament. Traction is made on the previously clamped and held transfixion ligature of the uterosacral ligament; by putting the ligament on tension, it is readily identified. The posterior peritoneum is reefed by a series of bites until the opposite uterosacral ligament location is reached. The suture passes through the right round ligament, the anterior peritoneum, and the left round ligament and is ready to be tied.

difference between a depth that may contain the patient's sexual partner and a shorter depth that may not (Fig. 10.50).

## CUL-DE-PLASTY

When there are strong uterosacral-cardinal ligaments, as usually seen with uterovaginal prolapse, with obvious shortening or telescoping of the vagina, the operator can confidently gain additional vaginal depth by fixing the vagina posterior to this ligament complex. One method of doing this is to use the McCall cul-de-plasty (22) or a modification of it.

In our modification most of the peritoneum of any coexistent enterocele is excised first, before the polyglycolic acid-type cul-de-plasty stitches are placed, eliminating the enterocele while reducing the size of the subsequent cul-de-sac (Fig. 10.51). An appropriate wedge should be removed from an unusually wide vault (Fig. 10.52) and the edges approximated. The cul-de-

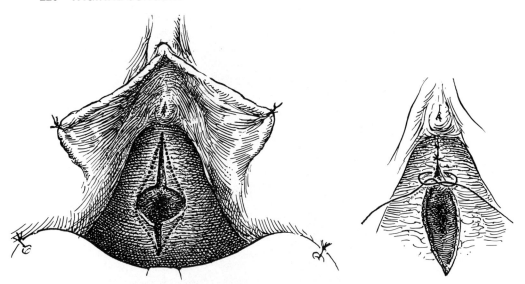

**Figure 10.46.** Before closing the vault of the vagina in a longitudinal direction, it can be narrowed, when desired, by excision of small wedges of tissue of a size as indicated by the *dotted lines,* converting the T-shaped incisions to a V shape, trimming only enough vaginal wall as to leave vaginal flaps that can be closed with subepithelial sutures without tension, everting the edges so as to avoid irregular overlapping or pockets of inverted epithelium.

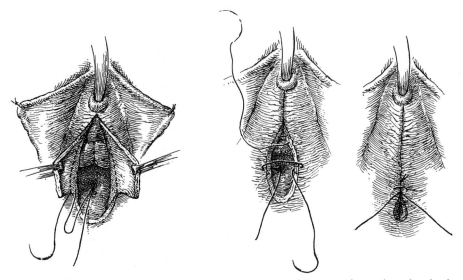

**Figure 10.47.** The amount of vagina to be removed by anterior colporrhaphy is shown by the *dotted lines*. One end of the tied peritoneal closure stitch is passed through each side of the vault of the anterior vaginal wall as shown. The anterior colporrhaphy is completed, and the peritoneal closure stitch end is tied, bringing the anterior vaginal wall to the site of the previous peritoneal closure, lengthening the anterior vaginal wall.

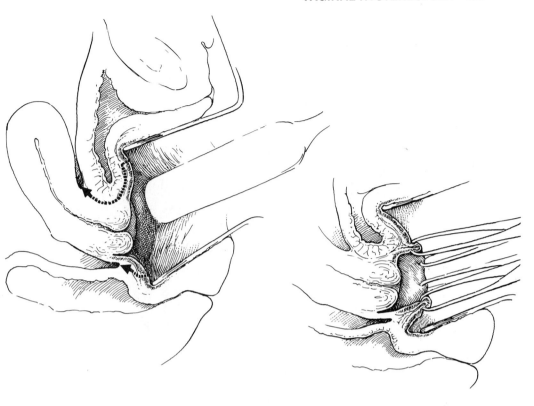

**Figure 10.54.** Partial vaginectomy with hysterectomy is depicted. The vagina and cervix are carefully exposed and thoroughly examined, and the amount of vagina to be removed with the specimen is determined with precision. The lines of proposed dissection are shown in the sagittal drawing on the *left*. Infiltration here by 1:200,000 adrenaline in 0.5% Xylocaine solution aids hemostasis and the later identification of the connective tissue planes and spaces. Distal to this point the vagina is grasped circumferentially by a series of single-toothed tenacula as seen on the *right*.

When the vagina after hysterectomy seems too short for marital comfort, anterior and/or posterior colporrhaphy can be performed if required and the Schuchardt incision closed. A sheath of mobilized peritoneum can be sewn to the distal cut edge of the vagina and the peritoneal cavity closed cranially (Fig. 10.57). An obturator should be worn postoperatively during the period of vaginal re-epithelialization. Distal length can be added by using the Williams vulvovaginoplasty (see Chapter 20), or a perineorrhaphy (see Chapter 21) if the perineum is deficient.

## A PLACE FOR THE SCHAUTA RADICAL VAGINAL HYSTERECTOMY

Despite the interest and efforts of enthusiastic American exponents (McCall, Barclay, Smale, and Crisp), the Schauta-Amreich radical vaginal hysterectomy is not often performed in most American clinics. As a result few are teaching this interesting operation. In Europe many of those accomplished in its technique are no longer in practice (Bastiaanse, Amreich, Mitra, Ingiulla,

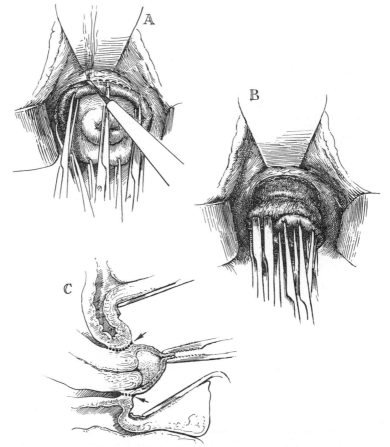

**Figure 10.55.** Partial vaginectomy with hysterectomy. Traction is applied to the tenacula and against countertraction supplied by the retractors. An incision is made by electrosurgical knife, scissors, or scalpel through the full thickness of the vagina *(A)*. The vagina is inverted as a sleeve over the cervix. An alcohol-soaked sponge is applied against the face of the cervix, the single-toothed tenacula are removed, and the anterior and posterior walls of the vagina are brought together by a series of Krobach mouse-toothed clamps, straight Kocher hemostats, or heavy sutures *(B)*. Sagittal section *(C)* further illustrates the line of sharp dissection to be followed to gain both anterior and posterior entry to the peritoneal cavity.

Navratil, and Tapfer). The operation has been kept very much alive, however, by Novak (25) of Yugoslavia, Reiffenstuhl (29) of Austria, and Carenza and Villani (6, 7) of Italy, among others.

At the present time Carenza considers the operation of benefit to individuals with earlier stages of invasive squamous cell carcinoma of the cervix (IA, IB, IIA) with negative lymphography. We occasionally find the operation suitable for the young patient in whom it is desirable to preserve ovarian function, for the very obese patient in whom exposure to the radical abdominal hysterectomy might be difficult, for the patient at high medical risk who cannot take a prolonged or deep general anesthetic, and for the patient with genital prolapse and a large and symptomatic cystocele and rectocele. In situ carcinomas of the cervix are better treated, when hysterectomy is desired, by simple total

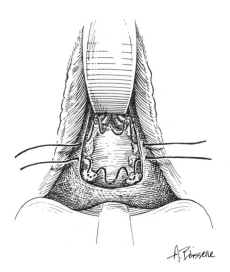

**Figure 10.56.** When there has been no coincident prolapse of the vaginal vault, depth may be preserved by closure from side to side as suggested by Durfee. A stitch of polyglycolic acid-type suture is passed through the full thickness of the lateral vaginal wall, the round ligament portion of the adnexal pedicle, a reefing of the anterior peritoneum, and the same structures in reverse order on the opposite side. A second stitch is placed through the full thickness of the posterolateral vaginal wall, the uterosacral ligament stump, a reefing of the posterior peritoneum, and the same structures in reverse order on the opposite side. Any gaps in the vaginal wall may be closed by interrupted sutures.

abdominal or vaginal hysterectomy, with the removal of an appropriate cuff of vagina if there is vaginal involvement by the tumor.

Radical vaginal hysterectomy is limited to those patients in whom careful preoperative study of biopsy or conization material indicates no evidence of lymphatic or vascular invasion. No matter how small the primary lesion, the likelihood of metastases should be inferred in those persons showing evidence of vascular or lymphatic invasion or penetration.

Evidence of actual or potential vascular involvement requires transabdominal lymphadenectomy as part of the initial surgical procedure. Negative preoperative lymphadenography is helpful, and detailed microscopic examination of the hysterectomy specimen postoperatively should include specific attention to recognition of any previously undisclosed evidences of lymphatic or vascular penetration. Should this be found, the patient must be given surgical pelvic lymphadenectomy or appropriate deep x-ray therapy to the pelvic lymph nodes. Postoperative endolymphatic therapy with radioactive isotopes is an attractive consideration but is of unproven value. Nodes whose

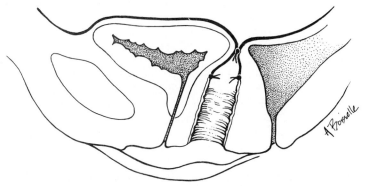

**Figure 10.57.** Proximal length can be added to a shortened vagina by attaching its cut edges to the margins of previously freed peritoneal flaps (8). The peritoneal cavity is securely closed by a separate cranially placed suture, as shown.

lymphatic pathways are totally obstructed by tumor might fail to receive the necessary radiation, although it is quite likely that adequate cancerocidal dosage can be delivered by this route to nodes partially infiltrated by metastatic disease and, quite possibly, to similarly involved lymph nodes that are surgically inaccessible.

Controversy concerning the importance of lymphadenectomy persists, although generally held present opinion favors lymphadenectomy. The possibility remains, however, that even when involved with early metastases the lymphatic system may play a protective role in the body's immunologic defense and the patient's survival against the propagation of a neoplasm. The possible importance of this factor continues to be emphasized by Crisp (8), echoing the convictions of Högler (12).

It is likely that the radical vaginal operation makes it possible to remove a greater amount of parametrium than is likely from the abdominal approach, but it is conjectural as to whether this will, in fact, provide a better prognosis. The radical vaginal hysterectomy also permits the removal of a predetermined amount of vagina or vaginal cuff at the time of the original operative procedure and under the direct vision and control of the operator. The exact amount of vagina to be removed should be determined by preoperative colposcopy and colposcopically directed biopsy and further demarcated by staining of the vagina with iodine solution at the time of surgery before the incision is placed in the vagina. In the hands of an experienced gynecologic surgeon the operation appears to be associated with a lower incidence of serious complications, particularly urinary fistulae, than does the abdominal counterpart.

At the present time we believe that for those women in whom vascular or lymphatic penetration has been established preoperatively by biopsy study or lymphography, certain advantages of a combined abdominovaginal hysterocolpectomy, including lymphadenectomy, can be seriously considered. The vaginal portion of the operation permits the widest possible excision of parametrium, rectal pillars, and uterosacral ligaments, and the abdominal lymphadenectomy, either extraperitoneal or intraperitoneal, completes the procedure. It would seem advisable, therefore, to plan an operative procedure that would combine the best features of both the abdominal and the vaginal operations into a single or composite operative procedure, which in the interests of shorter operating time, the patient's safety, and surgical efficiency might be accomplished by the simultaneous use of two operating teams.

There are several advantages of the radical-vaginal portion of the composite operation. Initial staining of the vagina with iodine assures that all of the vaginal tissues that might be involved will be removed with the cervix. The vaginal approach also assures vastly improved dissection of the paracolpium, the inferior portion of the horizontal connective tissue ground bundle, the inferior portion of the rectal pillars, and the vesicouterine ligaments. Ureteral exposure and dissection can best be accomplished during the vaginal portion of the operation. Meanwhile, through an appropriate incision, the abdominal team will have begun the bilateral extraperitoneal or intraperitoneal lymphadenectomy, which may be completed while the vaginal team is closing the Schuchardt incision. Combined synchronous operation has been reported by Mitra (23), Navratil (24), Howkins (13), and Vidakovic (32), among others, in various sequential modifications. The combined operation should be of particular value for those in whom vascular or lymphatic penetration has been established preoperatively by biopsy study or lymphography. However, it remains to be seen whether such a combined operation will provide an improved prognosis.

The technique of the Schauta-Amreich radical vaginal hysterectomy may be outlined as follows, including modifications of Novak, Carenza, and Barclay, which are concerned particularly with exposure of the ureter in the bladder pillar.

### Technique of the Radical Vaginal Operation

The perineal tissues to be incised by the Schuchardt approach and the vaginal tissues at the site of vaginal circumcision are thoroughly infiltrated by 0.5% lidocaine (Xylocaine) in 1:200,000 epinephrine (Adrenalin) solution (Fig. 10.58). When this has been thoroughly dispersed in the tissue to be incised, a Schuchardt incision is performed. The vagina is grasped in a circumferential fashion by a series of single-toothed forceps and is circumcised using either the cold scalpel or the electrosurgical unit (Figs. 10.59 and 10.60). The single-toothed tenacula are replaced with Krobach mouse-toothed clamps (Fig. 10.61), and by sharp and blunt dissection both anterior and posterior cul-de-sacs are exposed (Figs. 10.62 and 10.63). The left paravesical space is entered, and the ureter is palpated (Figs. 10.64 and 10.65). As Högler (12) has pointed out, the larger any cystocele, the greater the interureteric distance and the more lateral the location of the ureters.

The ureter is palpated in the bladder pillar between fingers placed in the paravesical space and a finger inserted in the vesicovaginal space. The "bladder pillar" is incised along its lateral edge, superficial to the ureter (Fig. 10.65), and the ureter is exposed. Skeletonization and ligation of the left uterine artery are accomplished (Fig. 10.66). The right paravesical space is developed, followed by identification (Fig. 10.67) and exposure of the right ureter and skeletonization and ligation of the right uterine artery. The bladder pillar is cut from the cardinal ligament at an appropriate spot. The cul-de-sac of Douglas is opened and the abdominal contents thoroughly and effectively displaced by an intraperitoneal pack. The peritoneum is carefully dissected from the medial side of the rectal pillar (Fig. 10.68), each rectal pillar is carefully cut from its

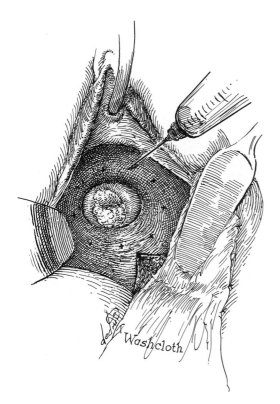

**Figure 10.58.** The Schauta radical vaginal hysterectomy is shown. A Schuchardt incision has been made and a gauze pack temporarily sewn into the incision. The vagina is being infiltrated by 0.5% lidocaine in 1:200,000 epinephrine solution. The *small crosses* mark the site of each needle penetration.

Washcloth

**Figure 10.59.** The circumference of the vagina has been grasped with single-toothed tenacula and an incision made directly into the vesicovaginal space.

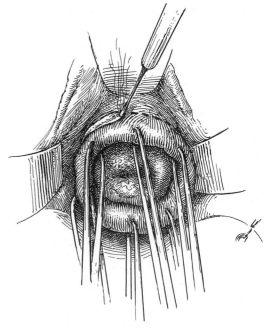

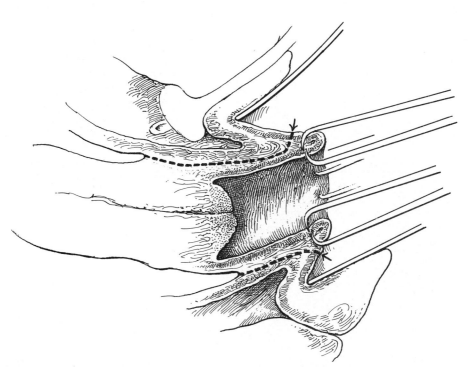

**Figure 10.60.** A sagittal view shows the cuff of vagina held by single-toothed tenacula. The pathway of incision and dissection is shown by the *broken line*.

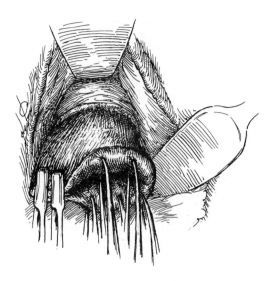

**Figure 10.61.** The single-toothed tenacula are replaced with Krobach mouse-toothed forceps.

attachment to the rectum, and each uterosacral ligament is divided. The anterior peritoneal cul-de-sac is opened, and appropriate retractors are inserted. Each cardinal ligament is clamped and cut close to the pelvic sidewall (Fig. 10.69), and the adnexa are examined and excised if necessary. Each broad and round ligament is clamped and cut, and the specimen is removed from the operative field. The peritoneum is closed, and the exposed undersurface of the bladder is reduced in size by raphing or gathering in a series of transversely placed interrupted mattress stitches, the lateral ones of which cover the ureter at the ureterovesical unction, burying this junction in a fold of the bladder wall. If a cystocele is present, the remainder of the anterior vaginal wall is incised in the midline to expose the urethrovesical unction. An anterior colporrhaphy with pubourethral ligament plication stitches (Fig. 11.16), with or without Kelly stitches (Fig. 11.13), is performed, and packing is introduced into the para-

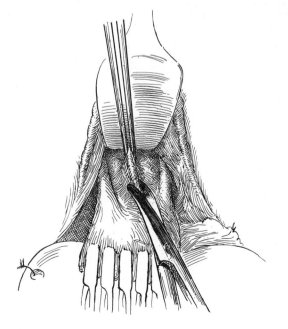

**Figure 10.62.** The connective tissue septum between bladder and cervix is cut by sharp dissection.

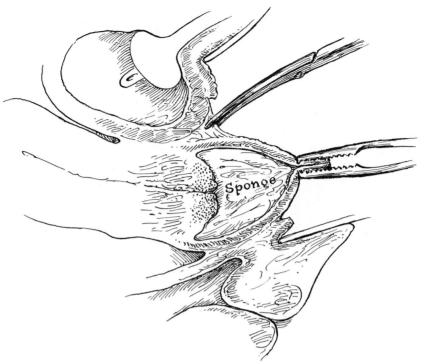

**Figure 10.63.** A sagittal view shows sharp dissection of the connective tissue beneath bladder and cervix. The handles of the scissors are elevated, directing the incision away from the bladder.

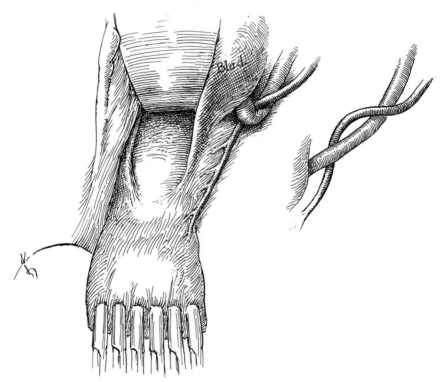

**Figure 10.64.** A phantom view shows the relationship between the ureter, bladder *(Blad)*, and uterine artery. When downward traction is applied *(left)*, the uterine artery brings with it the "knee" of the ureter. The relationship without traction is shown to the *right*.

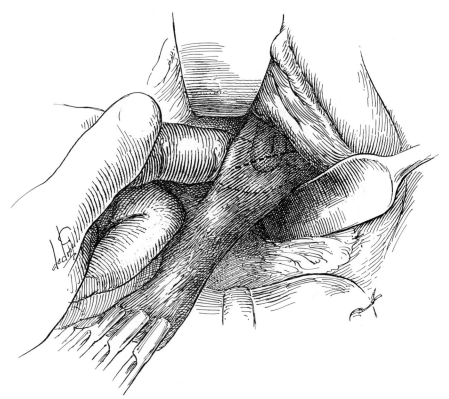

**Figure 10.65.** The paravesical and vesicovaginal spaces have been opened, and the ureter is palpated within the bladder pillar on the patient's left. An incision is made in the lateral margin of the bladder pillar along the side of the *broken line*.

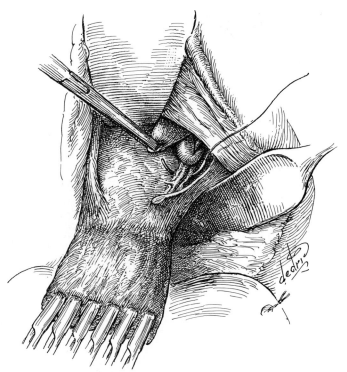

**Figure 10.66.** The left ureter has been exposed in the bladder pillar and the uterine artery skeletonized, preparatory to its ligation.

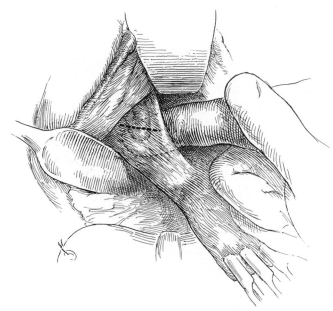

**Figure 10.67.** The right ureter is palpated and the bladder pillar will be incised in its lateral margin as shown by the *broken line*.

**Figure 10.68.** Both anterior and posterior cul-de-sacs have been opened. The peritoneum medial to the left rectal pillar is dissected free, in preparation for ligation of the pillar close to the rectum.

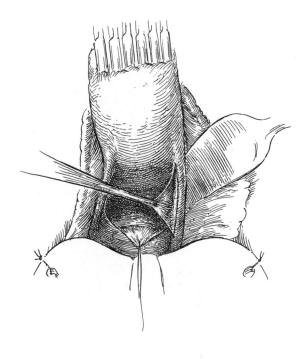

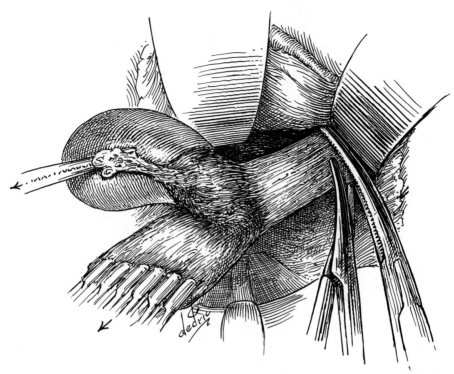

**Figure 10.69.** The uterine fundus has been brought through the anterior peritoneal opening and the vaginal cuff and cervix drawn sharply down, as shown. The cardinal ligament (parametrium) has been clamped close to the pelvic sidewall and will be cut free, as shown, first on one side and then on the other. The peritoneum will then be approximated and the Schuchardt incision closed.

rectal-paravesical spaces on each side. To aid in the preservation of vaginal length postoperatively, the cut edge of the vagina at its new vault may be sewn to the peritoneum by a series of interrupted sutures distal to its closure (Fig. 10.57). The Schuchardt incision is closed.

### References

1. Allen E: Discussion. *Am J Obstet Gynecol* 61A(Suppl):219, 1951.
2. Bandler SW: *Vaginal Celiotomy*. Philadelphia, WB Saunders, 1911.
3. Burnett L: Personal communication, 1987.
4. Candiani GB, Ferrari AG: *Isterectomia Vaginale*. Milano, Masson, 1986.
5. Capen CV, Irwin H, Magrina J, et al: Vaginal Removal of the Ovaries in Association with Vaginal Hysterectomy. *J Reprod Med* 28:589–591, 1983.
6. Carenza L: Attuali indicazioni alla colpoisterectomia allargata nel trattamento del cervico-carcinoma. *Patol Clin Obstet Ginecol* 1:3–8, 1973.
7. Carenza L, Villani C: Schauta radical vaginal hysterectomy. *Clin Obstet Gynecol* 25:913–937, 1982.
8. Crisp WE: The Schauta operation. *Obstet Gynecol* 33:453, 1969.
9. England GT, Randall HW, Graves WL: Impairment of tissue defenses by vasoconstrictors in vaginal hysterectomies. *Obstet Gynecol* 61:271–274, 1983.
10. Gitsch E, Palmrich AH: *Gynecological Operative Anatomy*. Berlin, Walter de Gruyter, p 9, 1977.
11. Gray LA: *Vaginal Hysterectomy*. Springfield, Charles C Thomas, pp 36–41, ed 3, 1983.
12. Högler H: *Schauta-Amreich's Radical Vaginal Operation of Cancer of the Cervix*. Springfield, Charles C Thomas, 1963.
13. Howkins J: Synchronous combined abdomino-vaginal hysterocolpectomy for cancer of the cervix-a report of fifty patients. *J Obstet Gynaecol Br Emp* 66:212–219, 1959.
14. Inmon WB: Pelvic relaxation and repair

including prolapse of vagina following hysterectomy. *South Med J* 56:577, 1963.

15. Janisch H, Palmrich AH, Pecherstorfer M: *Selected Urologic Operations in Gynecology*. Berlin, Walter de Gruyter, p 7, 1979.

16. Jaszczak SE, Evans TN: Vaginal morphology following hysterectomy. *Int J Gynecol Obstet* 19:41–51, 1981.

17. Käser O, Iklé FA, Hirsch HH: *Atlas of Gynecologic Surgery*. New York, Thieme-Stratton, ed 2, p 1220, 1985.

18. Krige CF: *Vaginal Hysterectomy and Genital Prolapse Repair*. Johannesburg, Witwatersrand University Press, 1965.

19. Malpas P: The choice of operation for genital prolapse. In Meigs JV, Sturgis SH (eds): *Progress in Gynecology*. New York, Grune & Stratton, vol 3, p 671, 1957.

20. Malpas P: Genital prolapse. In Claye A, Bourne A (eds): *British Obstetric and Gynaecological Practice*. London, William Heinemann, ed 3, p 655, 1963.

21. Mattingly RF, Huang WY: Steroidogenesis of the menopausal and postmenopausal ovary. *Am J Obstet Gynecol* 103:679–693, 1969.

22. McCall ML: Posterior culdeplasty: surgical correction of enterocele during vaginal hysterectomy: a preliminary report. *Obstet Gynecol* 10:595, 1957.

23. Mitra S: *Mitra Operation for Cancer of the Cervix*. Springfield, Charles C Thomas, 1960.

24. Navratil E: Radical vaginal hysterectomy (Schauta-Amreich operation). *Clin Obstet Gynecol* 8:676, 1965.

25. Novak F: *Surgical Gynecologic Techniques*. New York, John Wiley & Sons, 1978.

26. Philipp K: Ergebnisse der routinemaBigen entfernung der Ovarien und/oder Tuben im Rahmen der vaginalen Hysterektomie. *Geburtshilfe Frauenheikd* 40:159, 1980.

27. Pratt JH: Technique of vaginal hysterectomy. *Clin Obstet Gynecol* 2:1125, 1959.

28. Randall CL: The risks of gynecologic malignancies in older women. *Clin Obstet Gynecol* 7:545–557, 1964.

29. Reiffenstuhl G, Platzer W: *Atlas of Vaginal Surgery*. Philadelphia, WB Saunders, 1975.

30. Robinson RW, Cohen WD, Higano N: Estrogen replacement therapy in women with coronary atherosclerosis. *Ann Intern Med* 48:95–101, 1958.

31. Thompson JD, Lyon JB: Vaginal hysterectomy. *Clin Obstet Gynecol* 9:1033, 1964.

32. Vidakovic S: The vagino-abdominal approach to the extended operation. *Arch Gynakol* 186:420, 1955.

33. Werner P, Sederl J: *Abdominal Operations by the Vaginal Route*. Phildelphia, JB Lippincott, 1958.

# CHAPTER 11

# Anterior Colporrhaphy

Cystocele is primarily a consequence of damage to the vagina—either its supports or the vaginal wall itself. The primary site for reconstructive surgery at this site must therefore be directed to the vagina.

The urethra is maintained in position by two anatomic systems including suspension by the pubourethral "ligament" portion of the urogenital diaphragm and support by the vaginal wall and its attachments (see Chapter 1). Damage to either or both systems may alter its pelvic location and affect its function.

The bladder itself, on the other hand, is not effectively suspended but is intact, supported by the vagina and its attachments. The supports of the bladder causing cystocele are affected by damage to the vaginal wall itself, or the connective tissue to which the vagina is attached, or both.

It is a responsibility of the reconstructive surgeon to determine the specific sites and causes of damage for each patient as a part of determining a course of surgical action.

In preoperative patients, evaluation of the presence or absence of urinary stress incontinence generally denotes damage to the anterior genital segment. Inasmuch as various types of incontinence are often mixed, it is important to determine which particular components apply to a particular patient—whether the problem is primarily one of stress, overflow, urge incontinence, or a combination of these etiologic factors. A proper diagnosis is required for the identification and selection of an appropriate surgical remedy.

## TYPES AND ETIOLOGY OF CYSTOCELE

In examination and evaluation of the anterior wall (Fig. 11.1), the observer should have in mind that there are distinct types of cystocele that may be present. Cystocele has been described according to whether it is anterior to the interureteric ridge (anterior cystocele) or posterior to it (posterior cystocele) (3). Either or both conditions may exist and must be recognized and corrected if surgery is to be effective.

First, there may be only an anterior cystocele (pseudocystocele or "urethrocele"), in which situation a straining effort results in downward bulging or rotational descent of the urethra with or without a demonstrable tendency of the bladder to herniate behind the vesicourethral junction. The lower third of the anterior vaginal wall underlies the urethra. There is separation of the urethra from the urogenital diaphragm and the pubourethral "ligament" portion of the urogenital diaphragm that binds it to the pubis, or separation of the vagina from its intermediate connective tissue attachment to the arcus tendineus may permit rotational descent of the urethra with or without actual herniation of the bladder behind the vesicourethral junction. The rotational descent of the vesicourethral junction may be of varying degrees and is often associated with urinary stress incontinence.

With anterior cystocele (pseudocystocele or pseudourethrocele) the diameter of the urethra is unchanged (Fig. 11.2) except at its proximal end where it

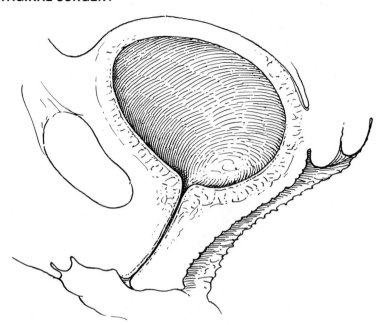

**Figure 11.1.**   The sagittal view of normal vesicourethral relationships is shown. Filling of the normally supported bladder has little or no effect upon the contour of its base.

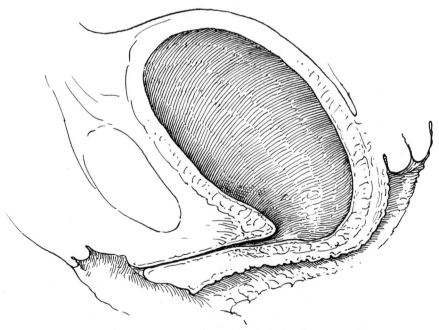

**Figure 11.2.**   Rotational descent of the vesicourethral junction is illustrated. Note the loss or straightening of the posterior urethrovesical angle.

## OBJECTIVES OF ANTERIOR COLPORRHAPHY

Considering the indications for repair, a well-informed gynecologist will first correlate the anterior vaginal wall damage with the patient's symptoms. He or she must consider the patient's history and carefully check for evidence of coexistent prolapse of the uterus, vaginal vault, enterocele, or rectum. Examination of the patient who is standing and bearing down will make this evident. It is also important to take into account a history of previous urinary stress incontinence that may have been relieved as the prolapse progressed, as emphasized by Symmonds and Jordan (31). The supports of the urethra, even though attenuated, may have more strength than those of the bladder due to their continuity with the urogenital diaphragm. Predictably, advanced progression of the bladder descent usually exceeds the accompanying urethral descent, resulting in an angulation or kinking of the urethra at its junction with the bladder. When a large cystocele is present, increases in intra-abdominal and intravesical pressure will be transmitted more to the dependent portion of the cystocele than to the attenuated vesicourethral junction. Hodgkinson (14) observed that within the bladder the hydrostatic pressure is always greater at the bottom of this column of water than midway up or at the top. This tendency, of course, is aggravated in the presence of a coexistent defect of the posterior vaginal wall. When there is no firm tissue layer beneath the sagging bladder, its elasticity when filling is relatively unrestrained by the absence of adequate posterior vaginal or perineal support.

## CHOICE OF OPERATION

The gynecologist must be mindful of the future functions and strains to which an anterior vaginal wall may be subjected—not only coitus, but future pregnancy and parturition, and not infrequently coincident heavy physical work. All of these factors must be correlated with current findings that may themselves be partially the result of earlier attempts at surgical repair. In particular, allowances must also be made for the atrophic changes that have occurred or are to be expected after the patient's menopause.

## RECURRENT CYSTOCELE

If a cystocele has recurred after an initial repair, the gynecologist contemplating another operation must first try to determine the reason for the unsatisfactory result after the earlier surgery. He should review the hospital surgical record of the previous operation and relate the earlier procedure with the current findings and then to the technique and suture choices now under consideration for this particular patient.

During the physical examination the gynecologist should check the position of the vaginal vault when the patient is standing and bearing down as by a Valsalva maneuver. This will disclose a coincident partial eversion of the vaginal vault, bringing the bladder with it.

When anterior sulci are absent, one should examine the patient for lateral detachment of the urethral paravaginal tissues. Baden and Walker (2) suggest that this can be suspected in a patient with relaxation of the anterior vaginal wall. When such a patient is instructed to tightly squeeze the pelvic muscles, a "holding" position, there is no response producing elevation of the anterior vaginal wall, suggesting that the connective tissue and vascular supports of the anterior vaginal wall have been detached from the arcus tendineus. The vagina is not attached directly to the arcus tendineus (5, 26, 34). The anterior vaginal fornix is attached to the arcus tendineus by a meshwork of intervening connective tissue (see Chapter 1) that may sustain various strains and stretching, or even unilateral or bilateral partial avulsion. This is usually a consequence of trauma from labor and delivery and is therefore seen more likely in parous patients. It may also be related to lifestyle and on occasion follow the pull of massive vaginal eversion, even in the nullipara. Therefore, *direct* surgical attachment of the vaginal fornix to the arcus tendineus (5, 28, 35, 36) may compensate and to some extent correct the widening of the anterior vaginal wall as seen with certain types of cystocele. Bilateral attachment is generally necessary when stretching or avulsion of the lateral supports is the cause of cystocele as suggested first by White (35). In our opinion, significant midline defects of the vaginal wall are much more common and will be remedied by the standard midline plications and colporrhaphy as will be described. Existence or coexistence of the less common lateral defects should be determined preoperatively for appropriate planning of surgical technique. It is essential to determine and surgically remedy any coincident prolapse of the vaginal vault that may be found. One should observe the presence and extent of rugae on the patient's anterior vaginal wall and compare them with those on the lateral vaginal walls. Rugae of comparable size in both sites suggest displacement cystocele, whereas diminished rugae on the anterior wall in the presence of good rugae on the lateral walls suggest distention cystocele. The surgeon must be certain to identify the etiology of recurrent cystocele as from either displacement, overdistention, or a combination of the two, with demonstrable defects in either the midline supporting structures, the lateral supporting structures, or both, and note the relationship of the cystocele to the urethrovesical junction or urogenital diaphragm.

Usually, there is little but a surgeon's ego to warrant consideration of repeating the same operative technique. It is probable that the initial repair was technically correct but inappropriately selected. The well-informed and responsible gynecologic surgeon, acquainted with the significant modifications of dependable operative procedures, will choose the best operation for a particular patient's problem. If an adequate operative procedure is completed in a technically correct manner, the operator's knowledge and skill should be rewarded with significantly few instances of postoperative recurrence.

The gynecologic surgeon should ever be alert to the possible correlation between postmenopausal bladder urgency and the probability of an atrophic "urethritis and trigonitis." Postmenopausal atrophic changes result in a significant thinning of the epithelial and subepithelial layers of the urethra and the bladder trigone, with a resultant oversusceptibility to stimulation and irritation. When this can be demonstrated or is even suspected, the patient is likely to benefit at least symptomatically and promptly from adequate estrogen replacement therapy. When a positive response is obtained, further consideration of the need for surgical repair should be deferred for a month or two until the beneficial results and symptomatology have stabilized and can be re-evaluated.

## ASYMPTOMATIC CYSTOCELE

There is very little to be said in favor of operating upon an asymptomatic cystocele unless it is coincident with other pelvic repair indicated for other reasons, or unless the gynecologist has observed over a period of time an unmistakable evidence of progression in the demonstrable protrusion of the vagina. Within limitations, the more advanced the progression of cystocele, the larger it becomes, the more complicated will be its repair, and the less certain will be the restoration of perfect bladder function, as there may be some permanent impairment of a properly balanced nerve supply. The desirability of appreciating a symptomatic progression is a primary advantage of re-examination by the same observer over a period of years. The individual observer can detect evidence of progression to a degree indicating need for operative repair and can make that recommendation before the patient's age precludes elective surgery because of increased medical risks. The examiner should record his or her impression of the size of the lesion in a manner permitting reliable comparison with the findings on subsequent re-examinations.

Appraisal of postmenopausal atrophy can often be determined by the degree of vaginal cornification demonstrable on cytologic examination. This index should at least roughly correlate with the persistence or absence of lateral wall rugal folds. If little cornification is present, an estrogen deficiency should be evident. The extent to which this is relevant should be estimated, and thought should be given to the desirability of estrogen replacement.

The gynecologic surgeon should be expected to know in detail the anatomy involved, the techniques of the recommended variations of anterior colporrha-phy, and the indications for possible modifications of one's usual techniques. Only with such information in mind will the operator maintain sufficient technical flexibility to assure accomplishment of the objectives recognized before surgery.

Once the gynecologist and patient have decided that the surgery is indicated, a primary objective is the restoration of normal anatomic relationships, with attention to contributing etiologic factors, all in a conscious effort to lessen the chances of recurrence in later years.

## TECHNIQUES OF COLPORRHAPHY

Many operations designed to restore a defective posterior urethrovesical angle will elevate the proximal urethra to a position once again responsive to changes in intra-abdominal pressure. It is only when these surgical changes affect the proximal urethra as well as the bladder that a significant aid to continence will have been restored (15).

The techniques for dissection and repair of the anterior vaginal wall must be varied, depending on many factors, including the presence of vaginal telescop-ing or coexistent vault eversion. The patient with a short vagina due to telescoping must be considered a candidate for its surgical lengthening by such an appropriate coincident procedure as vaginal hysterectomy or a Manchester operation, by shortening of the cardinal or uterosacral supports, by a trans-vaginal sacrospinous colpopexy, or by transabdominal sacrocolpopexy. Resto-ration of vaginal depth by bringing the vagina with bladder back into the pelvis is the essence of surgical treatment for the displacement type of cystocele. In procidentia, as defined by Ricci and Thom (27), the entire uterus is displaced and protrudes outside the pelvis. As a rule, the vagina is completely everted and an enterocele is present, but rectocele may be minimal or secondary. The displacement is greatest and most apparent in relation to the anterior vaginal wall and cervix, because the supporting vaginal and uterine portions of the cardinal ligaments have become markedly elongated and often attenuated. Because the anterior vaginal wall and cervix are attached by continuity to each other and to the pelvic sidewalls, they function as an anatomic unit. With massive prolapse, both suffer severe circulatory changes, not only as a result of stasis due to compression against the sides of the genital hiatus, but also congestion aggravated by gravity. The resulting degree of chronic congestion apparently stimulates significant lymphangiectasia that, in turn, stimulates considerable fibroblastic proliferation within the anterior vaginal wall. Chronic edema is followed by hypertrophy and fibrosis that thicken the anterior vaginal wall. With advancing years these tissues elongate and "sag" noticeably because they are deficient and defective in other components, especially elastic tissue. The gynecologist will want to mobilize the full thickness of the anterior vaginal wall, including epithelium and the underlying fibromuscular connective tissue layer, and can enter the desired plane most readily by opening directly into the vesicovaginal space (30).

The gynecologic surgeon should enter the proper pelvic spaces by sharp dissection. Development of the spaces by blunt dissection is used safely only after they have been entered. If dissection has been initiated in the wrong plane, it takes longer to locate the correct plane than to have found it correctly the first time. This direct approach to the vesicovaginal space is equally useful when initiating anterior colporrhaphy when a cystocele is to be repaired without coincident hysterectomy or cervical amputation, or in a patient in whom there has been previous hysterectomy or cervical amputation. A useful technique was described by Ricci and Thom (27):

"The anterior vaginal wall is placed on moderate tension by grasping each lip of the cervix with short tenacula and pulling the prolapsed vagina completely outward and downward. That part of the anterior vaginal wall above the point of fusion above the cervix is rolled or massaged between the index finger and thumb several times to accentuate planes of separation between bladder and cervix and vaginal wall. At the point where the fusion between the vaginal wall and the cervix ends and the avascular space begins, smooth and lacking in rugae, and usually about ¾ inch above the orifice of the cervix, the reduplicated layers of the entire thickness of the vaginal wall are grasped between two Allis clamps. The full thickness of the vaginal wall is cut between these two instruments with a curved scissors, the tip of the scissors pointing perpendicular to the axis of the cervix, exposing an avascular space and bringing the bladder musculature into view (Fig. 11.7). The cut surfaces of the vaginal wall are grasped with Allis clamps, and with a straight scissors the vaginal wall is cut upward exactly in midline. This incision is continued to the urethrovaginal junction where the cleavage plane ends. The bladder wall is displaced from both lateral flaps of the incised vaginal wall and cut from the cervix, exposing the vesicouterine peritoneal fold, which may be incised, the index finger introduced, and the pelvis explored."

Cystocele is commonly associated with a degree of uterine prolapse less than procidentia. A transurethral Foley catheter is inserted, and the bladder is emptied. Incision into the avascular space through the full thickness of the anterior vaginal wall may be accomplished alternately by an inverted T-shaped incision at the point where the vagina meets the cervix. The midpoint of the anterior vaginal cuff incision is grasped between two forceps and incised exactly in the midline and directly into the avascular vesicovaginal space. The incision is then carried superiorly to the point of fusion of urethra with vagina.

If any resistance to the passage of the catheter is noted, a urethral stricture should be suspected. In such a circumstance one must be careful to avoid urethral plication at this point, making the stricture worse. In fact, one might well dilate such a urethra while the patient is still asleep in the operating room. If the patient is postmenopausal, postoperative vaginal estrogens may be of considerable help in reversing the effects of atrophy.

The remainder of the suburethral anterior vaginal wall is incised in the midline to within 1 or 1½ cm of the external urethral meatus. The degree of bolstering of the vesicourethral unction will be determined by the extent of the earlier damage to the supports of the vesicourethral junction, the degree of attenuation, and the relative integrity of the tissue available for plication.

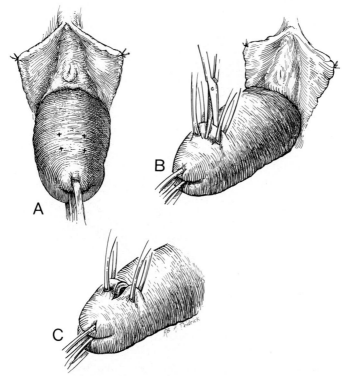

**Figure 11.7.** A procidentia is noted in *(A)*, and the points to be included within the grasp of the Allis clamps are noted by the *small crosses*. They overlie the vesicovaginal space that separates the bladder from the thickened anterior vaginal wall that is incised by the scissors placed perpendicular to its surface *(B)*, opening directly into the vesicovaginal space as seen in *(C)*.

In the performance of anterior colporrhaphy, the surgeon should reconstruct the full length of the anterior vaginal wall, including the vesicourethral junction and the supports of the urethra. This reconstruction will involve separating the urogenital diaphragm from the vagina and, after its plication, reattaching it to the vagina. This may be associated occasionally with some temporary postoperative difficulty in voiding. This is far preferable to an occasional iatrogenic urinary stress incontinence from having straightened out the neck of the bladder and obliterated the urethrovesical angle (Fig. 11.8). One must be mindful that the patient is being operated upon in the lithotomy position and under anesthesia. The different tissue relationships that will prevail when the postoperative patient is conscious and standing must be thoughtfully judged. Vulnerability to urinary continence is greatest when the fully conscious patient is in the standing position.

Surgical repair of a large hypotonic "decompensated" cystocele probably restores some intravesical pressure, lowering the incontinence. Surgical support of the vesicourethral junction should strengthen the anatomic and physiologic factors favoring postoperative continence.

By sharp dissection, using either scissors or scalpel according to the preference of the operator, the full thickness of the anterior vaginal wall should be separated from the bladder laterally and anteriorly as far as the lateral limits of the vesicovaginal space, sometimes almost to the pubic rami, in a line of cleavage that preserves the attachment between the subepithelial fibromuscular

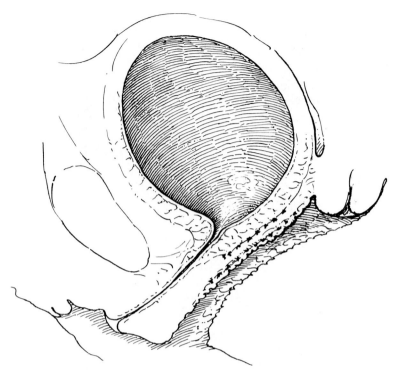

**Figure 11.8.** Overcorrection of cystocele has straightened the vesicourethral angle.

connective tissue layer and the vaginal epithelium. As the dissection proceeds laterally, it is often possible to free up a possibly incomplete but identifiable musculoconnective tissue between the connective tissue left attached to the vaginal epithelium and independent of the predominantly musculature layer of the bladder wall. Hopefully, such lines of cleavage can be established without compromising the blood supply of these supporting tissues, but greatest care must be taken to open along tissue planes and not simply slice tissue into arbitrary layers at the expense of tissue planes that usually harbor blood supply (Fig. 11.9).

A simpler technique that does not dissect and thereby disturb the vaginal blood supply leaves the entire thickness of the vaginal wall unsplit and retains the attachment of all musculoconnective tissue to the vaginal epithelium. A most carefully measured ovoid or wedge of the redundant *full thickness* but thinned vaginal wall is excised (30). Unless the entire full thickness of the anterior vaginal wall has been correctly mobilized, an excision of the superficial epithelial layer alone could be as inadequate an operative procedure as to treat an inguinal hernia by simple excision of an ellipse of overlying skin without having reduced the hernia, excised the sac, and adequately repaired the underlying thinned tissues accounting for the defect.

In most instances the fibromuscular connective tissue capsule of the bladder itself should be narrowed by plication with a running locked 2-0 polyglycolic acid-type suture that extends from the connective tissue capsule at the vault of the vagina all the way to the urogenital diaphragm.

A most common error in the technique of anterior colporrhaphy is illustrated in Figure 11.9, bottom row: the vaginal epithelium has been separated from the fibromuscular layer of the vagina, but the vesicovaginal space has not been

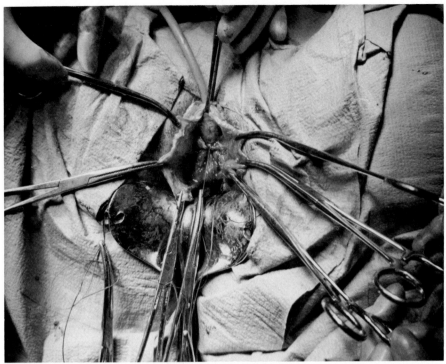

**Figure 11.19.** Tying of the stitches shown in Figure 11.17 is photographed.

stitches are placed in the periurethral supporting tissues, they may in addition to correction of funneling, unintentionally approximate the paraurethral portions of the posterior pubourethral ligaments. Pubourethral ligament sutures, on the other hand, being placed more laterally, are inserted directly into the urethral attachment of the posterior pubourethral ligament portion of the urogenital diaphragm, as noted by Halban (13) and Martius (19). This placement seems to explain our greater degree of success with this procedure.

Because the optimal place for the use of Kelly plication stitches is in the presence of funneling or vesicalization of the urethra and bladder neck, there are times when one might choose to use pubourethral plication stitches *and* Kelly plication stitches in a particular clinical situation, i.e., rotational descent of the urethrovesical junction coexistent with urethral funneling. The merits of these techniques for each case must be decided individually.

 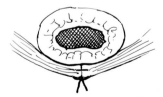

**Figure 11.20.** Suture plication directly into the urethral wall will narrow the urethral lumen as seen in the illustration at the *left*. When this has not been a goal of surgery, a urethral stricture may be produced. By contrast, pubourethral "ligament" plication, illustrated on the *right*, may elevate and support the urethra but not permanently alter the size of the lumen. Occasionally both types of stitch will be used.

It is obvious there are other important factors contributing to urinary stress incontinence, including the effects of an attachment of the pubococcygeus to the lateral paraurethral and paravaginal connective tissues, as has been pointed out by Muellner (23). When there is insufficient paraurethral tissue strength demonstrable to indicate success with pubourethral ligament stitches, supplemental transvaginal methods of support should be considered. Such methods include the bulbocavernosus fat pad transplant where blood supply is needed (See Chapter 18), the pubococcygeus muscle transplant when a strong pubococcygeal muscle is present, or lateral paravaginal reattachment. These alternatives will be described later.

After placement of the pubourethral ligament sutures, the ends are tied and then held for sewing to the underside of the trimmed anterior vaginal wall later in the procedure. Additional paraurethral plication stitches can be placed in the tissue lateral to the midurethra to provide additional support by plication of attenuated intermediate pubourethral ligaments without constriction of the urethral lumen, which could result if such stitches were placed directly into the wall of the urethra.

When stress incontinence is the sole problem, a buried nonabsorbable suture may be used in the plication of pubourethral ligaments, being meticulously careful that the suture not penetrate the lumen of either urethra or bladder lest it form a nidus for future infection or stone. When the vesicourethral junction has been elevated to a spot cranial to the inferior margin of the pubis, any appreciable funneling of the bladder neck or urethra should be corrected by plication with interrupted sutures of 2-0 absorbable sutures placed directly in the wall of the urethral funnel itself. These can be placed from side to side by the mattress-type suture of Kelly. The stitches of Royston and Rose (29) will shorten a pathologically elongated trigone.

As a first step in correcting cystocele, the operator may longitudinally plicate the whole length of the connective tissue capsule of the bladder by a series of running or interrupted 2-0 or 3-0 absorbable sutures. Care must be taken not to overcorrect the cystocele lest one unintentionally but effectively obliterate the posterior urethrovesical angle and, by making the urethra the most dependent portion of the bladder, favor a postoperative stress incontinence (31).

When anterior colporrhaphy has been immediately preceded by vaginal hysterectomy, the residual inverted T-shaped flaps of the upper vagina should be carefully trimmed to an inverted V. In removing or trimming the vaginal flaps in a manner designed to provide a desirable contour for the vault of the vagina, it must be remembered that the greater the amount of anterior wall flap removed, the lesser the amount of posterior flap that can be removed. Otherwise the additional narrowing of the vault with high posterior colporrhaphy will result in a narrowed vagina, and dyspareunia may follow.

The overenthusiastic or careless excision of too much anterior vaginal wall will simply narrow the vagina without appreciable improvement of incontinence. When united under any appreciable tension, the closure of the vaginal membrane may separate or slough postoperatively, thereby inviting recurrence. If flap tension is evident, simple longitudinal "relaxing incisions," at the vaginal three- and nine-o'clock positions that undermine 1 cm of the full thickness of the lateral vaginal walls, will release the tension and increase the caliber of a narrowed vagina (See Chapter 20). Such lateral relaxing incisions may be left open and allowed to granulate in, and they usually will be re-epithelialized within 2 to 3 weeks (Fig. 20.2). We recognize that in colporrhaphy it is the reapproximation of the subepithelial fibromuscular tissues that will produce the desired repair and not the reapproximation of the superficial vaginal skin.

Sometimes a satisfactory long-term result can be accomplished by separating a thin layer of connective tissue from the vaginal membrane and by mobilization and plication, often as the result of multiple and somewhat incomplete rows of fine synthetic absorbable or nonabsorbable suture. The redundant sling of the fibromuscular tissues is shortened and strengthened by duplication, as the supporting layer of vaginal membrane will be found to fit the newly formed plane of the anterior vaginal wall with much less excision of vaginal membrane than would have been thought necessary.

Aldridge (1) has suggested that full-thickness vaginal wall approximation, after removal of a properly sized, somewhat V-shaped wedge from the vaginal flap beneath the urethra, is more important in supporting the urethra than plication of the urethral wall itself. The suburethral vaginal wall should be closed by running or interrupted 2-0 absorbable stitches, placed subcuticularly if the operator desires, through the full thickness of the underlying fibromuscular layer. The first stitch starts near the urethral meatus. If the repair has been immediately preceded by hysterectomy, the ends of the tied peritoneal closure stitch are sewn to the undersurface of the now trimmed upper vault margins of the anterior vaginal wall near the attachment of the "bladder pillars" to the vaginal wall, thus assuring maximal elongation of the anterior vaginal wall when these stitches have been tied. Tying is best accomplished by sliding the index finger down the suture strand to a point below the knot while bringing the vaginal wall to the point of peritoneal closure. Because the peritoneal closure stitch, as described, actually includes and has also approximated the uterosacral ligaments, this effectively, even though indirectly, attaches the anterior vaginal wall to the uterosacral ligaments and helps to lengthen the anterior vaginal wall and direct the vaginal axis posteriorly (Fig. 10.45). As the reconstitution of the anterior vaginal wall continues, subcuticular stitches are placed approximately 1 cm apart. If not previously accomplished, the ends of the pubourethral ligament suture may be sewn and tied to the undersurface of the vaginal wall at the site of the previous attachment of the vagina to the urogenital diaphragm as indicated in Figure 11.16, thus re-establishing the fusion normally found in this area between the vaginal wall and urethra. The remainder of the full thickness of the vaginal wall beneath the urethra is closed with subcuticularly placed 00 absorbable sutures.

## SIMULTANEOUS PERINEORRHAPHY

Because the lower anterior wall rests upon the perineal body for the length of the urethra, it follows that adequate perineal support should also be provided whenever urethral support has been the major objective of any vaginal reconstruction (see Chapter 12). The results of coincident perineorrhaphy will not only reinforce the external genital sphincter system but have improved our long-term results of repair for the cure of urinary stress incontinence.

We do not recommend the Watkins-Wertheim interposition type of operation for the treatment of cystocele because of the eventual risk of bleeding from the retained uterus. Should pathology develop that would indicate hysterectomy, the operation is made appreciably more difficult as a result of the extensive adhesions to the uterine fundus and the proximity of the lower ureters and the bladder trigone to the adherent fundus. Rarely transposition using the Ocejo modification (see Chapter 18) may be used (10) if the vaginal wall is very thin and the uterine cervix is well supported.

# ALTERNATE TRANSVAGINAL METHODS OF SUPPORT OF THE VESICOURETHRAL JUNCTION

When traction upon the Kocher hemostat applied to the paraurethral tissue shows no evidence of pubic fixation of the tissue to which the hemostat has been applied (as by failure of it to move the patient a small bit), there has either been avulsion or detachment of the paraurethral or paravaginal tissues on one or both sides of the pelvis. Insufficient pubourethral ligament support for confident reconstruction requires consideration of alternate methods of support. The pubococcygeus muscle transplant may be employed (4, 7, 16).

## PUBOCOCCYGEUS MUSCLE TRANSPLANT OF INGELMAN-SUNDBERG

The finger-thick medial pedicle of the pubococcygeus on each side should be isolated by dissection and transected in the midportion of the vagina at the level of the vesicourethral unction. It is sewn by transfixion suture to the similar pedicle from the opposite side. Such transplanted muscular fibers also provide useful support after repair of a urethrovaginal fistula, especially one occurring at the vesicourethral junction in which instance, without such transplant, subsequent postoperative urinary stress incontinence would be a probability.

### Technique

The vagina may be opened in the midline, and the full thickness of the walls are mobilized laterally almost to the pubic rami, through the lateral limits of the vesicovaginal space if necessary. Palpation of the upper two-thirds of the lateral vaginal wall will permit identification of the medial borders of the pubococcygei that, with a little dissection, can be visualized. Alternately, an inverted U-shaped incision can be made through the full thickness of the anterior vaginal wall. This will expose the full length of the urethra, most of the bladder, and, laterally, the pubococcygei at the point where they cross the urethra and the vagina.

A finger-sized pubococcygeus is mobilized and separated laterally from the remainder of the muscle (Figs. 11.21 and 11.22). When transected posteriorly, this muscle graft will be suspended by its continuity with the superior extremity of the rest of the muscle. The length of the portion mobilized should be chosen so as to permit the ends of the pedicle of each side to be united snugly but without tension using a series of transfixion sutures placed in a side-to-side fashion beneath the vesicourethral junction.

The free segment of posterior pubococcygeus from which the upper muscle had been cut is now sewn by a mattress suture to the main body of the levator ani on its respective side to prevent its retraction and loss of support; or if a prominent rectocele is present, these fibers may be mobilized and fixed beneath the posterior vaginal wall during the subsequent posterior repair. After assurance of the effectiveness of the transposition, the anterior vaginal wall is closed in the usual manner with fine polyglycolic sutures.

When midline plication is not an effective answer for the treatment of rotational descent of the vesicourethral junction, another choice is lateral or paravaginal fixation on one or both sides as necessary. If a patient has both a lateral defect and a midline lesion that should have been diagnosed preoperatively, a midline incision in the anterior vaginal wall provides operative exposure for the repair of each of these elements, i.e., pubourethral ligament plication and paravaginal fixation.

Attachment of the paraurethral connective tissue to the arcus tendineus on

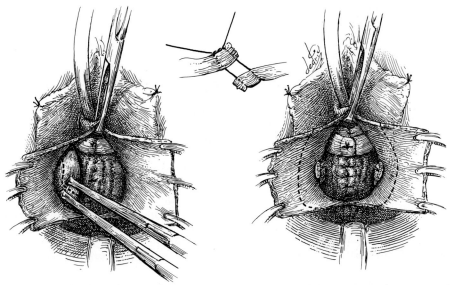

**Figure 11.21.** Pubococcygeus muscle transplant is depicted. The full thickness of the anterior vaginal wall has been opened for its full extent and reflected laterally as far as the pelvic diaphragm. The pubourethral "ligaments" have been plicated beneath the vesicourethral junction, and the bladder capsule has been plicated by a series of interrupted mattress sutures. The medial border of the pubococcygeus muscle has been identified and exposed. A finger-thick pedicle has been transected and freed laterally along the *dotted line* shown in the illustration at the *left*. A similar step is accomplished on the opposite side, and the muscle bellies are overlapped and approximated by one or more mattress sutures as shown in the drawings to the *right* and in the *center*. The transected posterior muscle bundle of pubococcygeus may be fixed to the vaginal wall, and the excess vagina removed as shown by the *dotted line*. The colporrhaphy is completed and the anterior vaginal wall closed from side to side.

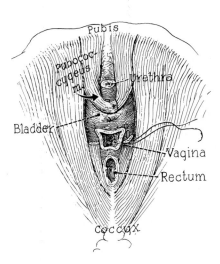

**Figure 11.22.** The important new relationships of the pubococcygeus muscle are shown diagrammatically. The ends of a medial pubococcygeus sling are attached to one another beneath the vesicourethral junction.

the undersurface of the pubis adjacent to the symphysis has been employed successfully. This is an interesting, effective approach first advocated by others (2, 5, 28, 35, 36). A transvaginal technique is shown in Figures 11.23–11.25.

## PLASTIC SYNTHETIC MESH SUPPORT

When a large cystocele is associated with an abnormal thinning of the vaginal wall, it is possible to use a single-layered, porous plastic mesh insert. The plastic mesh favors reformation of an adequately strong but satisfactorily functional vaginal wall (21, 25).

A layer of Mersilene mesh gauze is sewn into the vesicovaginal space so as to cover the entire surface of the exposed bladder surface that had previously been in contact with the anterior vagina. We have used this type of foreign material only on postmenopausal or previously sterilized patients. The anterior vaginal wall, fixed and infiltrated densely by fibroblastic connective tissue as occurs after implantation of the mesh, probably would not tolerate the stretching and dilation of labor without avulsion of the mesh after disruption of its attachments.

Mersilene mesh seems particularly effective in this use because it is flexible, permanent, porous, and only a single layer in thickness. Perhaps most importantly, the mesh is readily infiltrated by connective tissue, forming a permanently thickened vaginal wall. It is placed in a similar manner as the Tantalum patch, introduced for the same purpose by Moore et al. (22). Correspondence with Moore has determined, however, that he has abandoned the use of tantalum because of fragmentation of this material in an area where it was so susceptible to bending. We have subsequently found Mersilene to be most helpful because of its permanence as well as its flexibility. [A somewhat similar but absorbable collagen mesh prothesis was employed successfully by Friedman and Meltzer (8).] Supplemental reinforcement and insulation of this patch by the vaginal lapping operation (Chapter 18) or by a wide bulbocavernosus fat pad transplant (19) should be performed. Mersilene stimulates development of added thick pliable tissue layer between the mesh and the undersurface of the vagina.

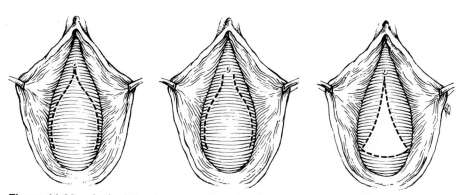

**Figure 11.23.** An incision for correcting simultaneous midline and lateral defects of vaginal support is shown by the *dotted line* in the drawing to the *left*. In the *center* drawing bilateral incisions for correcting lateral defects of support are shown, and in the drawing to the *right* an incision for correcting midline defects is shown. Excess vaginal wall will be excised as shown by the *striped lines*.

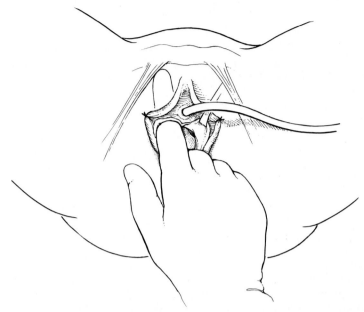

**Figure 11.24.** An opening has been made through the anterior vaginal wall and the operator's index finger, sweeping the bladder and urethra medially, palpates and by blunt dissection exposes the arcus tendineus of the levator ani.

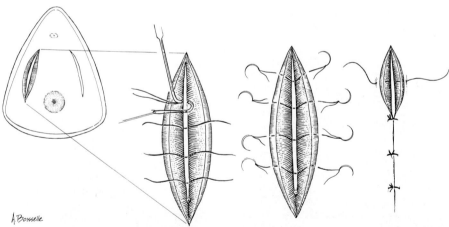

A. Boisselle

**Figure 11.25.** White's method (35) of transvaginal paravaginal fixation is illustrated. The vagina is shown to the *left* of the illustration. The urethra is at the twelve-o'clock position, and the cervix or vaginal vault at the six-o'clock position. Bilateral incisions are made through the full thickness of the wall of the vagina at a site overlying the arcus tendineus, as shown. Using the Deschamps ligature carrier a number of sutures are placed in the arcus tendineus, as shown. Each free end is passed through the full thickness of the vaginal wall as indicated in the illustration to the *right*, and when all have been placed, they are tied as shown in the illustration in the *far right*, fixing the vagina to the arcus tendineus. If nonabsorbable sutures are used, they should be placed in the subcuticular portion of the vaginal wall and the knots buried.

## Technique

After the vesicovaginal space has been opened and the full thickness of the anterior vaginal wall has been reflected from the midline laterally for the full extent of the vesicovaginal space, a pattern of sterile cardboard is cut to fit the estimated size of the defect. This serves as the pattern from which a rhomboid-shaped piece of Mersilene gauze can be fashioned. The mesh is then tacked to the capsular connective tissue underlying the bladder by three or four sutures on either side along the lateral margins of the vesicovaginal space, from as high in the vaginal vault as can be reached to the area beneath the vesicourethral junction (Fig. 11.26). In unusual cases, one can, if desired, extend the patch anteriorly to reinforce the urethra as well. Sutures should also be placed anteriorly into each pubourethral ligament. Laterally, the mesh can be attached to the firm tissues of the lateral wall of the perivesical spaces, to the obturator fascia, and to the pelvic diaphragm. The prosthesis should be insulated by the addition of the vaginal lapping procedure (Fig. 11.27) or a bulbocavernosus fat pad transplant.

It is important to remember that use of this type of mesh should be limited to placement as a subepithelial prosthesis. Inmon (17) has successfully buttressed the vesicourethral unction when supporting tissues are defective by imbedding a short hammock of Mersilene mesh transvaginally, sewing it to the urethrovesical supporting tissues of first one side and then the other. However, the material must always be carefully buried beneath a two-layered closure and not be allowed to contact an epithelial surface.

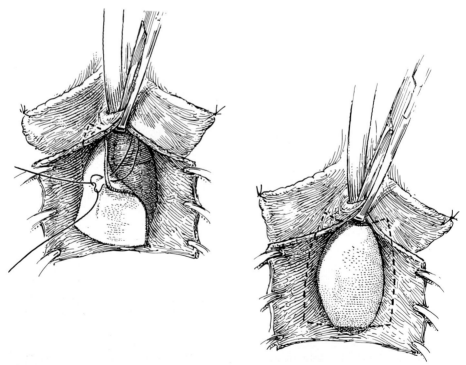

**Figure 11.26.** The pubourethral "ligaments" have been plicated, as shown in the drawing on the *left*, and the Mersilene patch has been fixed in position, as shown by the *dotted line* on the *right*. The colporrhaphy is then completed, excess tissue of the vaginal wall is excised, and the vagina is closed from side to side.

intra-abdominal pressure, a factor more often evident as atrophic changes decrease the elasticity of the vaginal wall and the integrity of the supporting tissues during a patient's postmenopausal years.

A relaxed perineum may or may not coexist with a demonstrable rectocele. A relaxed perineum is due rarely to an inadequate nerve supply to the muscles contributing support of the two components of the perineal body. More commonly, there is a defect acquired as a result of overdistention during parturition or, occasionally, the result of inadequately repaired or unrepaired obstetric laceration of the perineum. When this is the sole or major site of damage, virtual absence of the perineal body provides a pathologic degree of exposure of an otherwise normal posterior vaginal wall, accounting for the appearance known as pseudorectocele (Fig. 12.1). When such an explanation is suspected, insertion of the examining finger into the rectum will demonstrate no abnormality in the caliber of the rectum and no irregular distensibility of the anterior rectal wall. Symptoms are usually minimal, and the patient is often considered a candidate for perineal reconstruction or perineorrhaphy only when other surgery is indicated, such as vaginal hysterectomy or anterior colporrhaphy.

Congenital absence of the perineum exposes the posterior vaginal wall simulating the appearance of rectocele, which need not be present. This condition, too, may be termed a pseudorectocele. Proper treatment requires surgical reconstruction of the defective perineum, using whatever tissues are at hand. When an acquired defect is repaired, the tissues to be reapproximated were previously in apposition, and normal innervation can be expected to be present, unlike the tissue building necessary to repair a congenital defect when connective tissues and muscle must be appropriated from the nearest fibromuscular layers.

### True Low Rectocele

True low rectocele is usually the result of obstetric forces accounting for a major disruption of the attachments of the levator ani fascia and the bulbocavernosus muscles to the perineal body. Either injury may occur independently without production of a midvaginal or high rectocele and is most frequently the result of a shearing off of the lower attachments of the rectovaginal septum and the fascia of Denonvilliers from their attachment along the superior portion of the perineal body. When additional etiologic factors are

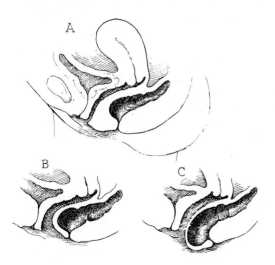

**Figure 12.1.** A normal relationship between vagina, perineum, and rectum is depicted in *A*. A major perineal defect is seen in *B*, there is no rectocele, but restoration of the perineal body is indicated. A major perineal defect with rectocele is shown in *C* and, in this circumstance, perineorrhaphy should be accompanied by an appropriate posterior colporrhaphy.

present, such as a defective or absent fascia of Denonvilliers, a coexistent mid- or high vaginal rectocele may develop. Marked gaping and eversion at the introitus will then be noted. Although a relaxed posterior wall removes some support to the sides of the urethra, bladder function will be only slightly disturbed unless the urogenital diaphragm has also been damaged. Any tendency to constipation will be aggravated because of the decreased effectiveness and correspondingly increased bearing-down effort during defecation.

## Midvaginal Rectocele

Midvaginal rectocele, whereas also due to postobstetric damage, is usually not related to damage involving the levator ani, as the vaginal attachment and effective support of the pelvic diaphragm is below this area of involvement. There may have been pathologic stretching and laceration of the connective tissues between vagina and rectum so that not only is this tissue pathologically thin, but also the rectal and vaginal capsules and the rectovaginal septum have often become fused to one another by adhesions. Such fusion tends to deprive both the rectum and the vagina of their desirable capability of independent function. The contour of one must follow the functional contour of the other. A bearing-down sensation, discomfort after a bowel movement, and inability to empty the bowel completely are usual symptoms. Midvaginal rectocele often coexists with high rectocele and, if one is to be repaired, both should be repaired.

## High Rectocele

Upper vaginal or high rectocele usually is also the result of a pathologic overstretching of the posterior vaginal wall. Here, the anterolateral attachments of the cardinal ligaments (hypogastric sheath) bind the vagina and cervix together to such an extent that the cervix functions almost as a part or extension of the anterior vaginal wall. The length of the anterior vaginal wall plus the diameter of the cervix normally equals the length of the posterior vaginal wall. The cranial envelope of the rectovaginal space terminates at the most caudal portion of the cul-de-sac of Douglas. This assures both flexibility and mobility and, with the rectovaginal space, forms a more or less frictionless inclined plane down which the structures anterior to the rectovaginal space can slide without disturbing those primarily rectal structures posterior to the rectovaginal space. Classic procidentia, therefore, although beginning as an eversion of the upper vagina, usually permits the entire uterus and much of the bladder to extend outside the bony pelvis. A coexistent enterocele develops along which the cervix, uterus, and bladder may drop as though in a sliding hernia, and all of this occurs not infrequently without an accompanying rectocele. Such a descensus, noticeably involving the bladder, has been regarded as evidence of primarily anterior segment damage and is usually the result of chronically increased intraperitoneal pressure, but it could be due to damage sustained during the first stage of labor, as when there have been bearing-down efforts or attempts to accomplish delivery before full dilation of the cervix. Therefore, anterior segment damage per se may not be mechanistically related to damage to the levator ani or its sheath.

### Etiology of High Rectocele

The peritoneal fusion fascia of Denonvilliers is missing from the posterior vaginal wall covering an enterocele, with consequent loss of support to the anterior rectal wall as well as to the posterior vaginal wall in this area, thus predisposing to high rectocele.

In discussing enterocele, Malpas distinguishes prolapse of the vault of the vagina with an obvious peritoneal sac, the bulge usually containing omentum or a loop of intestine. The posterior wall of the sac is formed by the upper rectum, and high or upper rectocele may coexist. Upper rectocele may also coexist with congenital deepening of the pouch of Douglas, as in this situation too, there is no fascia of Denonvilliers to provide support to the anterior rectal wall. With uterovaginal or sliding prolapse, on the other hand, the high rectum is not involved, so the peritoneal descent involves only the anterior wall of the cul-de-sac of Douglas usually without dilation of the peritoneal sac. Because uterovaginal prolapse may not compromise the integrity of the rectum itself, the major objective of repair will be to shorten the cardinal-uterosacral ligament complex and reattach it to the vault of the vagina; whereas in total vault prolapse, a high posterior colporrhaphy with careful excision of all of the peritoneal pouch is an essential supplement. When cardinal-uterosacral ligament strength is lacking, sacrospinous colpopexy may be used to support the vaginal vault (Chapter 16).

Damage may be present in the upper, middle, or lower portions of the posterior vaginal wall in any combination. Damage in the upper vagina may be noted either as an enterocele, a potential enterocele, a high rectocele, or a widened posterior fornix that might be subsequently narrowed. Damage to the midvagina, which has been referred to as the rectal portion of the posterior vaginal wall is perhaps the most common condition. Not infrequently, this may be the only lesion indicating repair. Reconstruction in this area should be designed to preserve or restore independent movement of the vaginal and the anterior rectal walls. This can be accomplished by the careful identification and preservation of the relatively avascular tissue relationships comprising the rectovaginal space.

If the anterior rectal wall becomes fused to the posterior vaginal wall, either by accident or by design, the possibility for normally independent movement of the walls of these adjacent viscera will be lost. When adhesion occurs, the vaginal wall must not only follow the contour of the rectal wall but must, to some extent, participate in rectal function as well. This is likely to result in persistent difficulties with constipation and defecation. Along with Bullard and Goff (4), we would like to emphasize that it is desirable to preserve the normal independence of these two passageways. Only at the level of the perineal body should the vaginal and rectal walls become fused in the reconstruction of the posterior vaginal wall.

## POSTERIOR COLPORRHAPHY AND THE RECTOVAGINAL SEPTUM

An unexpectedly shortened and persistently uncomfortable vagina after posterior colporrhaphy can result in dyspareunia. To minimize this complication, some years ago we decided to abandon the standard Hegar-Halban levator plication for correction of weakness in the posterior vaginal wall. In selected cases, we now often employ a full-length posterior vaginal wall reconstruction following the suggestions of Jeffcoate (6) and Porges (9) that the need for and the extent of a posterior vaginal wall repair now is determined preoperatively by examination of the unanesthetized patient.

Utilizing full-length posterior vaginal reconstruction immediately after vaginal hysterectomy, it has become apparent that when the operator's finger is inserted into the "avascular rectovaginal space" the progress of such blunt finger dissection is consistently obstructed at the vaginal apex near the cut edge of the vaginal vault by a thin but firm membrane. This membrane usually requires a distinct incision for penetration. The membrane has been studied in more detail to determine whether it has surgical significance.

Tobin and Benjamin (12) had concluded that the tissue described by Denonvilliers in the male included two layers, the ventral peritoneal fusion layer with which we are at the moment concerned and a dorsal or posterior layer composed of rectal fascia. A gynecologic contribution to this discussion may be found in the 1957 paper by Uhlenhuth and Nolley (13) written in a rebuttal of a 1954 opinion expressed by Ricci and Thom (10). These provocative studies reached almost diametrically opposed conclusions, which may perhaps be explained by differences in methodology. Ricci's cited evidence, which led him to deny the existence of "fascial tissue" in the integrity of the vaginal walls, was based entirely on the study of hematoxylin and eosin-stained histologic preparations and involved no correlation with gross anatomic dissections. Uhlenhuth, on the other hand, based his conclusion solely on gross dissection with no attempt at histologic correlation or confirmation. Reconciliation of these controversial reports was the objective of the simultaneous study of both the gross anatomy and related histologic specimens reported with Milley and Nichols in 1968 (8). We believe our studies have demonstrated a rectovaginal septum that can be identified as a distinct and relatively strong connective tissue layer between the vagina and the rectal walls, extending in a curved coronal plane, somewhat in conformity with the curvature of the bony pelvis. This septal structure is attached cranially to the caudal peritoneum and the rectouterine pouch of Douglas, and it extends inferiorly to its caudal fusion with the perineal body. The tissues of this septum were always adherent to the posterior aspect of the vaginal connective tissue but may easily be separated from it by blunt dissection. The demonstrable adherence to "vaginal wall" would seem to explain at least partially why the existence of a septum has, at times, been denied.

In transverse and coronal dissections, this septum was found to curve posterolaterally, paralleling the course of the paracolpium and blending laterally with the parietal layer of the pelvic fascia. It varies in character from a thin, readily perforated, translucent membrane to a tougher layer of almost leathery consistency.

Histologic studies have demonstrated this septum to consist of a fibromuscular elastic tissue, including dense collagen, abundant smooth muscle, and coarse elastic fibers, all readily separable from the fibromuscular elastic tissue recognizable as the posterior vaginal wall. In sections stained by orcein for elastic fibers, the area of the rectovaginal septum contained larger and coarser fibers than were demonstrable in the connective tissue within the vaginal wall proper. It is possible that such differences in elastic tissue fibers give the septum its demonstrable integrity during dissection. Appropriate tissue stains are needed to demonstrate the presence of a septum. We have concluded that the difficulty in demonstrating a rectovaginal septum histologically, using standard hematoxylin and eosin staining and the adherence of this septum to the connective tissues of posterior vaginal wall, explains why the existence of this important structure had often been denied.

We believe these observations are of more than academic interest, because the strength and integrity of this membrane is clinically significant and surgically useful. Earlier surgeons attempted to maintain the functional independence of the posterior vaginal and the anterior rectal walls. With one examining finger in the vagina and one in the rectum, the walls of the passageways can normally be shown to move independently, each exhibiting a surprising degree of freedom. The rectovaginal septum normally facilitates the independent mobility of the rectal and vaginal walls and, as a result, assures their functional independence. The rectovaginal septum also acts as a protective barrier of resistance to the spread of neoplasia or infection between the rectum and the vagina, as was suggested by Uhlenhuth and Nolley (13).

Note in Figure 1.25 that the rectovaginal septum normally curves posterolaterally as it becomes attached to the fascia overlying the levator ani. Decreasing the vaginal width by approximating the cut edges after excision of a midportion of the septum will, therefore, increase the pull on the lateral attachments of the septum that tend to direct the vagina posteriorly toward the sacrum. This will tend to restore the original and proper upper horizontal vaginal axis. The excision of the upper vaginal wedge of tissue may help accomplish a similar purpose.

In the repair of obstetric or surgical episiotomy, restoration of the rectovaginal septum as a distinct layer at the apex of the wound will not only permit better support but will assure better function and increased comfort.

This can be readily accomplished by the substitution of the usual through-and-through epithelial stitches with a running subcuticular layer. Not only is the postoperative and postpartum discomfort less, but epithelial inclusion cysts are effectively prevented.

A pathologic thickening of the rectovaginal septum, caused by the development of scarring within the posterior avascular rectovaginal space, can usually be broken down with ease during the preliminary dissection. Its presence can be recognized and is usually demonstrable during a preoperative rectovaginal examination, if the examination is designed to demonstrate limited mobility in terms of the inability of the vaginal wall to be moved independently of the anterior rectal wall. Rupture of the septum, even in the presence of an apparently intact vagina, may result in adhesions and fixation of the vaginal wall to the underlying rectal wall. This injury can lead to the development of midvaginal rectocele. Under such circumstances, uninhibited distention of the rectum must result in distention of the posterior wall of the vagina with consequent high and/or midvaginal rectocele formation and symptomatic interference with function.

If a patient has developed a weakness and thinning throughout the posterior wall of the vagina and the operator elects to repair only the lower part of that weakness by a standard technique of perineorrhaphy without colporrhaphy, the persistence of disturbed function or an early recurrence is predictable, probably with a troublesome exacerbation of symptoms.

Secondary connective tissue hypertrophy of the uterosacral ligaments should often be regarded as one evidence of the body's compensatory response to incipient pelvic floor damage, and full-length posterior colporrhaphy may be desirable whenever this observation has been made. If the full length of the posterior vaginal wall has been opened after vaginal hysterectomy, the vault may be sewn to a uterosacral fixation stitch, and the stitching continued downward, reapproximating side to side the cut edges of the vagina.

The rectovaginal septum appears to have been recognized and carefully restored in the New York Woman's Hospital type of repair as described by Goff (4) and later in Bullard's modification of Goff's technique of posterior colporrhaphy. However, a septum as such was not emphasized by Goff as an identifiable or significant structural entity. A possible explanation for this lack of emphasis or recognition is suggested in the following quotation from Uhlenhuth and Nolley (13):

"It has been mentioned that the rectovaginal septum adheres closely to the vagina; it is, therefore, probable that the surgeon, in performing a posterior colporrhaphy, does not get into the space between the vaginal fascia and rectovaginal septum, but into the space between the rectovaginal septum and rectal fascia."

As the experience of the gynecologic surgeon increases, it becomes apparent that the tissues normally supporting the upper third of the vagina are different from those to which the middle and lower thirds are attached. A low colporrhaphy and perineorrhaphy cannot be expected to provide an anatomically adequate repair of a weakness in the upper third of the vagina.

Harrison and McDonagh (5) wrote that "by far the most commonly neglected step in vaginal plastic procedures is reconstruction of the upper posterior vagina." When high rectocele and enterocele coexist, which is not infrequent, each must be recognized and repaired separately.

## POSTERIOR COLPORRHAPHY WITHOUT PERINEORRHAPHY

When the defect to be repaired involves only the perineal body, reflection and mobilization of perineal skin and vaginal membrane should stop at that point, and the gynecologist should proceed to repair only the defective perineum and perineal body. When there is coexistent rectocele of the mid or upper vagina, however, this herniation also should be approached at this time by extending the reflection of vaginal membrane by dissection into the rectovaginal space to a point above the bulge of the rectocele. Any adhesions binding the anterior wall of the rectum to the full-thickness flap of posterior vaginal wall should be divided by blunt and, when necessary, sharp dissection.

From time to time, an individual who has previously had an otherwise adequate perineorrhaphy demonstrates a symptomatic rectocele which may not have been evident at the time of initial surgery (Fig. 12.2). This may appear to be an enterocele. Under such circumstances, above an adequate perineal body, the operator may simply open the posterior vaginal wall directly into the rectovaginal space through either a transverse or longitudinal incision into the vagina (Fig. 12.3). This can be performed without denuding or opening the perineum.

With lateral traction on sutures or clamps at the hymenal margin, the operator may open the rectovaginal space and establish a line of cleavage between anterior rectal wall and the connective tissues of the rectovaginal septum, taking care not to open the often attenuated or thinned-out rectal wall.

**Figure 12.2.** A perineorrhaphy may hide an unrepaired midvaginal rectocele. Effective repair must always begin proximal to the point of weakness.

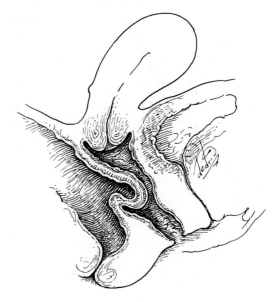

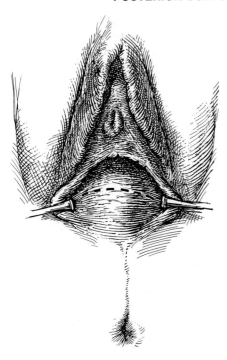

**Figure 12.3.** When posterior colporrhaphy without perineorrhaphy is desired, the rectovaginal space may be entered through a transverse incision through the posterior vaginal wall proximal to the perineal body.

When there is excessive scar tissue resulting from episiotomy repairs, preliminary insertion of the operator's double-gloved finger into the rectum may be advisable for identification and guidance.

The dissection freeing the rectum from the posterior vaginal wall and the septal tissues adherent to it should be carried to a level somewhat superior or cranial to any demonstrable rectocele (Fig. 12.4). The amount of vaginal membrane to be removed is determined by estimating the amount of excess vaginal wall; just enough should be excised to permit a normal three-fingerbreadth vaginal introitus and vaginal caliber without demonstrable tightness and stenosis. The amount of vagina removed should take the patient's endocrine age into account, anticipating some future postmenopausal shrinkage and loss of elasticity. DeCosta (3) has called attention to the desirability of leaving the introitus of the older woman a little "loose", anticipating that the rigidity of her husband's erection may not be as firm as in his younger years. It is, in general, better to err on the side of leaving too much vaginal skin when a multilayered repair technique is being used. With this in mind, it is important not to excise any suspected excess of vaginal membrane until the repair is essentially complete, at which time the supposed excess of vaginal epithelium will often fit surprisingly well over the restored rectovaginal septum.

With a high rectocele, the apex of the vaginal incision as well as the identification and mobilization of the connective tissue that is to become the rectovaginal septum should be carried to the very apex of the vagina. It may be necessary to cut through the edge of the vaginal cuff to the attachment of the upper portion of the rectovaginal septum to the cul-de-sac. If the upper margin of the portion of the vaginal wall to be removed proves to be higher than the attachment of the rectovaginal septum to the bottom of the cul-de-sac of Douglas, the latter will likely be opened. This actually is an advantage, however, because it permits identification and facilitates shortening and the suturing together of the uterosacral ligaments. This can be effected under direct

**Figure 12.4.** Sagittal section demonstrating the initial line of dissection exposing the full perineum and rectocele. Above the perineum the dissection enters the rectovaginal space and continues proximal to the highest point of the rectocele.

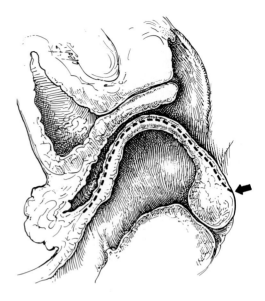

vision, incorporating the ligaments in the top of the posterior colporrhaphy. It provides an opportunity to estimate and excise any excess peritoneum before closing the cul-de-sac. This is particularly appropriate treatment whenever there are relationships such as excessive width of the vault suggesting a predisposition to the development of enterocele.

## RECTAL PILLARS (DESCENDING RECTAL SEPTA)

The so-called rectal pillars (Fig. 16.8) are essentially bilateral concentrations of connective tissue extending alongside the rectum from the lower margin of the uterosacral ligament to the perineal body at the level of its attachment to the levator ani. They separate the rectovaginal space from the pararectal space on either side and contain many elastic fibers within a connective tissue network with both lymphatic and vascular channels.

Enterocele frequently coexists with high rectocele. With enterocele, the posterior vaginal wall has less support from the fascia of Denonvilliers; and under such circumstances, support for the rectovaginal septum often can be developed by approximation of the rectal pillars, bringing them together in the midline anterior to the rectum. If the uterus has not been removed, the uppermost of these approximating sutures may well incorporate the uterosacral ligaments and the posterior aspect of the uterine cervix for additional strength and stability. In performing sacrospinous colpopexy (Chapter 16), it will always be necessary for the operator to penetrate the right rectal pillar as he or she proceeds from the rectovaginal space to the pararectal space in the direction of the right sacrospinous ligament.

Although ballooning of the anterior rectal wall appears to be the result of rectocele rather than the cause, it may be reduced with one or more layers of running locked 2–0 or 3–0 absorbable suture, which may be continued downward posterior to the level at which the perineal body will be reconstructed (Fig. 12.5). The full thickness of the posterior vaginal wall is closed from side to side, the perineal body is reconstructed, and the perineal skin is closed.

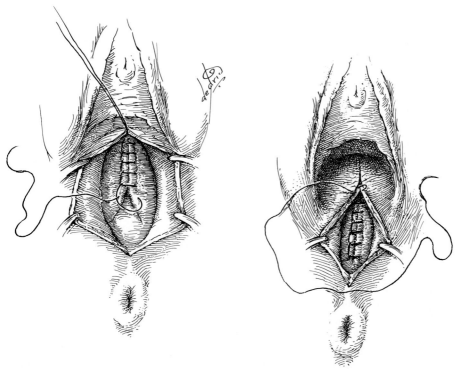

**Figure 12.5.**   Any ballooning of the anterior rectal wall may be corrected by one or more layers of running, locked, fine absorbable suture commencing proximal to the defect and continuing distally for its full length. Reconstitution may be carried posterior to the site of the new perineal body, yet to be restored. Side-to-side closure of the full thickness of the posterior vaginal wall is accomplished to the proximal margin of the perineal body and fixed at its cranial margin by suture to the tissue of the rectovaginal septum. In addition, reconstruction of the perineal body may be indicated.

## CLASSICAL TYPE OF POSTERIOR COLPORRHAPHY

At about the three- and nine-o'clock positions, an adequate bite of the hymen and its subcutaneous tissue is picked up by a clamp or suture to provide for lateral traction and expose the vaginal side of the perineal body. Used only for retraction, these lateral sutures or clamps are to be removed during the final steps in reconstruction. A narrow V-shaped or wider U-shaped incision is made through the perineal skin, depending on how large a perineal defect is to be repaired.

After the initial V-shaped opening through the perineal skin, a somewhat triangular segment of skin is dissected from the thus exposed structures of the perineum and perineal body and continued upward by undermining beneath the full thickness of the posterior wall. Adhesions tending to thicken the normal attachments of vaginal membrane may be the result of earlier obstetric damage, and all such attachments should be freed. The vaginal membrane must be freed of all appreciable fixation by scar tissue. In an older patient, when there is atrophy and narrowing of the tissues and skin of the perineum, but when coital ability is to be preserved, only an initial midline skin incision that exposes the subcutaneous tissue of the perineum may be desirable (Fig. 12.6). Occasionally, an inverted T-shaped incision may be made in the posterior vaginal wall to facilitate access to the rectovaginal space. In all repairs of a rectocele it is essential that the vaginal membrane be separated from any and all pathologic adhesions to the perineal body and the rectal wall, to a point well above any demonstrable rectocele. The perineal skin flaps are then undermined and freed up, exposing the surfaces of what is usually a distorted or irregularly deficient perineum, displaying the defective segments that are to be reconstructed into a more normal perineal body.

After entering the rectovaginal space, as previously described, any anterior ballooning of the rectum may be readily corrected by one or more layers of running, locked, fine absorbable interrupted sutures placed in the muscularis and connective tissue of the anterior rectal wall, from points both above and below the extent of the area of demonstrable rectocele.

The rectum may be displaced posteriorly by a retractor; and after incision of the estimated excess of vaginal membrane, the cut edges of the full thickness of the posterior vaginal wall, including the still adherent fibers of the rectovaginal septum, are brought together by a running subcuticular suture of 0 or 00 absorbable suture. At the apex, this suture might well include a generous bite of the lateral vaginal connective tissue of the paracolpium, and possibly even the most inferior portion of the uterosacral ligaments (Fig. 12.7) if the incision and dissection have been carried into this area. The running subcuticular suture or sutures should carefully and purposefully avoid attachment to the fascia over the levator ani but should be continued to end in the cranial border of the perineal body. When, on occasion, the vaginal wall seems unusually thin and it may not appear desirable to employ subcuticular suturing, a running locked suture through the full thickness of the posterior vaginal wall, if so placed as to avoid invagination of the cut edges, may be used to reunite the vaginal membrane in the midline. If the vaginal membrane is noticeably thin, as is often

**Figure 12.6.** When there is atrophy and narrowing of perineal skin, an initial midline perineal incision may be desirable to expose the base or inferior surface of the perineal body.

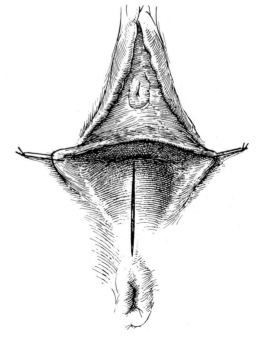

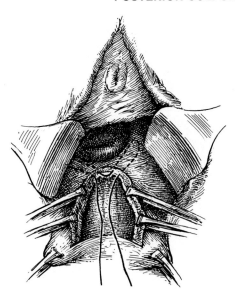

**Figure 12.7.** The suture closing the posterior vaginal wall might, at its apex, include a generous bite of the lateral vaginal connective tissue and, when possible, the uterosacral ligaments.

seen in a postmenopausal vagina, the stimulus of several weeks of preoperative estrogen therapy may increase blood loss during the operation. However, the resulting vaginal membrane is thicker to close and seems to heal more rapidly. Particularly in the closure of vaginal membrane, it is important, first, that sutures bring the tissues together without tension and, second, that knots not be tied so tightly as to blanch the tissues appreciably. The risk of such strangulation is particularly great when interrupted mattress type sutures are being tied. This classical type of posterior colporrhaphy was described by Goff (4).

In our modification of the frequently used Goff technique, a wedge or segment of what is estimated to be the proper size and shape is excised from the whole length and full thickness of the posterior vaginal wall, while leaving the septal layer attached. It is important to have carefully estimated preservation of sufficient vaginal circumference for satisfactory sexual function. The amount of vaginal wall to be retained, and, therefore, the size of the vagina after colporrhaphy, varies according to the age of the patient, her parity, and the presence or amount of estrogenic hormones.

The lateral cut edges of the vagina, to which the rectovaginal septum has remained fused, are then approximated by intravaginal subcuticular or interrupted sutures (Fig. 12.8), leaving the rectum and its facial investments uninvolved in this suturing and capable of natural independent movement. At the completion of this phase of a posterior repair, the operator should be able to insert a finger between the anterior rectal wall and the reconstituted rectovaginal septum throughout the full length of the repair, demonstrating restoration of the functional independence of the rectal and vaginal walls and the absence of iatrogenic fixation of the rectal wall (Fig. 12.9). The attenuated levator fascia may have been united only in the lower half or third of the vagina, thus permitting a more normal horizontal tilt to the upper vagina. The subvaginal portion of the perineal body is restored by interrupted sutures, and the suture line is continued down the vaginal wall and over the perineal body and back to the hymenal margin.

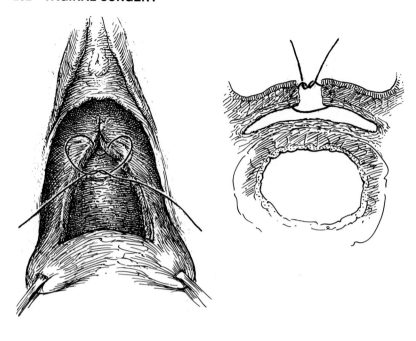

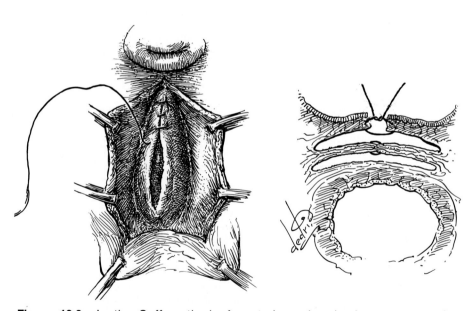

**Figure 12.8.** In the Goff method of posterior colporrhaphy, an appropriate full-thickness wedge of posterior vaginal wall has been excised and the tissues, including the fused rectovaginal septum, are closed from side-to-side as noted in the upper portion of the illustrations. A subcuticular suture is preferred. The Bullard modification is shown *below* in which the rectovaginal septum has been dissected from the posterior vaginal wall and closed as a separate layer between rectum and vaginal membrane. When this has been accomplished, excess vaginal membrane is trimmed, and the sides are brought together by interrupted suture. A running subcuticular suture may be used.

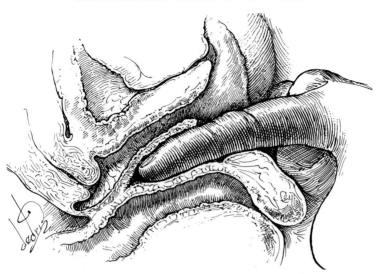

**Figure 12.9.**    At the completion of the posterior colporrhaphy and before starting the perineorrhaphy, the operator should be able to insert an index finger freely between the posterior vaginal wall to which the rectovaginal septum is attached and the anterior surface of the rectum, demonstrating the desired freedom of the space.

## POSTERIOR COLPORRHAPHY BY LAYERS

The Goff technique of posterior colporrhaphy usually will assure an anatomically acceptable result, but it may not be as certain to restore the integrity and function of a rectovaginal septum as can be assured by the layering technique of Bullard. This layering technique essentially consists of: (a) separation of the septal tissues, first from the anterior rectal wall, and second from the overlying vaginal membrane, and (b) thickening of the resulting layer of loosely arranged musculoconnective tissue and restoration of an appreciable layer of septum by several plicating sutures of fine suture.

The dissection and repair should involve the following principles:

1. The posterior vaginal wall should be incised in the midline to a point well above the rectocele, as far as the apex of the vagina when a high rectocele and/or enterocele is present.
2. The rectovaginal space is then identified and the rectal wall separated by blunt dissection from the overlying connective tissue of the rectovaginal septum, usually without difficulty.
3. Using curved Mayo scissors, by spreading the points in demonstrable planes of cleavage more than by cutting into or through tissue layers, the vaginal membrane may then be reflected anteriorly and away from the connective tissue.

There results: (a) a thinned and bulging anterior rectal wall readily identified; (b) a loose and somewhat thinned posterior vaginal wall that appears excessive for the caliber of the vagina that is to be restored; (c) a loosely incomplete, somewhat fragmented, and partially detached layer, often only sections of intervening connective tissues, all of which should be carefully preserved and should be incorporated by plication with fine suture material into a restoration of a demonstrably stronger rectovaginal septum.

The tissues of the carefully identified rectovaginal septal layer, throughout a width approximating 3 cm and a length of 5 to 6 cm, are united in the midline. Although thickened by a few plicating sutures, this septum is not attached by suture to either the underlying rectal wall or to the overlying posterior vaginal membrane.

When demonstrating this technique, it was Bullard's habit, after a few sutures had thickened the rectovaginal septum and the edges of the vagina had been trimmed and reunited in the midline (but before suturing to restore the perineal body), to demonstrate the integrity of this rectovaginal septum and its nonattachment to either the vaginal or rectal walls. He would do this by simultaneous insertion of two fingers into the space available on either side of the septum, one finger between septum and vaginal wall, the other between septum and rectal wall. Reduced adhesion between the layers of repair will favor independent mobility of the vagina and the rectum, which we believe should be an important objective of a posterior vaginal repair.

We believe it should be axiomatic that, as a surgeon might not capriciously discard viable tissue that can be incorporated in the repair of a herniating viscus, the gynecologist need not excise tissue usable in restoring a recto-vaginal septum simply because it is adherent to an assumed excess of posterior vaginal wall that will probably be excised. Rather, the gynecologist might carefully identify a line of cleavage that separates connective tissue from the redundant posterior vaginal membrane and, after thickening by fine plicating sutures, this layer may well serve to restore the integrity of a significant rectovaginal septum, which becomes interposed between the anterior rectal wall and the posterior vaginal membrane. Restoration of a recognizable septal layer is an objective and the distinctive characteristic of Bullard's modification of Goff's technique of posterior colporrhaphy.

At the completion of a vaginal repair, there is critical need for an objective evaluation of the result. If the result is not satisfactory and a satisfactory vaginal depth and axis have not been achieved, this is the optimal time for any needed correction or modification. If the patient's condition permits, prolongation of this initial operation is certainly preferable to bringing the patient back for a second operation. A vaginal caliber that is tight at the end of surgery cannot be expected to enlarge after healing is complete. As a matter of fact, if any change occurs, and particularly as the patient grows older, a tight vagina tends to become smaller.

If it is found that, in spite of the operator's intention, the repair has resulted in a vaginal caliber obviously or even suspiciously tight, appropriate relaxing incisions may be made through the thickness of the lateral vaginal walls (Fig. 20.2); but when this has been done, the vagina should then be rather tightly packed for a longer period than 24 hours. When necessary, full-thickness grafts may be sewn into incisions parallel with the axis of the vagina made at the point or points of constriction, utilizing vaginal membrane previously resected from either the anterior or the posterior vaginal wall. With this possibility in mind, when portions of the vaginal membrane have been excised, they should be kept wrapped in moist, saline-soaked sponges on the nurse's instrument stand until the conclusion of the operation.

When a suture or sutures are palpated or visualized within the lumen of the rectum, that portion of the suture within the rectal lumen should be immediately cut in order to lessen postoperative pain and the chance of rectovaginal or rectoperineal fistula. The cut ends will promptly retract up and out of the rectal lumen. The effectiveness of the repair should not be jeopardized by the loss of the effect of that single suture.

To minimize oozing and collection within the spaces between layers, we sometimes pack the vagina lightly with 2-inch plain or iodoform gauze, which we prefer to remove the morning of the day after surgery.

As a result of our studies and experience with these operative techniques, it appears to us that the apparently divergent conclusions of Uhlenhuth and Nolley (13) and Ricci and Thom (10) can now be reconciled. The marked degree of natural fusion of the rectovaginal septum to the posterior vaginal wall makes its histologic demonstration difficult except by special connective tissue staining. During dissection, on the other hand, a septum can be readily identified in a most consistent manner, but only when definite effort to do so has been made. Because for a number of years we have been identifying the septum in the manner described and have been pleased with the results of the technique as described, we recommend these procedures for the consideration of others.

## DEFECTS IN THE PERINEUM

An inadequate or defective perineum may result in such an exposure of the midportion of the posterior vaginal wall as to constitute a pseudorectocele (Fig. 12.1) as noted by Richter (11). Careful digital examination of the rectum will allow differentiation of pseudorectocele from true rectocele. Pseudorectocele is characterized by normal rectal caliber, angulation, and tone, and the posterior vaginal and anterior rectal walls are independent. When a true rectocele has developed, however, the adjacent vaginal and rectal walls will often be joined together with a loss of vaginal rugae over the rectocele and a tendency of the rectum to form a pouch. The pouch can be demonstrated easily when the examiner's finger flexes and extends anteriorly. This ballooning segment can become a pathologic pocket that may trap fecal material, causing incomplete bowel movements as well as postevacuation discomfort.

Defects in the perineum are usually the result of obstetric damage, either from unrepaired or inadequately repaired laceration, or from an ill-timed or incompletely repaired episiotomy. Incomplete repair results in lateral retraction of muscles that are normally attached to the perineal body. Detachment or interruption of the transverse perinei and the bulbocavernosus must be recognized and corrected. Not only will the repair aid in the support of the anterior wall of the rectum, but it will also add considerable support to the anterior wall of the lower vagina and urethra. In this connection, it should be remembered that the length of the perineal body effectively approximates the length of the female urethra, in part because of the passage of the medial portion of the pubococcygeus muscle along the sides of the vagina, urethra, and rectum. This sends slips of connective tissue to fuse with the capsule tissue investing every one of these hollow organs. When indicated, appropriate and adequate perineorrhaphy effectively complements the support of the anterior vaginal wall and the urethra.

In examination of the patient before posterior colporrhaphy, it is important to recognize, as emphasized by Davies (2), that:

"Any perineal laceration which permits the labia minora to retract laterally and expose a gaping vagina harbors the divided and retracted origin of the bulbocavernosus muscle. Such a lesion lowers the efficiency of the voluntary urethral sphincter and should be considered as an etiologic basis for stress incontinence in the female."

The operator should also carefully note the position of the patient's anus in relation to the most dependent portion of the buttocks, the tip of the coccyx, and the ischial tuberosities. Posterior displacement of the anus strongly suggests detachment of the anal sphincter from the perineum. This may also be noted with a defect of the levator ani, either because of an intrinsic fault of the muscle or as a result of defective innervation of this voluntary muscle. In either instance, regardless of etiology, straining during defecation may, in effect, produce elongation and funneling of the levator ani, with the anus descending to an even more dependent position. The harder the patient strains, the narrower the stool must become, and the more difficult to defecate. Obstipation is often the result. Barrett (1) proposed an incision be made posterior to the rectum, with attachment of the separated levators to each other and to the rectal wall. This technique is considered in the description of retrorectal levatorplasty in Chapter 13.

It should be remembered that, historically, the objective of perineorrhaphy was to improve the patient's ability to retain a pessary. Unfortunately, all too often this concept has been extended to an erroneous comparison to a cork plugging the neck of an inverted bottle. This inadequate but popular concept visualizes a good perineal repair as not only preventing progression of upper vaginal prolapse, but also as a factor preventing the development of genital prolapse in general. We disagree with this concept and would refer skeptics to the observation that genital prolapse is uncommon among women with unrepaired third and fourth degree obstetric lacerations who had long suffered a complete loss of any support the perineal body would have offered the uterus, cervix, and upper vagina.

## PERINEAL BODY

In the woman, the perineal body is a structure of considerable anatomic and physiologic importance. The basic objective of perineorrhaphy, therefore, is to restore an effective perineal body, with realignment of muscles and connective tissues to a degree that will assure normal relationships and encourage normal, comfortable function.

It must be remembered that the principal portion of the levator ani concerned with support of the lower vagina and birth canal attaches to the sides of the vaginal connective tissue through the fibers of Luschka rather than to the muscular tissues of the posterior vaginal wall itself. Although the levator ani may be lengthened, displaced laterally, and sometimes detached as a result of perineal laceration or other obstetric trauma, damage to the levator ani may also produce only a midvaginal rectocele cranial to the perineal body. When examining such a patient, it is important to note whether external hemorrhoids are present because weakness of the perineum and anal sphincter may contribute to their development. When there is prolapse of the upper vagina and cervix, however, the distention of the genital hiatus by the protrusion may have lessened the tone of the introitus musculature by much the same mechanism as the dilating wedge of an enterocele in this area may widen the pelvic outlet. Much of the tone of the lateral vaginal walls will be regained after an effective repair, largely as a result of the removal of a major causative factor (the prolapsing cervix, uterus, or enterocele).

Most so-called levator stitches result only in increased approximation of thinned or separated layers of the perineal body and do not usually result in a buildup of the levator itself. If placed far enough laterally to include only the fascia of the pelvic diaphragm, they may reinforce a defective pelvic diaphragm; but if placed directly into the belly of the levator muscle, these sutures may actually destroy portions of the muscle, eventually resulting in a shelf-like ridge of nonelastic fibrous tissue within the introitus and immediately beneath the posterior vaginal wall. It is preferable to place superficial, side-to-side stitches because they will usually reconstitute the perineal body and draw the fascia of the pubococcygeal muscles closer to the upper lateral sides of the perineal body. This will effectively narrow the widened genital hiatus.

The extent to which reconstruction of a very loose vaginal outlet will contribute to coital satisfaction has been undoubtedly overemphasized. A consensus of the more thoughtful gynecologists recognize that a noticeable looseness of the vagina is not a common cause of marital incompatibility; and as a result, prophylactic "tightening up" of the introitus will not necessarily improve marital relations that are frayed more often by nonanatomic factors. More realistic considerations of domestic satisfactions must take into account the several factors that are to be involved. However, indicated correction (but not overcorrection) of a damaged or relaxed perineal body can be expected to improve coital satisfaction within an otherwise compatible domestic relationship.

The caliber of the premenopausal or estrogen-maintained vagina with respect to the accommodation of an erect penis has wide limits of compatibility, as vaginal elasticity permits the vagina under normal circumstances to grasp or contain the male organ much as an expansile rubber glove grasps a finger. Thus, the normal-sized vagina can adapt comfortably and adequately to a large male organ as well as to a small one. The elasticity of the vagina is, therefore, important in preserving coital harmony, and unnecessary surgical procedures that tend to result in fibrosis and rigidity should be avoided.

The argument as to which muscle bundles do or do not penetrate the perineal body is, in large part, more academic than practical. The gynecologic surgeon should not regularly attempt to bring muscle bundles into the perineal body that were not there to begin with and should not try to incorporate them in the repair, because such displaced bundles are more likely to be replaced by fibrosis, with a resulting loss of elasticity and persistent tenderness. To understand the objective of repair, we should start with a fairly definite concept of normal fibromuscular attachments and relationships of the perineal body. Making allowance for individual variation, we must also recognize the function of each component and attachment if our effort to restore the more essential relationships is to succeed.

The perineal body may be visualized as roughly pyramidal, and a repair must restore the body in all three dimensions. The base of the pyramid is situated beneath and parallels the perineal skin. The anterior, posterior, and two lateral surfaces all converge superiorly to the most inferior limit of the rectovaginal space, fusing with the lowermost margin of the rectovaginal septum (Chapter 1).

Although the perineum has been likened to the keystone of an arch, such an analogy is inappropriate. The base of such a keystone would be its widest part, thus gravity would pull it down and out of position rather than wedging it more firmly in place.

## TECHNIQUE OF PERINEORRHAPHY

Reconstruction of the perineal body begins with uncovering the perineal body along its base beneath the perineal skin and on the vaginal (anterosuperior) side. Excess vaginal wall and skin is mobilized, and then the reconstruction is performed. This is often accomplished by side-to-side reapproximation of denuded tissues both deep and superficial. The upper portion of this side-to-side reapproximation of the perineal body should pull the pubococcygei closer without actually including them in the sutures. As a result, the genital hiatus is narrowed. Lower placed stitches also help to reconstruct the lower portion of the urogenital diaphragm, bringing the transverse perinei together. Similar sutures reattach the bulbocavernosus muscles to the perineal body.

## OPERATIVE PROCEDURE

A transverse incision for perineorrhaphy carries with it not only the potential of providing incomplete exposure of the inferior surface of the base of the perineal body, but adds the additional risk of facilitating creation of a ridge-like "dashboard perineum" with the probability of associated dyspareunia. This undesirable result is so likely because an inadequate incision directs the surgeon's attention to reconstructing only the anterior and upper portion of the perineal body, because that is the only area he has exposed or denuded, leaving the equally important mid- and posteroinferior portions of the perineal body unexposed and not involved in the repair.

For this reason, a "standard" transverse incision is not recommended unless a significant perineal body reconstruction is not planned, and when the surgeon's intent and efforts are to be directed to the repair of a rectocele well above the perineal body.

After clamps or traction sutures have been applied to the hymenal margin on either side, we prefer to make a V-shaped incision (Fig. 12.10) in the perineal skin layer (U-shaped for especially large perineal defects). The width of the

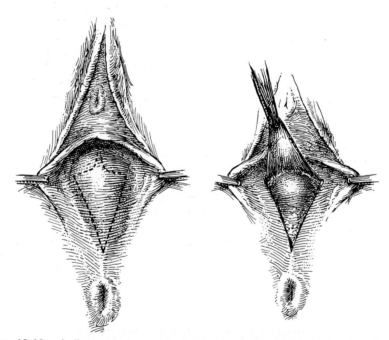

**Figure 12.10.** A diamond-shaped piece of tissue of an appropriate width has been carefully estimated in the drawing on the *left*. The amount of perineal skin to be removed is determined by the quantity of excess tissue, just enough being excised to permit a normal three-fingerbreadth vaginal introitus without stenosis. It is better to err on the side of leaving a little too much tissue than too little. The dissection is carried superiorly into the vagina, exposing the full site of the future perineal body. If rectocele is present, the rectovaginal space is entered, and the dissection freeing rectum from vagina is carried to a level above any rectocele which is present.

base of this triangle, in relation to the hymenal margin, should be estimated in accordance with the desired size of the resultant vaginal introitus. The greater the amount of epithelium removed, the smaller will be the caliber of the resulting vaginal orifice. A V-shaped incision in the perineal skin will assure better access to more of the tissues of the perineal body than would be possible with the usual transverse incision along the posterior hymenal margin.

It is important to place the lateral traction sutures or clamps on the hymenal ring and not on the labia minora. This placement prevents obstruction from a superficial transverse ridge or dashboard-like perineum, which may result if the retracting forceps or sutures are too lateral.

Scar tissue is freed by sharp dissection (Fig. 12.11).

It is of utmost importance that any detachment of the connective tissue of the rectovaginal septum from the cranial or uppermost portion of the perineal body be remedied by surgical reattachment that will assure restoration of normal function, particularly as regards the role of the perineum and its continuity with the rectovaginal septum during the act of defecation. Because considerable scarring from previous trauma may be found in this vulnerable area, dissection through indistinct cleavage planes should proceed with caution, to avoid entering the rectum. After this reattachment and restoration, incomplete bowel movements may be relieved and a recurrence will be unlikely.

During reconstruction of the lower third of the vagina in advanced cases, when there is little tissue with which to work, it may be necessary to provide better support to the rectal ampulla (Fig. 12.12) to bring the medial margins of the puborectalis or pubococcygei muscles together by a small series of superficially placed and loosely tied interrupted sutures, which, in turn, may at their insertion be attached to a sagging ampulla. Although at times highly desirable, it is important that such support be accomplished without production of troublesome and inevitably tender ridges beneath the posterior vaginal wall. After each stitch is placed, the ends of the suture should be crossed before

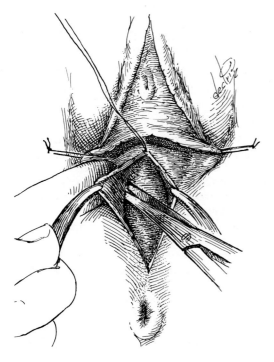

**Figure 12.11.** Scar tissue attached to introital skin is carefully freed by sharp dissection, so that the tissue from which a perineal body will be built can be mobilized readily.

**Figure 12.12.** In occasional instances of extreme perineal defect, it may be desirable to bring the fascia of each pubococcygeus together in the midline in front of the rectum; palpable ridges of tissue must be carefully avoided.

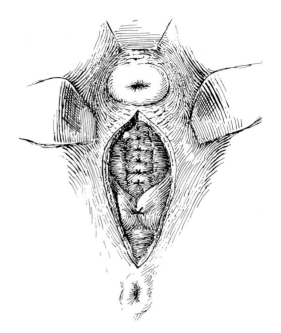

tying and traction applied. If a ridge is palpated, the stitch should be promptly removed and replaced, usually closer to the rectum. When perineal surgery is performed under local anesthesia, the voluntary muscle bundles may be more readily identified.

The retracted ends of often long-separated bulbocavernosus muscles should be first identified then reattached to the perineal body. Separated segments of the transverse perinei should also be reunited if the medial edge of the levator ani and the puborectalis can be identified. For correction of a low rectocele, the adjacent fascia of the pelvic diaphragm is attached to the posterolateral surface of the vagina, duplicating the original attachment of the fibers of Luschka, fixing and holding the vagina in place (Fig. 12.13). The smooth muscle of the perineal body should then be brought together by a few interrupted horizontally placed perineal sutures not tightly tied (Figs. 12.14 and 12.15), helping further to re-establish its integrity.

Although not a common result of perineal injury during childbirth, when posterior displacement of the anus occurs, it is essential that it be repaired. It is necessary to reattach the capsule of the external sphincter ani to the perineal body, for example using a figure-eight suture (Fig. 12.16), as described by Kennedy and Campbell (8). This step stabilizes the perineum in a way similar to reattachment of the spokes to the hub of a wheel (perineal body).

Operative compression of the veins communicating with hemorrhoids will often temporarily aggravate hemorrhoids that may have been present; but as postoperative edema subsides, a new tissue equilibrium is usually established after which the hemorrhoids may undergo involution and improvement, especially if any sphincter weakness has been corrected. For this reason, hemorrhoidectomy should not be done at the same time as a posterior colporrhaphy. The need for hemorrhoidectomy can better be evaluated postoperatively after several months.

The superficial perineal fascia may be brought together using running or interrupted sutures, and then the perineal skin may be closed with running or interrupted sutures. Subcuticular sutures should be used in the closure of both the vaginal epithelium and the perineal skin, taking care to avoid irregularities

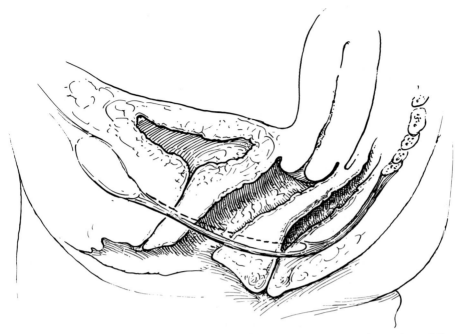

**Figure 13.1.** Sagittal section of the pelvis shows elongation and sagging of the levator plate. The usual angle between the anal canal and the rectum has been lost, as well as the horizontal axis of the rectum and the upper vagina.

labor, as well as subsequent lifelong establishment of good bowel habits and even the use of a mild laxative or suppository, if necessary, with increased bulk in the diet. Increased water intake (remembering that some degree of systemic dehydration is more common coincident with the diminution of thirst that grows greater with aging), and regular pubococcygeal isometric resistive exercises are helpful.

With perineal descent constipation may appear as an early symptom due to loss of the integrity of an intact pelvic diaphragm during bearing down efforts. As this phenomenon of voluntary bearing down becomes more regular and intense, the pudendal nerve may be damaged by stretching (11, 12, 23, 24), disturbing the innervation of both the pelvic diaphragm and the external anal sphincter with resultant partial paralysis and atrophy of these muscles.

This may sometimes produce perineal prolapse with first obstipation and later rectal incontinence if the protective internal sphincter mechanism becomes overburdened. When perineal prolapse also correlates with a decreased perception of subjective feelings of rectal fullness, there may be degeneration of some of the neuromuscular receptors within the levator ani. This, in turn, may correlate with a less favorable prognosis after anatomic surgical reconstruction.

Bowel function is to a large extent a phenomenon of habit, and the gastrocolic reflex pattern regularly assists. Providing there is content in the sigmoid colon, defecation is achieved by voluntarily first relaxing the pelvic diaphragm and external anal sphincter, unlocking the colic valve letting normal intestinal peristalsis take over with relaxation of the involuntary internal anal sphincter. Movement is then aided by modest increases in intra-abdominal pressure as by voluntary bearing down. A disorder of any of these steps may predispose to constipation.

It is possible that reconstruction of a damaged levator muscle with an intact nerve supply may produce a functionally more favorable result than when the nerve supply has been significantly defective, whatever the cause.

The levator plate, formed by fusion of the bellies of the pubococcygeus muscles, for the most part posterior to the rectum, extends to the insertion of these muscles upon the coccyx and lower portion of the sacrum (2, 22). When the plate is intact, it is more or less horizontal in position; but when markedly attenuated, it becomes a loose hammock (Fig. 13.2). As the plate sags it tips and with increases in intra-abdominal pressure, may permit those structures that lie upon it to literally slide downhill. The latter structures, principally the vagina and rectum, in addition to descending, on occasion may exhibit telescoping when their respective axes are in the direction of increases in intra-abdominal pressure.

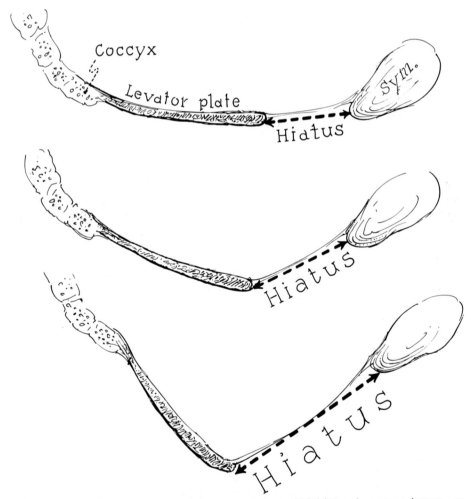

**Figure 13.2.** As the levator plate sags, the genital hiatus becomes larger, as shown. In addition, the pull of gravity and the forces of intra-abdominal pressure accentuate the strain upon the pelvic suspensory system. *Sym.,* symphysis pubis. (After Berglas B, Rubin IC: Study of the supportive structures of the uterus by levator myography. *Surg Gynecol Obstet* 97:672–692, 1953.)

Uniting the medial portions of the pubococcygei between the vagina and rectum and anterior to the latter does thicken the tissues of the perineum by interposition of a muscular layer not initially well developed here. However, this neither shortens the muscles, nor restores the defective axis of the plate itself, nor corrects the pathologic descent of the anus and rectum (Fig. 13.3). To achieve the latter goals, the literature has not recorded much surgical technique or experience, although lengthening of the levator plate has been described by the transperineal approach of Lange (16) and by transabdominal surgery using various modifications of the operation of Roscoe Graham (6, 8, 9).

Although it is possible to plicate the pubococcygeal muscles posterior to the rectum using a transabdominal approach, the exposure is difficult and deep within the pelvis, and pathologic vaginal displacements with associated cystocele and rectocele cannot be approached satisfactorily through the same operative exposure. Barrett (1) suggested a transperineal approach by incision and dissection between the anus and vagina, "posteriorly to the rectum in properly selected cases and the separated levator reunited with attachment of the rectal wall to this muscle," but apparently did not document pursuit of his idea.

Clinical interest in the Kraske or sacral transperineal approach to some surgical lesions of the rectum has reaffirmed the safety of this route (3, 4, 9, 13–15, 17, 18, 21, 30), and we have described a procedure using this approach to correct the levator deficiencies described above (19, 20). This transperineal retrorectal approach shortens the pubococcygei and puborectalis as necessary, and unites the medial bellies of these muscles in the midline posterior to the rectum, thus lengthening the levator plate and advancing the genital hiatus anteriorly. The posterior rectal wall is attached to the internal periosteum of the

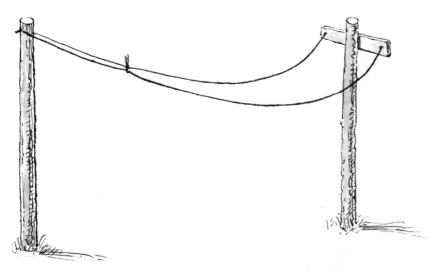

**Figure 13.3.** Pathologically elongated pubococcygei may be represented as a sagging clothesline suspended between two fixed poles. Tying one side to the other, as shown, will bring each side closer to the other but will not shorten the lines nor reduce the sagging. For this reason, perineorrhaphy, per se, is ineffective in the treatment of the anal and perineal prolapse that is secondary to pathologic elongation of the pubococcygeal portion of the pelvic diaphragm. The clotheslines (as well as the pubococcygei) can effectively be shortened only by decreasing their length.

lower sacrum by a series of interrupted sutures re-establishing or constructing a relatively horizontal axis to the rectum and to the vagina overlying it. This procedure permits suspension of the elongated rectum (5, 14, 26) and, by the addition of appropriate supplemental anterior and posterior colporrhaphy (25, 28), the correction of any coexistent cystocele and rectocele. Any enterocele should be excised (31 ).

Significant individual variation in the strength and length of the anococcygeal raphe and the rectococcygeus muscle or ligament has been noteworthy.

The essential steps of the operation are as follows:

The patient is positioned in the Kraske jackknife position (Fig. 13.4), although the standard lithotomy position may be used in those patients with plenty of room and on whom coincident colsorrhaphy will be performed. A midline incision is made from the sacrum to the site of the external anal sphincter. The anococcygeal raphe is identified and separated from the coccyx; the latter is grasped in a towel clip but is not removed. Fat is displaced identifying the undersurfaces of the pubococcygei and the levator plate, which is usually incised in the midline, separating the right muscle belly from the left. The rectum is identified and separated from the levator muscles and plate. The rectococcygeal muscle or ligament is identified, if present, and transected, the retrorectal (or presacral) space thoroughly explored (Fig. 13.5), and the undersurface of the sacrum cleansed of fat and loose connective tissue, exposing the periosteum.

Three plication stitches are placed in the posterior rectal wall 1 cm apart and are tied but not cut (Fig. 13.6). Using an overglove, a rectal examination is done to determine any suture penetration of the rectal mucosa, which if found would require replacement of the suture. These sutures are then sewn to the presacral fascia (Fig. 13.7). Polyglycolic acid-type sutures (Dexon or Vicryl) are used throughout the operation. A large dental mirror and fiberoptic headlight are

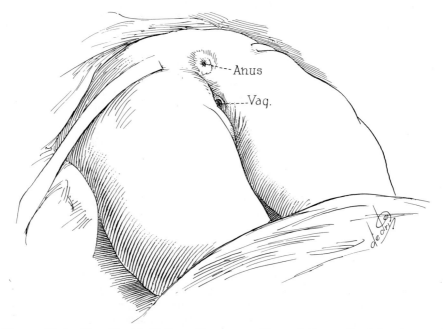

**Figure 13.4.** The "jackknife" or Kraske position of the patient is shown. A sandbag has been placed beneath the hips, and the gluteal muscles are pulled apart by wide strips of adhesive tape fastened to the edges of the operating table.

tologic Society, Cleveland, OH, June 1966.

11. Henry MM, Swash M: Assessment of pelvic floor disorders and incontinence by electrophysiological recording of the anal reflex. *Lancet* 17:1290–1291, 1978.

12. Henry MM, Swash M: *Colpoproctology and the Pelvic Floor.* London, Butterworths, 1985.

13. Jenkins SG, Thomas CG: An operation for the repair of rectal prolapse. *Surg Gynecol Obstet* 114:381–383, 1962.

14. Klingensmith W, Dickinson WE, Hays RS: Posterior resection of selected rectal tumors. *Arch Surg* 110:647-651, 1975.

15. Kraske P: Zur Extirpation Hochsitzender Mastdarmkrebse. *Vehr Dtsch Ges Chir* 14:464–474, 1885.

16. Lange F: Intestinal and anal surgery. Quoted in Hadra BE (ed): *Lesions of the Vagina and Pelvic Floor.* Philadelphia, McMullin & Co, 1888.

17. Lockhart-Mummery JP: Rectal prolapse. *Br Med J* 1:345–348, 1939.

18. Mason AY: Trans-sphincteric surgery of the rectum. *Prog Surg* 13:66–97, 1974.

19. Nichols DH: Retrorectal levatorplasty for anal and perineal prolapse. *Surg Gynecol Obstet* 154:251–254, 1982.

20. Nichols DH: Retrorectal levatorplasty with colporrhaphy. *Clin Obstet Gynecol* 25:939–947, 1982.

21. O'Brien PH: Kraske's posterior approach to the rectum. *Surg Gynecol Obstet* 142:412–414, 1976.

22. Parks AG: Modern concepts of the anatomy of the anorectal region. *Postgrad Med J* 34:360–366, 1958.

23. Parks AG: Anorectal incontinence. *Proc Roy Soc Med* 68:681–690, 1975.

24. Parks AG, Swash M, Urich H: Sphincter denervation in anorectal incontinence and rectal prolapse. *J Br Soc Gastroentol* 18:656–665, 1977.

25. Redding MD: The relaxed perineum and anorectal disease. *Dis Colon Rectum* 8:279–282, 1965.

26. Romer-Torres R: Sacrofixation with marlex mesh in massive prolapse of the rectum. *Surg Gynecol Obstet* 149:709–711, 1979.

27. Sharf B, Zilberman A, Sharf M, et al: Electromyogram of pelvic floor muscles in genital prolapse. *Int J Gynaecol Obstet* 14:2–4, 1976.

28. Sullivan ES, Leaverton GH, Gary H, et al: Transrectal perineal repair; an adjunct to improved function after anorectal surgery. Proceedings of American Proctologic Society, New Orleans, Louisiana, April 1967.

29. Taverner D, Smiddy FG: An electromyographic study of the normal function of the external anal sphincter and pelvic diaphragm. *Dis Colon Rectum* 2:153–160, 1959.

30. Turner GG: Ideals and the art of surgery. *Surg Gynecol Obstet* 52:273–311, 1931.

31. Wiersema JS: Treatment of complete prolapse of the rectum by the vaginal approach. *Arch Chir Neerl* 28:25–31, 1976.

# CHAPTER 14

# Repair of Old Laceration of the Perineum

Howard Kelly once observed (1) that genital prolapse was only rarely observed when there had been a complete and unrepaired perineal laceration. Because the principal effectiveness of the pubococcygei and levator ani is exerted posterior to the rectum, where their fusion forms the levator plate, a laceration through the anterior rectum, perineal body, and posterior vagina is not likely to have been due to forces simultaneously exerted to a point of overstretching the major sources of the uterine support. Although the injury disrupted the anal sphincter, many of these patients will, by vigorously exercising the pubococcygeus over a long period of time, produce an actual hypertrophy that results in a side-to-side spincter-like action that helps hold the sides of the fistula in opposition and accomplishes a semblance of anal continence. Although this mechanism will not regain a control of flatus, continence of the stool may be regained, particularly if the patient is careful to maintain a helpful degree of constipation.

A patient will present herself for repair of a complete perineal laceration at any time, even years after the original injury. Miller and Brown (3, 7) have emphasized three fundamental principles essential to successful repair: (*a*) evidence of a good blood supply, (*b*) absence of infection in the tissues to be involved, plus (*c*) closure of the repair with no tension on the sutures as the tissues are reapproximated. It is equally important to excise all scar tissue in order to assure tissues similar to those of a fresh fourth-degree laceration. Layer-by-layer reconstruction of rectal wall perirectal connective tissue, anal sphincter, and rectovaginal septum before closure of the overlying vaginal floor should be accomplished by terraced rows of fine absorbable suture, but there is a tendency for such a repair to break down with formation of rectovaginal fistula. Such a discouraging result is particularly likely in the postmenopausal patient whose tissues are atrophic and with reduced blood supply.

Intestinal peristalsis is reduced by age, particularly in the postmenopausal years. It also may be reduced indirectly by nicotine withdrawal of someone who has stopped smoking. The best results are obtained when an obstetric laceration is properly repaired immediately after delivery, when the vascularity of the perienum and perivaginal tissues favors rapid healing. On the occasion of a later secondary repair, scar tissue is appreciable, wound healing is poorer, and recurrence of the fistula from a breakdown of the repair is more likely.

A method of repair providing an optimal chance of a good result with the first repair is obviously a procedure of choice. The Noble-Mengert-Fish anterior rectal flap operation has often been recommended, and primary healing with restoration of function also usually follows the Warren-Miller-Brown vaginal flap operation.

The choice between the Noble-Mengert-Fish (2, 4) rectal flap operation and the Warren-Miller-Brown (3, 7) operation can often be made on the basis of the size of the vagina. The vaginal flap operation makes the vagina measurably smaller and, therefore, would be used when this is a desired goal, whereas the rectal flap operation can be used in a patient with a smaller vagina, as it does not remove vaginal membrane. The rectal flap operation is particularly useful if an old fourth-degree laceration extends no more than 3 or 4 cm into the anal canal. Freeing up and pulling down the anterior rectal wall and placing anchoring sutures near the edge of the mobilized segment of anterior rectal mucosa to the anal sphincter and perineal skin outside of the former anal canal will cover the area where postoperative disruption of sutures not protected by such a flap will often occur. In principle and usefulness this procedure is not unlike the mucosal flap operations for rectovaginal fistula, as described in Chapter 19, but it is indicated preferentially when external anal sphincter integrity has been disturbed.

The technique of the rectal flap [Noble-Mengert-Fish (2, 4)] procedure may be accomplished after a preoperative bowel preparation as follows: The scarred edge of the anterior rectal wall is grasped with several Allis clamps along the inverted U-shaped defect in which the anal membrane has by scar become fused to the posterior vaginal wall. A transverse semilunar incision is made across the posterior wall of the vagina immediately above this scar tissue, and the rectovaginal space is entered (Fig. 14.1). Once this space has been identified, the separation of the rectum from the vagina is accomplished by blunt dissection. With a guiding finger in the rectum and Allis clamps supported in the palm of the same hand, separation of tissue planes can extend all the way to the vault of the vagina and then is carried laterally the full width of the rectovaginal space. The Allis clamps attached to the anterior rectal will provide gentle traction and permit some sliding and gentle stretching of the now

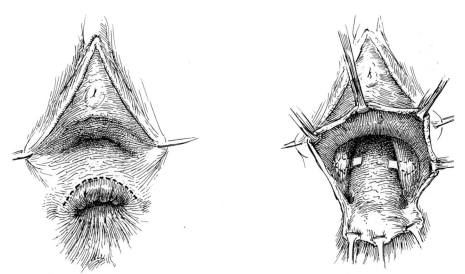

**Figure 14.1.** The rectal flap operation (Noble-Mengert-Fish) is depicted. The mucocutaneous incision needed for the Noble-Mengert-Fish operation to restore the anal sphincter is identified by the *dotted line* in the drawing to the *left*. The edges of the incision are grasped by Allis clamps and dissection carried upward to the rectovaginal space. Pararectal connective tissue is separated from the antero-lateral surface of the rectum as shown by the *arrows* in the drawing to the *right*.

mobilized anterior rectal wall until it may readily reach the site where it is to be anchored to the anal sphincter and perineal skin. Use a "Bovie" electrosurgical needle electrode to aid hemostasis. Its brief electrical stimulation also will help identify a striated muscle. The retracted ends of the anal sphincter are then sought at the site of the identifying dimples and freed if possible. The partially mobilized ends of the sphincter are grasped by Allis clamps and the ends of the sphincter pierced by two mattress sutures of 2–0 delayed absorbable synthetic suture, to be tied after the sutures restoring the perineal body have been placed and tied. If the retracted ends of the sphincter cannot be isolated because they have become deeply buried in the scar tissue and have lost recognizable identity, there need be no concern as long as the operator brings the scar tissue (which can be demonstrated by traction to contain the sphincter ends) together in the midline before completion of the associated perineorrhaphy.

The suitably denuded and mobilized lateral soft tissues necessary to form a reconstructed perineal body are then united in the midline by a series of interrupted 0 polyglycolic acid-type absorbable sutures in the fashion of an extensive perineorrhaphy, over the intact portion of the mobilized anterior rectal wall (Fig. 14.2). Ridges and shelving of tissues are to be avoided by careful suture placement. These sutures are then tied without strangulation of the tissue, and excess skin and mucosa are appropriately trimmed. The lower edge of the flap of the anterior rectal wall is fixed to the skin of the perineum by several interrupted 2–0 absorbable polyglycolic acid-type sutures placed not more than 1 to 2 cm apart. An occasional stitch should include a superficial bite of the anal sphincter.

The reconstructed anal canal should admit one fingerbreadth comfortably; if not, due to retraction and shortening of the anal sphincter fibers, the paradoxical sphincter incision described by Miller and Brown (3) can be performed. Such an incision should be made between the four- and five-o'clock position, cleanly through the perineal skin and anal sphincter and perpendicular to the muscle fibers of the sphincter (Fig. 14.3). The sphincter remains relaxed and

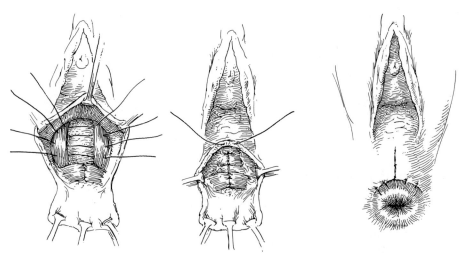

**Figure 14.2.** The ends of the external anal sphincter have been united and stitches placed in the pararectal tissues as shown in the drawing to the *left*. They are tied as seen in the *middle* drawing, and the posterior vaginal wall will be closed from side to side. A perineal body has been reconstructed with interrupted sutures. The vaginal and perineal skin has been closed, and the result after the excess flap has been trimmed is seen in the drawing to the *right*.

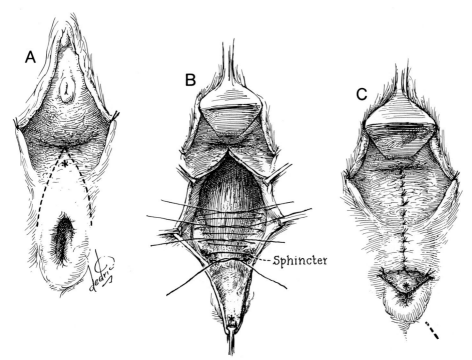

**Figure 14.3.** The vaginal flap operation (Warren-Miller-Brown) is shown. An inverted V-shaped incision is made through the full thickness of the vagina and skin of the perineum *(A)*, opening into the rectovaginal space. Traction is applied to the vaginal skin overlying the rectum at the site noted by the *asterisk*. This is freed laterally from the surrounding scar tissue, exposing the site of the perineal body and the ends of the anal sphincter. These are united from side to side with a series of interrupted stitches *(B)* of absorbable polyglycolic acid-type sutures. When the perineal body has been restored and the sphincter ends approximated, the posterior vaginal wall and skin of the perineum are closed by a series of interrupted stitches. The excess and flap skin may be trimmed now, or be permitted to remain *(C)* and the excess trimmed later as an outpatient procedure after the perineum and perineal skin have fully healed. This will retard undue shrinkage and retraction of this flap during the healing phase. If the reconstructed anal canal does not admit one fingerbreadth generously, the paradoxical sphincter incision of Miller and Brown can be performed. (See text, the site shown by the *dotted line* at the *bottom right* of C.

ultimate continence is reduced until healing in effect reunites the sphincter ends with scar tissue restoring a degree of functional competence. It requires between 8 and 12 weeks for this to take place, and the patient should be so informed.

Incompetence of the anal sphincter is almost invariably the result of obstetric laceration, the integrity of the sphincter generally having been interrupted in the midline near the twelve-o'clock position. The anterior wall of the rectum may or may not have been torn as well. When total healing has not taken place after repair of the fresh injury, various combinations of healing may occur: (*a*) The rectal tear may have healed but not the sphincter or perineal body. Sphincter incontinence results. (*b*) The perineal body and skin may have healed but not the rectal laceration. (*c*) The sphincter repair or some part thereof may or may not have healed. (d) A rectovaginal fistula is present, with or without sphincter incontinence.

When the healing process has been stabilized after injury or previous repair, and any raw areas have become epithelialized, planned reconstruction whould take place provided the patient is symptomatic and desires a restoration.

## TECHNIQUE OF THE VAGINAL FLAP OPERATION

After preoperative cleansing of the bowel by enemas until clear, an inverted V-shaped incision is made in the posterior vaginal wall of such a width that when the sides of the vagina are subsequently united, the introital width will be of the desired caliber (3, 7; Fig. 14.3). The base of this vaginal flap is continuous with the margin of the anterior rectal wall.

By sharp dissection through any scar tissue, the avascular space between the rectum and vagina is developed for several inches, mobilizing the anterior rectal wall. Stretching it by traction may bring it and the V-shaped vaginal flap to beneath the site of the external anal sphincter.

The buried ends of the sphincter are grasped, and appropriate mattress sutures of 2–0 long lasting but absorbable suture (polydiaxanone or PGA) are placed without tying.

The perineal body is reconstituted by several side-to-side sutures that are tied. Then, the anal sphincter stitches are tied and the perineal skin closed from side to side.

The undersurface of the vaginal flap is sewn to the external anal sphincter and perineal skin, and the excess is trimmed and removed.

## RESTORATION OF CONTINENCE BY REPAIR OF A LACERATED ANAL SPHINCTER

This operation [as suggested by Novak (5)] is designed to restore sphincter integrity and anal continence to a patient in whom this has been lost by laceration, most commonly after a fourth-degree obstetric laceration, and often one in which the rectal laceration may have healed after its repair at delivery but there was postoperative breakdown of the anal sphincter repair and occasionally of the perineum. The operation provides good exposure to the critical areas, particularly the ends of the lacerated anal sphincter as well as the tissue from which the perineum will be reconstructed. An essential step is one whereby the stitches that are placed reinforcing or restoring the integrity of the perineal body take much of the tension from the ends of the recently approximated external anal sphincter, splinting or bracing this repair and aiding in the integrity of its healing. If this tissue has been adequately identified and mobilized, it is not necessary to bring the medial borders of the pubococcygei together in front of the rectum, thus lessening the chance for painful ridges in the newly approximated tissue and subsequent dyspareunia. Polyglycolic acid-type suture is used, size 0 or 00. When the perineum has "disappeared," it must be mobilized and reconstructed as an integral part of the repair, which will effectively take much of the strain off the sphincter repair during its healing phase.

Symptoms of anal sphincter insufficiency are those of rectal incontinence, i.e., inability to control rectal gas and/or feces, especially when liquid. At times, soiling may precipitate a troublesome vaginitis.

The gynecologist must be mindful of the anorectal incontinence produced also by nerve damage, often the pudendal, sufficient to essentially denervate the pelvic diaphragm and the external anal sphincter (6). This can be suspected

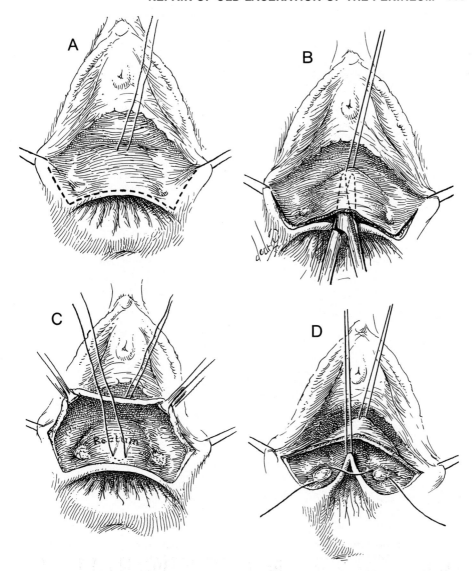

**Figure 14.4.** Sphincterplasty (Novak) is depicted. The perineal defect has been displayed by the three traction sutures as shown. An initial incision along the mucocutaneous border is followed by incisions lateral to the dimples identifying the ends of the torn anal sphincter *(A)*. The configuration of this is not unlike the letter W. The rectovaginal space is identified and entered *(B)* and the vagina carefully separated from the rectum by sharp dissection that extends lateral to the divided ends of the anal sphincter. A traction suture has been placed in the anterior wall of the rectum *(C)*. When upward traction has been applied to the rectal traction stitch, the tone ends of the sphincter stand out even more clearly *(D)*. They are grasped with Allis clamps and freed from the surrounding tissue by sharp dissection, and a stitch is placed in each end of the torn sphincter. Any previous laceration of the anterior rectal wall is approximated from side to side with two layers of interrupted stitches if the mucosa is intact, otherwise the traction suture of the rectal wall has to be placed higher up, the laceration totally excised, and the freshened rectal wound approximated with two layers. (*continued*)

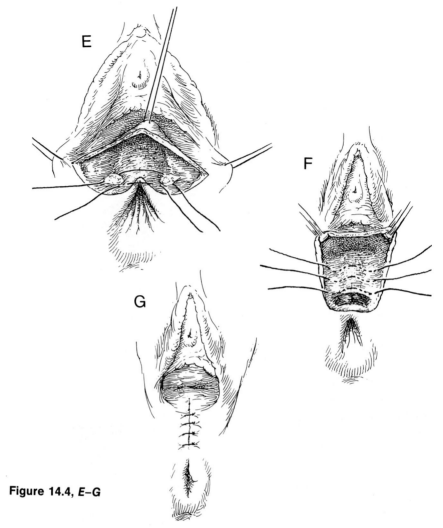

**Figure 14.4,** *E–G*

The ends of the torn anal sphincter *(E)* are approximated by tying the previously placed stitch, and an additional reinforcing mattress stitch or two are placed in the sphincter muscle and tied. The perineal body is reconstructed by a series of interrupted stitches *(F)* approximating it from side to side. The skin of the vagina and perineum is closed vertically *(G)*. (After Abram C in Novak F: *Surgical Gynecologic Techniques.* New York, John Wiley & Sons, pp 164–170, 1978.)

during the preoperative pelvic examination when the patient cannot voluntarily contract her pubococcygei and her external anal sphincter. The diagnosis can be confirmed by electromyography. This nerve damage, when acquired, is probably the consequence of straining at stool or from difficult or prolonged labor. Myoplasty will tighten a loose external sphincter system; but if the muscles have been denervated, the prognosis for functional improvement is guarded. Residual postsurgical function will be improved in the patient with unilateral or partial residual innervation remaining. Rectal continence will be aided by a good internal (involuntary) sphincter system.

Other less common causes include peripheral neuropathy as in some diabetics, diseases of the central nervous system or spinal cord or cauda equina, and postsurgical trauma as after laminectomy. It may be associated with the perineal descent syndrome (see Chapter 13). Some persons complaining of chronic diarrhea may really harbor an underlying undiagnosed sphincter incompetence secondary not only to sphincter laceration but also to sphincter denervation. Rectal sphincter weakness is usually not effectively treated by a sphincter plication in a patient who has not sustained a previous sphincter laceration. Medical treatment including loperamide hydrochloride (Imodium) may be helpful.

## TECHNIQUE OF OPERATION FOR RESTORATION OF ANAL SPHINCTER COMPETENCE

The bowel should be cleansed preoperatively by enemas until clear. Three traction stitches are placed as shown in Figure 14.4A (5). The damaged tissues must be dissected and mobilized carefully and scar tissue freed by sharp dissection. None of the tissue need be discarded. The torn ends of the sphincter will be buried in scar tissue and are identified by the subcutaneous dimples as shown. An incision resembling the letter W is made with the knife through the skin margin between the vagina and rectum and extended upward *lateral* to the cut ends of the sphincter. The rectovaginal space is entered and the vagina carefully separated from the anterior wall of the rectum up to the site of the previously placed traction suture, as shown in Figure 14.4B.

Allis forceps grasp the cut edge of the vagina. Scar tissue is freed by both sharp and blunt dissection with wide mobilization of vagina from rectum. The caudal portion of the rectovaginal space and site of the perineum are clearly exposed. A traction stitch is placed in the muscularis of the anterior rectal wall, as shown in Figure 14.4C. When upward tension is applied to this latter suture, the dimpling identifying the scar of the torn edges of the external anal sphincter will be more noticeable, and the edges may be grasped with Allis clamps or Kocher forceps. The scarred ends of the sphincter may be excised from the surrounding scar tissue by sharp dissection and a polydiaxanone or polyglycolic acid-type suture placed in the retracted scarred ends of the sphincter, as shown in Figure 14.4D. If the freed sphincter is long enough, the ends can be overlapped. For recurrent cases a suture of a permanent monofilament, Prolene or Surgilene, can be used provided it can be buried effectively.

If there is a V-shaped defect in the anterior anal wall, it is approximated by interrupted submucosal polyglycolic acid-type sutures (Fig. 14.4E), and a second reinforcing layer is placed to take the tension off the first layer.

The perineal body is reinforced or reconstructed by a series of horizontally placed interrupted sutures (Fig. 14.4F), the stitch in the anal sphincter is tied, a second and perhaps third reinforcing mattress suture is placed in the muscle itself and tied, and the perineal skin is closed vertically (Fig. 14.4G).

## POSTOPERATIVE CARE

Postoperative care for all of these procedures is otherwise much like that after repair of any type of rectovaginal fistula. Stool softeners are given for a month postoperatively. A clear liquid and nonresidue diet should be employed for 5 days, during which period constipation is to be encouraged. A rectal tube, however, may be used for short intervals to overcome any difficulty in expelling flatus. Stool softeners are started the third postoperative day and a gentle laxative the fourth, at which time a gradual return to house diet is initiated. An initial bowel movement is usually desirable by the seventh postoperative day, after which softening of the stool should be maintained for the following 2 or 3 weeks.

## References

1. Kelly HA: *Operative Gynecology.* New York, D Appleton & C., Vol I, p 211, 1898.
2. Mengert WF, Fish SA: Anterior rectal wall advancement. *Obstet Gynecol* 5:262–267, 1955.
3. Miller NF, Brown W: The surgical treatment of complete perineal tears in the female. *Am J Obstet Gynecol* 34:196–209, 1937.
4. Noble GH: A new operation for complete laceration of the perineum designed for the purpose of eliminating danger of infection from the rectum. *Trans Am Gynecol Soc* 27:357, 1902.
5. Novak F: *Surgical Gynecologic Techniques.* New York, John Wiley & Sons, pp 164–170, 1978.
6. Swash M: New concepts in incontinence. *Br Med J* 290:4–5, 1985.
7. Warren JC: A new method of operation for the relief of rupture of the perineum through the sphincter and rectum. *Trans Am Gynecol Soc* 7:322, 1882.

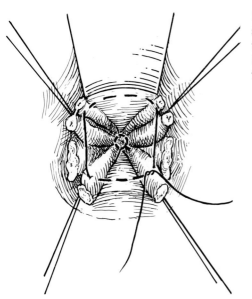

**Figure 15.6.** A first purse-string stitch has been tied, closing the peritoneal cavity. A second purse-string has been placed 1 cm distal to the first. It, too, will be tied.

type of suture placement but do not disturb the course of the ureter. They are especially useful when there is no vault prolapse present. They can be placed after either transabdominal or transvaginal operations (Fig. 15.7), but it must be remembered that neither effectively supports a poorly or unsupported vaginal vault.

Enterocele with prolapse of the vault posterior to the cervix in the patient whose uterus has been fixed by a Gilliam suspension or ventral fixation is treated transvaginally by high ligation of the neck of the sac. This includes a deep bite or two into the lower posterior part of the cervix or lower uterine segment, then excision of the sac.

Midline approximation and shortening of the uterosacral ligaments is performed if they are strong; and repair of any coexistent cystocele and rectocele, the latter including the high full-length posterior colporrhaphy. If eversion of the upper vagina coexists and cardinal and uterosacral ligament strength are insufficient to support the vaginal vault securely it may be sewn to the right sacrospinous ligament (see Chapter 16).

Transabdominal procedures include excision of redundant cul-de-sac peritoneum with approximation of uterosacral ligaments, longitudinal obliterative sutures of the Halban type (4) (Figs. 15.8 and 15.9), or circumferential obliterative sutures of the Marion-Moschowitz (9, 12) type. If there is a wide voluminous posterior vagina, this should be narrowed by wedging as suggested by both Waters (18) and Torpin (17). This can be done either transabdominally or transvaginally and will tend to approximate the uterosacral ligament attachments closer to the midline. The McCall transvaginal cul-de-plasty (11) may be useful if there are palpably strong uterosacral ligaments, as with the uterovaginal or "sliding" type of prolapse.

When coexistent eversion of the vagina is present and the abdomen is open, transabdominal colposacropexy might be considered to preserve vaginal length, although it must be remembered that any coincident cystocele and rectocele must be repaired by a separate procedure at a later date. When any transabdominal procedure is performed which, changes the vaginal axis to a more vertical direction, such as the Marshall-Marchetti-Krantz (10) or the

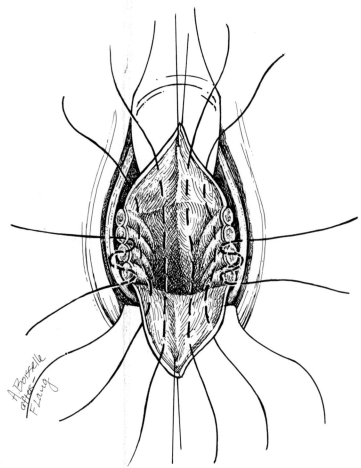

**Figure 15.7.** Sagittal obliteration of the cul-de-sac may be performed after vaginal hysterectomy as shown.

Burch (3) procedure, or ventral suspension or fixation (see Chapter 16), the cul-de-sac of Douglas should be adequately protected by surgical obliteration of the peritoneum-lined cul-de-sac anterior to the rectum. The increased exposure, vulnerability, and risk of enterocele if a deep anterior or posterior cul-de-sac is not obliterated should be more widely recognized. An anterior enterocele that develops after hysterectomy probably is best treated by transvaginal resection of the sac and redundant peritoneum, with restoration of the normal upper vaginal axis and correction of any defect in the levator plate.

Pudendal or lateral enterocele may be approached transvaginally if the margins of the neck of the sac are distinguishable and can be readily identified. If they are vague and ill defined, either a combined vaginal-abdominal or an abdominal approach should be considered.

The simplest treatment of true rectal prolapse with or without coexistent genital prolapse is the insertion of Thiersch wires to reinforce the anal sphincter. More radical procedures for recurrence are the transperineal resection of Altemeier et al. (1) or, better yet, the transabdominal operation of Ripstein and Lanter (16), which uses a sling-like pararectal replacement of synthetic plastic material to replace or supplement attenuated rectal supports.

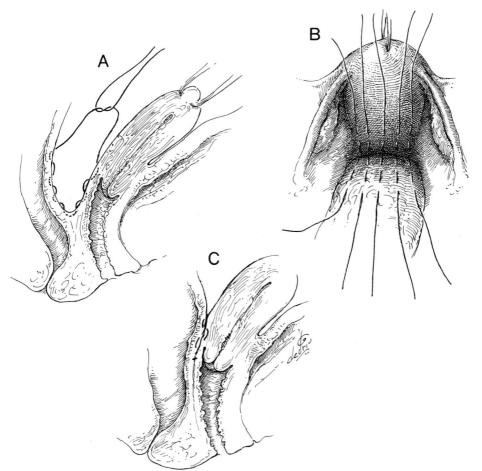

**Figure 15.8.** The cul-de-sac is being obliterated by a series of interrupted stitches placed from front to back. The placement of the stitches is shown in sagittal section in *A,* as viewed from the abdomen in *B,* and after tying in *C.* If the uterus is no longer present, similar stitches are placed in the posterior wall of the vagina. (Reproduced with permission of JB Lippincott from Nichols DH: Repair of enterocele and prolapse of the vaginal vault. In Barber H (ed): *Goldsmith's Practice of Surgery,* 1981.)

Coincident genital prolapse should be treated by appropriate surgical reconstruction. Anal prolapse may be treated by retrorectal levatorplasty as described in Chapter 13.

It is essential that the gynecologist recognize enterocele and any potential likely to result in an enterocele and correlate this with cause, symptoms, progression, and other coexistent pelvic damage. An enterocele may be any one of the following types: congential, pulsion, or traction, and, occasionally, iatrogenic, spontaneous, or acquired. A pulsion enterocele may be followed by a cystocele and rectocele, whereas a traction enterocele is preceded by a cystocele and rectocele. An enterocele may occur with or without eversion of the vagina and with or without prolapse of the rectum. The location of the hernia will be determined by its cause. The etiology, symptoms, and principles of surgical treatment are considerably different for each of the various sites.

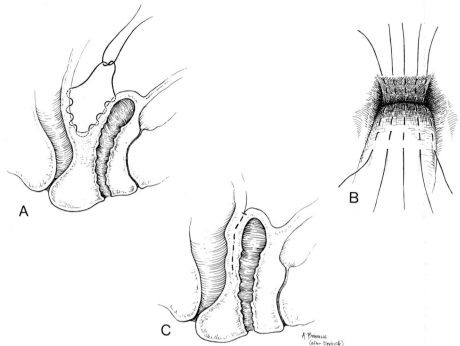

**Figure 15.9.** Similar obliteration of the cul-de-sac may be performed after transabdominal hysterectomy.

There is no one standard corrective operation. A choice of the possible operative procedures should be made on a rational, correlative basis in accordance with the principles that have been suggested (Table 15.1).

### References

1. Altemeier WA, Hoxworth PI, Giuseffi J: Further experiences with the treatment of prolapse of the rectum. *Surg Clin North Am* 35:1437–1447, 1955.
2. Anderson WR: Pudendal hernia. *Obstet Gynecol* 32:802–804, 1968.
3. Burch JC: Urethrovaginal fixation to Cooper's ligament for correction of stress incontinence, cystocele, and prolapse. *Am Obstet Gynecol* 81:281–290, 1961.
4. Halban J: *Gynäkologische Operationslehre.* Berlin, Urban and Schwarzenberg, 1932.
5. Hawksworth W, Roux JP: Vaginal hysterectomy. *J Obstet Gynecol Br Commonw* 63:214–228, 1958.
6. Lash AF, Levin B: Roentgenographic diagnosis of vaginal vault hernia. *Obstet Gynecol* 20:427–433, 1962.
7. Lenzi E: *L'Ernia Vaginale del Douglas O Elitrocele.* Pisa, Edizioni Omnia Medica, 1959, pp 65-69.
8. Litschgi M, Käser O: The problem of enterocele. *Geburtshilfe Frauenheilkd* 38:915–920, 1978.
9. Marion J: Quoted by Read CD. Enterocele. *Am J Obstet Gynecol* 62:743–753, 1951.
10. Marshall VF, Marchetti AA, Krantz KE: The correction of stress incontinence by simple vesicourethral suspension. *Surg Gynecol Obstet* 88:509–518, 1949.
11. McCall ML: Posterior culdeplasty: Surgical correction of enterocele during vaginal hysterectomy, a preliminary report. *Obstet Gynecol* 10:595–602, 1957.
12. Moschowitz AV: The pathogenesis anatomy and cure of prolapse of the rectum. *Surg Gynecol Obstet* 15:7–21, 1912.
13. Nichols DH: Types of enterocele and principles underlying the choice of operation for repair. *Obstet Gynecol* 40:257–263, 1972.
14. Pirogoff (Fig. 4, Plate XXI) in Hart DB: *Atlas of Female Pelvic Anatomy.* Edinburgh, W & AK Johnston, 1884.
15. Read CD: Enterocele. *Am J Obstet Gynecol* 62:743–757, 1951.
16. Ripstein CC, Lanter B: Etiology and surgical therapy of massive prolapse of the rectum. *Ann Surg* 157:259–264, 1963.

17. Torpin R: Excision of the cul-de-sac of Douglas for the surgical sure of Hernias through the female caudal wall: Including prolapse of the uterus. *J Med Assoc Ga* 36:396–406, 1947.

18. Waters EG: Vaginal prolapse. *Gynecology* 8:432–436, 1956.

19. Weed JC, Tyrone C: Enterocele. *Am J Obstet Gynecol* 60:324–332, 1950.

20. Wilensky AV, Kaufman PA: Vaginal hernia. *Am J Surg* 49:31–41, 1940.

21. Zacharin RF: *Pelvic Floor Anatomy and the Surgery of Pulsion Enterocele*. New York, Springer-Verlag, 1985.

# CHAPTER 16

# Massive Eversion of the Vagina

## SCOPE OF THE PROBLEM

There are few maladies in feminine life more disturbing to its quality than that of massive eversion of one's vagina. It is specific, dramatic, obvious, frustrating, embarassing, and progressive. It may occur with or without the presence of the uterus, as prolapse of the latter is the result and not the cause of the eversion. The malady is surgically curable, with relief of symptoms, and restoration of normal anatomic relationships.

Primary sacrospinous colpopexy immediately after vaginal hysterectomy in a patient with uterine prolapse, without surgically useful strong uterosacral cardinal ligament support (general prolapse, see Chapter 3) is not common but is surpisingly easy to accomplish. This is because there has been no previous surgery to alter tissue planes and spaces. It can be added to the primary procedure by an experienced vaginal surgeon within an additional 15 minutes of operating time between the steps of peritoneal closure and the posterior repair.

Massive eversion of the vagina is a complex disorder. Cystocele, rectocele, and enterocele may or may not coexist, and the distinction is surgically important as each, when present, should be repaired. Comfort and normal vaginal function can be restored by carefully selected surgery.

More women are living longer and there is much interest in maintaining a self-image of femininity and the capacity for sexual activity beyond the menopause.

Although some cases of massive eversion of the vaginal vault occur in the nullipara, probably related to congenital pelvic tissue weakness, defective innervation, or unusual trauma, the majority are seen in parous women. Among these women the incidence might be reduced by obstetrically skillful management of labor and delivery. In various childbirth settings, there is less frequent use of timely and anatomically repaired episiotomy and babies may be delivered by persons other than skilled obstetricians. With some resurgence of interest in home delivery, we should expect to see an increase in the incidence of genital prolapse as well as other gynecologic consequences of unattended childbirth.

That a ''dropped uterus'' is the result and not the cause of genital prolapse has not always been appreciated. ''Routine'' abdominal hysterectomy has been performed for uterine prolapse in the mistaken belief that in the condition of dropped uterus: no uterus, no dropping. The vaginal vault prolapse persists whether or not the uterus is present, and these patients are seen in consultation some time after their primary surgery, frequently referred by the initial surgeon.

In taking the patient's history, one should carefully note whether or not there was a previous urinary stress incontinence when the patient was younger and which symptoms were relieved as the vaginal vault descended, suggesting a kinking of the urethra coincident with the prolapse. Such a patient is very likely to develop a recurrent urinary stress incontinence when the vagina has been repositioned within the pelvis unless special appropriate steps are accomplished with the anterior colporrhaphy to lessen the likelihood of this possibility.

The chronically increased intra-abdominal pressure that was so often the cause of massive eversion of the vagina may also promote the development of a coincident hiatal hernia. Such a patient will often give a history of heartburn when lying down.

The patient should be examined when she is fully awake and when she is standing. One should replace the vault and reobserve any possible cystocele, rectocele, and enterocele. A notation should be made as to the positive findings on examination, that appropriate repair may be scheduled and remembered as part of the definitive surgery.

Generally, if weaknesses in these areas are present, even of minor degree, they all should be simultaneously repaired. This will improve the overall surgical success of a reconstructive procedure and decrease the necessity for a separate future secondary operation.

When a decision has been made for repair of genital prolapse, a skilled surgeon should have several surgical techniques from which to choose. As Charles Mayo said, "one should make the operation fit the patient, not make the patient fit the operation." Although a surgeon tends to concentrate on operations that he or she performs best, various combinations of damage necessitate thoroughly learning the various techniques, that one may choose that which will best fit the need of the individual patient. There are significant preventive aspects concerning recurrent prolapse that we can encompass in the operating room during our day-to-day practice of surgical gynecology.

Posthysterectomy vaginal vault eversion is related to the adequacy of support of the vaginal vault. Prevention of eversion is directly related to recognizing the strength and length of the patient's uterosacral ligaments at the time of surgery. If they are strong and long, they should be shortened before they are attached to the vaginal vault. A wide vaginal vault should be surgically narrowed, and the cul-de-sac obliterated or any enterocele excised. Sewing the uterosacral ligaments together at the time of posthysterectomy peritonealization is useful, and the New Orleans or McCall culdeplasty can be used. When cardinal-uterosacral strength is lacking, the surgeon must use an alternate method of colpopexy.

The surgeon should attempt to restore normal vaginal depth and axis particularly after any vesicourethral pinup operation such as the Marshall-Marchetti-Krantz or the Burch modification (4) that pulls the vagina anteriorly. Many times, this can be achieved by a perineorrhaphy and posterior colporrhaphy.

Although massive eversion of the vagina is more common in the postmenopausal patient, it also can occur in the young and the uterus may or may not be present. It is more common in the white patient than in the black patient for reasons not totally understood. Progressive unrepaired uterine prolapse will often progress to procidentia in which there is displacement of the entire uterus outside of the pelvic cavity. Surgically usable cardinal-uterosacral ligament strength may be absent in the patient with total genital procidentia, and colpopexy to a nongynecologic structure such as the sacrospinous ligament may be required to restore vaginal depth.

Because there are various etiologic factors, different surgical procedures are required for correction. Figure 3.7 shows an obvious protrusion of cervix beyond the vulva. Notice the rectocele and cystocele, but no enterocele. This condition represents general prolapse, usually postmenopausal, and includes weakness of the pelvic supporting tissues with consequent descent of the cul-de-sac. All the internal genitalia have dropped, but the relationship between the anterior rectal wall and the back of the uterus is unchanged. This relationship is the same as when the uterus and rectum were higher in the pelvis. Although the cul-de-sac is displaced, it does not dissect between the rectum and vagina as would be true of enterocele (3). One must make this distinction because both etiology and surgical therapy of prolapse with enterocele, shown in Figure 3.6 are entirely different. The cervix is outside the pelvis, and there is cystocele and enterocele but no rectocele. The relationship between the cervix and the anterior wall of the rectum is changed because the cul-de-sac and its peritoneum have dissected between the rectum and vagina, and the latter actually slides along the anterior wall of the rectum, the vaginal counterpart of rectal prolapse.

Amreich (1) indicated the importance of preserving vaginal depth after hysterectomy. If, after removal of the uterus, the vagina is otherwise well supported and sits upon an intact levator plate, intra-abdominal pressure applied to the vagina will be countered by pressure from the pelvic diaphragm. The vagina will be compressed between these two pressures and remain in place. But if the vagina is short after hysterectomy, it may telescope upon itself, becoming even shorter as intra-abdominal pressure is directed in the axis of a vagina which ends anterior to the levator plate (Fig. 16.1). An exception is the patient who has had a Wertheim or Schauta radical hysterectomy, in which the scarring in this area is so great that very little will disturb it. Preserving vaginal depth is an important prophylactic feature of all genital surgery.

After total hysterectomy, the uterosacral ligament complex is detached from the uterus and, if not reattached to the vaginal vault, undergoes atrophy. After a few months or years it may no longer be sufficiently strong to be of much use in surgical reconstruction of the future vault eversion.

There are partial degrees of eversion which, if ignored at hysterectomy or otherwise left unattended, will generally progress (Fig. 16.2).

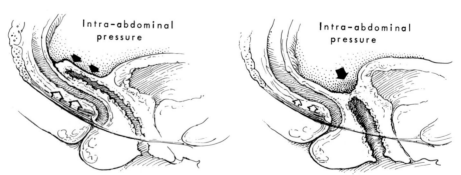

**Figure 16.1.** A deep vagina after hysterectomy tends to be sqeezed or "sandwiched" in place between the forces of intra-abdominal pressure from above (*black arrows*) and the resistance of the levator place below (*white arrows*), as shown on the left. When the vagina is so short as to end anterior to the levator plate, intra-abdominal pressure will be exerted in the axis of the vagina, tending to telescope it and make it even shorter, as seen in the drawing on the right. (After Amreich J: Aetiologic und Operation des Scheidenstumpf prolapses. Wien Klin Wochenschr 63:74–77, 1951.)

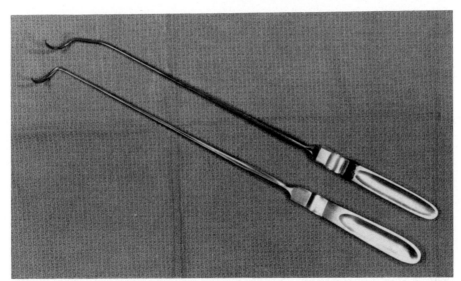

**Figure 16.12.** Long Deschamps ligature carriers are shown. An angled Deschamps ligature carrier (modeled after one modified by Rosenshein) noted at the top, is useful when the sacrospinous ligament is unusually deep. The handle must be swung through a wide arc. These instruments are available on special order from Codman & Shurtleff, Custom Device Dept., New Bedford, MA 02745, or Mr. William Merz, American V. Mueller, Chicago, IL 60648.

at the nine- or three-o'clock position and notes the position and size of the right sacrospinous ligament. During the progress of the surgeon's path from the rectovaginal space into the pararectal space, the descending rectal septum should be penetrated by either sharp or blunt dissection *closer to the undersurface of the vagina* than to the rectum, aiming directly at the site at which the ischial spine has been palpated.

The operator perforates the right rectal pillar at a spot overlying the ischial spine and proceeds from the rectovaginal space into the right pararectal space (Fig. 16.11). This penetration can be made bluntly with the fingertip if the pillar is thin or weak, or with scissor tips or a long hemostatic forceps, such as a tonsil forceps. A forceps tip may be inserted through this window into the right pillar, and the forceps or the tips of the Mayo scissors opened and spread, enlarging the penetration and exposing the superior surface of the pelvic diaphragm. A long and preferably straight retractor of suitable size (Figs. 8.10, 8.16, 8.17) is inserted deeply into the wound, displacing the rectum to the patient's left; another displaces the cardinal ligament and ureter anteriorly. Similar exposure, although with less facility, can be obtained by three narrow Deaver retractors, but the curve of the Deaver offers no advantage and one must be especially careful not to let the tip of the retractor be pushed across the anterior surface of the sacrum, lest it risk damage to the sacral veins.

Direct adequate illumination of this deep area is essential and can be provided by a spotlight just over the operator's shoulder or by a suitable bright fiberoptic forehead lamp. Loose areolar tissue is pushed to one side, exposing the superior surface of the pelvic diaphragm, and the blunt dissection easily proceeds to the ischial spine. The superior surface of the coccygeus muscle is clearly identified, running posterolaterally from the ischial spine. Areolar tissue may be pushed from the surface of the right coccygeus muscle containing the sacrospinous ligament, if desired, using a "rosebud" or wisp sponge. Bleeding within the pararectal space exposure is uncommon, and is usually of anomalous venous origin, and can be controlled readily by medium-sized vascular clips.

If one is to use the right sacrospinous ligament, the middle finger of the left hand should be placed on the medial surface of the ischial spine and under direct vision the tip of the long-handled Deschamps ligature (Fig. 16.12) carrier penetrates the coccygeus muscle-sacrospinous ligament at a point 1 ½ to 2 fingerbreadths medial to the ischial spine. The carrier tip is pushed through (not around or under) the ligament. Considerable resistance is usually encountered and this must be overcome by persistent forcefulness in the process of rotating the handle of the ligature carrier. Gentle traction to the handle will actually move the patient on the table, confirming proper placement. If no resistance is encountered, the ligature carrier could be either in front of the ligament or around the ligament rather than through it, exposing the structures behind the ligament to potential injury. Therefore, if no resistance is encountered as the ligature carrier is passed through the structure, the operator should remove the ligature carrier and reinsert it through the substance of the ligament. Obvious resistance should be encountered as the tip of the ligature carrier is being passed through the ligamentous tissue.

Early in one's experience, the surgeon will wish to expose the area of fixation for suture placement to his or her direct vision, requiring appropriate anatomic dissection. Suture loop or needle retrieval must always be under direct

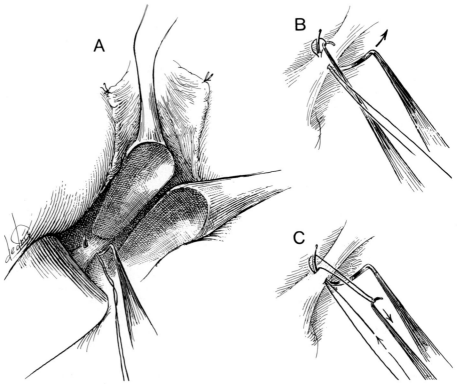

**Figure 16.13.** *A.* An upper retractor holds the transverse cervical ligament out of the way, and a similar retractor on the right displaces the rectum. The right sacrospinous ligament has been exposed and penetrated by the ligature carrier. *B.* The loop of suture within the ligature carrier is caught by the hook. *C.* Traction upon the hook brings the free end of the suture through the ligament, and the ligature carrier can be withdrawn.

visualization, however, the muscle and the ligament within can often be grasped in the tip of a long Babcock clamp that helps to isolate the tissue to be sutured from any underlying vessels or nerves. The sutures in the Deschamps ligature carrier or needle should be inserted directly into the ligament 1 ½ to 2 fingerbreadths medial to the ischial spine (Fig. 16.13). With increased experience and through a smaller incision into the septum, the tactile sense can be developed without compromising the accuracy of suture placement at a point 1 ½ to 2 fingerbreadths medial to the ischial spine. If the window made through the descending rectal septum is smaller than 3 cm in diameter and difficulty is encountered in exposing the surface of the muscle and the operator is certain that the rectum has been displaced medially, it is possible to pursue an alternative approach to penetration of the ligament. The tip of the operator's left middle finger is inserted through the window and along the inner surface of the pelvic diaphragm until the tip of the ischial spine and the sacrospinous ligament are identified. Keeping the lateral surface of the tip of the middle finger adjacent to the tip of the spine, the tip of the long-handled Deschamps or the modified Deschamps ligature carrier (Figs. 16.11, 16.12) holding its suture is directed along the undersurface of the operator's left index finger until it reaches the sacrospinous ligament-coccygeus muscle complex. At a point clearly 1 ½ to 2 fingerwidths medial to the spine, and well away from the underlying pudendal nerve and vessels, the tip of the ligature carrier is rotated and made to penetrate the sacrospinous ligament. The fingers of the left hand are withdrawn, the retractors suitably repositioned, and the tip of the ligature carrier is visualized at this point, the suture grasped, the carrier removed, and the operation proceeds in the usual fashion. (Rarely, the nearby sacrotuberous ligament will be found to be stronger and more convenient than the sacrospinous, in which case suture to the sacrotuberous ligament may be substituted.)

The suture material is grasped at the tip of the ligature carrier (Fig. 16.13B) and held with the hook and the loop pulled through 2 or 3 inches, and the Deschamps carrier is removed slowly and carefully in a counterclockwise fashion. The blunt point of the Deschamps ligature carrier is less apt to lacerate nearby blood vessels than is the sharp point of the conventional needle. The latter, being brittle because it is made of extruded wire, might break, and the broken tip hard to find and possibly lost. A second suture is similarly placed 1 cm medial to the first, and held. Alternatively, it seems quite permissible after pulling the first suture through, as shown in Figure 16.13C, while retaining both free ends, to cut the loop in its center, pairing each end of the cut loop with its respective free suture end, thus, obtaining two sutures through the ligament but with only one penetration by the Deschamps carrier (Fig. 16.14).

Postoperatively, the vault of the vagina deviates to the side of the patient to which the attachment was made, but this produces neither dyspareunia nor dysfunction.

The depth of the vagina to be realized after sacrospinous colpopexy is dependent upon the distance from the vulva to the point at which the vagina is fixed to the sacrospinous ligament.

The vagina normally is much wider at the vault. This is particularly evident when the vagina has turned inside-out, as from massive posthysterectomy prolapse. Whether or not a colpopexy should be unilateral or bilateral depends upon the width of the vaginal vault. If it is wide and the operator intends to keep it that way, the colpopexy should be bilateral. If the vault is narrow or if the operator has deliberately made it narrow, then the colpopexy should be unilateral. If a wide vault is attached unilaterally, the unattached side will gradually descend, unless it is surgically narrowed.

Usually, equally good results are obtained if a unilateral colpopexy is performed and a wide vault is resected to convert the shape of a vagina from

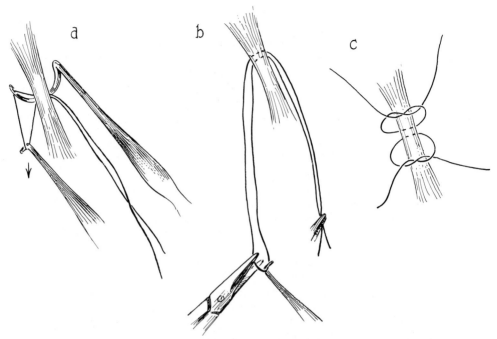

**Figure 16.14.** After the suture, doubled, has been passed through the ligament and caught by the hook *(a)*, the ligature carrier is removed. The loop may be cut in the center *(b)* and each end paired with its respective free suture, as shown, thus obtaining two sutures through the ligament *(c)* but with only one penetration by the Deschamps ligature carrier.

one resembling a lightbulb to that of a cylinder of uniform diameter-as it is now an instrument of coitus, not parturition.

The free end of the sutures through the ligament are sewn to the underside of the vagina, but not yet tied. If an anterior colporrhaphy has not yet been performed, a full-length repair of the anterior vaginal wall is usually done now. The upper part of the posterior colporrhaphy is begun, and when the upper 2 inches of posterior vaginal wall have been approximated, traction is made to the free end of the pulley stitch, all slack is taken up, and it and each of the other colpopexy stitches are tied, fixing the vaginal vault in the hollow of the sacrum, and the remainder of the posterior colporrhaphy and perineorrhaphy are completed.

If a narrow vault is attached bilaterally, the undersurface of the vagina cannot reach the surface of the coccygeus muscle-sacrospinous ligament complex without suture bridges. If these are absorbable sutures, the scar will be weak and recurrence of the prolapse likely. If they are of nonabsorbable Prolene or Surgilene, the vault will stay in place.

The vagina ideally should be sewn to the muscle-ligament as a firm tissue-to-tissue approximation. One method of bringing the soft movable vagina to the surface of the coccygeus muscle and ligament might be described as a "pulley." After the stitch has been placed in the ligament, one end of the suture is rethreaded on a free needle and sewn and tied by a single half-hitch to the full thickness of the fibromuscular layer of the undersurface of the vaginal apex, while the free end of the suture is held long. Traction to the free end of the suture at the proper time will pull the vagina directly onto the muscle and ligament (Fig. 16.15), where a square knot will fix it in place. When the vagina is thin or if greater vaginal length is desired, each end of the colpopexy stitch

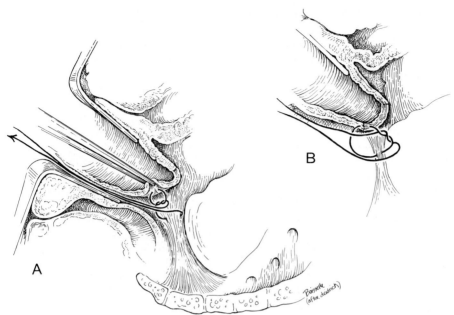

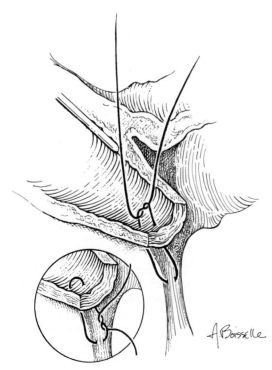

**Figure 16.15.**   *A.* The ''pulley'' stitch is illustrated. One end of the suture through the sacrospinous ligament has been sewn to the undersurface of the cut edge of the vaginal vault. Traction to the other end of the suture draws the vagina up and laterally to the surface of the ligament, and the ends are tied together, fixing the vagina to the ligament at this point. A second ''safety'' stitch similarly placed through the ligament is sewn to the subepithelial tissues of the vaginal wall and tied *(B).*

**Figure 16.16.**   When the vaginal wall is thin, its full-thickness may be sewn to the surface of the coccygeus muscle-sacrospinous ligament complex as shown, leaving the knot of an absorbable suture within the lumen of the vagina. If a monofilament nonabsorbable suture has been used, the knot is buried beneath the vagina, as shown in the inset.

may be inserted *through* the vagina, as shown in Fig. 16.16. This should be done after the excision of an appropriate segment of posterior vaginal wall as part of the posterior colporrhaphy, and side-to-side approximation with a running subcuticular stitch of polyglycolic acid suture has united the sides of the upper half of the vagina. Tying the fixation stitch before this latter step reduces visibility for exposure of the vaginal vault, making suture of the colporrhaphy more difficult. It is essential that the pulley stitch be tied snugly so there is no void or gap between the vagina and the ligament (Fig. 16.17). Such a gap would be called a "suture bridge" and should be avoided, because once the suture is absorbed there would be less in the way of strong scar tissue to hold the vagina to the ligament, and should the vagina pull away, the prolapse may recur. We now use no. 2 size polyglycolic acid type (Dexon or Vicryl) for this suture, as too fine a suture in this ligament might act somewhat like a saw and actually cut through the ligament with tying. This no. 2 size thickness has good knot-tying strength, and being of controlled slow absorbency, will last for several weeks. This is in contrast to catgut, which retains its maximal strength and continuity for only 7 to 10 days. A monofilament synthetic nonabsorbable suture such as size 0 Prolene or Surgilene may be

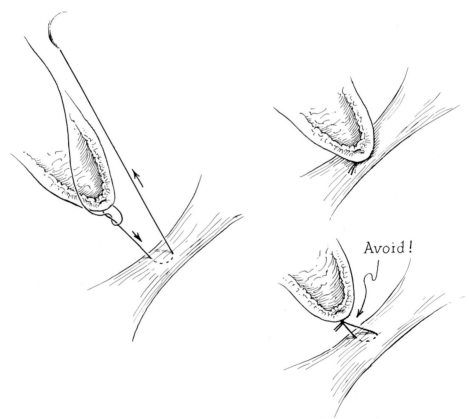

**Figure 16.17.**   A suture has been passed through the sacrospinous ligament and a firm bite taken into the tissues of the vaginal wall to which it is fixed at this point by a single half-hitch as shown on the *left*. Traction to the opposite free end of the suture will use the point of passage through the firm tissue as a pulley, bringing the movable tissue to this point, where the two tissues are now in direct contact with one another and a conventional knot is tied, fixing the new relationship, seen in the upper right. A suture-bridge, as shown on the lower *right,* should be avoided.

added, particularly in the patient with significant chronic respiratory disease or with recurrent prolapse, though care should be taken that the knot of any nonabsorbable suture be buried beneath the vagina.

Permanent sutures such as monofilament synthetic nonabsorbable suture Prolene or Surgilene size 0 can be recommended as the principal colpopexy stitches in the following circumstances:

1. Recurrent vaginal vault eversion;
2. A patient with chronic respiratory disease;
3. A patient with a short vagina of insufficient length to reach the ischial spine; in this circumstance, one may create a deliberate suture bridge between the top of the vault of the short vagina and the surface of the coccygeus muscle-sacrospinous ligament;
4. A patient who will be required to perform heavy lifting after her convalescence.

Figure 16.18 shows the effect on the vesicourethral junction of bringing an everted vault of the vagina back into the hollow of the sacrum.

This pulley stitch need be done with only one of the suture pairs. The second or "safety" stitch can be inserted through the muscular wall of the vagina but not tied until the pulley stitch has brought and tied the vagina securely to the sacrospinous ligament. The second or safety stitch is later readily tied with a simple square knot (Fig. 16.15B). Any needed anterior colporrhaphy is now accomplished.

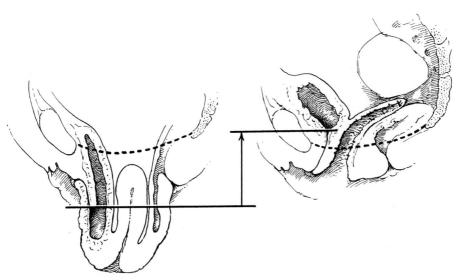

**Figure 16.18.** The relationship of the vesicourethral junction to the pubis and pelvis is illustrated in sagittal section. The usual location of the pelvic diaphragm is indicated by the *dotted line*. The vesicourethral junction is indicated by the *solid line*. On the *left,* advanced genital prolapse is depicted showing that eversion of the vagina may pull on tissues supporting the vesicourethral junction, exteriorizing the latter. The effects of restoration of vaginal depth and axis are shown on the *right.* Repositioning of the vagina has provided upward traction to tissues of the vesicourethral junction, helping to restore them once again to a position within the pelvis. (Reproduced with permission of Harper & Row from Nichols DH: Effects of pelvic relaxation on gynecologic urologic problems. *Clin Obstet Gynecol* 21:1766, 1978.)

It is now time to tie the sacrospinous fixation stitches. By traction to the free end of the stitch (opposite to that which had been fixed to the undersurface of the vagina), the vaginal wall is drawn to rest squarely upon the surface of the sacrospinous ligament-coccygeus muscle complex, and the knots are tied. The posterior colporrhaphy and perineorrhaphy are then completed. The whole operation is shown in Color Figures 16.1-16.8. The vault of the vagina will be found to lie in its normal horizontal axis, although deviated slightly to the patient's right. The vagina can be packed lightly with iodoform gauze for 24 hours. Because the right rectal pillar is now compressed between the vagina and the right sacrospinous ligament, immediate postoperative examination will show the rectum to be pulled to the patient's right. Within a few weeks the pillar must elongate, for by then the rectum can again be found to be in the midline. Postoperatively, many patients observe a transient mild discomfort or pulling sensation deep in the right buttock, without transmission of discomfort to the thigh, but as the edema subsides this regresses within a few days or weeks. Examination usually shows excellent vaginal depth and axis (Fig. 16.8B), and increased intra-abdominal pressure serves to press the vagina against the levator plate and accentuates the restored horizontal axis of the vagina. To date, no patient has complained of dyspareunia after this type of vaginal fixation.

## OPERATIVE COMPLICATIONS

### Penetration of a Viscus

If a needle tip penetrates the lumen of any adjacent viscus (the rectum would be most likely), the needle should be withdrawn. If a laceration is encountered it should be repaired by a standard two-layered closure. If at any time during the procedure it has been determined by a rectal examination that a suture has transgressed the wall of the rectum, the suture should be promptly removed and replaced in a proper position outside the rectal lumen.

Pudendal on sciatic trauma, a rare complication of sacrospinous colpopexy, is recognized by immediate severe postoperative gluteal pain running down the posterior surface of the affected leg. It should be treated promptly by deligation and medial reposition of the fixation sutures.

In spite of the *full-length* anterior colporrhaphy usually done, a mild but usually transient urinary stress incontinence has been noted in an occasional patient, probably the result of temporarily straightening the posterior urethrovesical angle. It tends to disappear after several months as a new posterior urethrovesical angle becomes established. Kegel perineal resistive exercises are helpful. Rarely, suprapubic vesicourethral suspension may be recommended.

Recurrent but asymptomatic cystocele without stress incontinence is the most frequent complication of colpopexy and most will become evident within the first 3 months postoperatively. They rarely require treatment. Some are probably the result of progression after under-repair at the time of surgery, some are the result of natural progression of the disease, and some the result of unrecognized and unrepaired lateral (paravaginal) attenuation or avulsion. The presence and degree of the latter, when recognized preoperatively or intraoperatively, can be repaired as part of the reconstructive surgery (see Chapter 11).

### Transabdominal Surgery

There are some abdominal approaches to the solution of this difficult problem, but success of these procedures is variable. Ventral fixation of the uterine fundus to the anterior abdominal wall was once popular. Although the

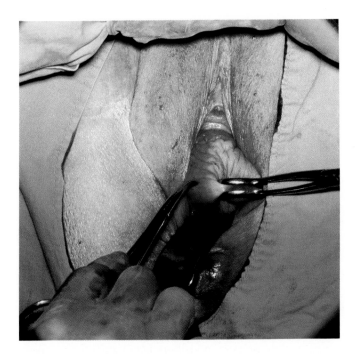

**Color Figure 16.1.** The scar at the apex of the vagina has been grasped by a sponge forceps. The hemostat marks a small dimple; this is the site at which the right uterosacral ligament was attached to the vagina at hysterectomy almost 30 years earlier. (Photograph by Lester V Bergman, courtesy LTI Medica and The Upjohn Company. Coyright 1982 by Learning Technology Incorporated.)

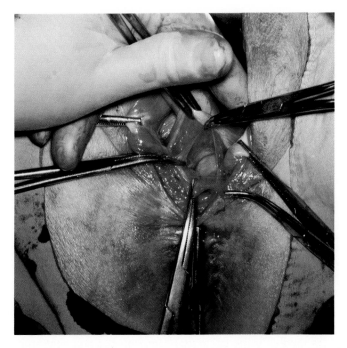

**Color Figure 16.2.** An enterocele has been identified, opened, and mobilized before resection. (Photograph by Lester V Bergman, courtesy LTI Medica and The Upjohn Company. Copyright 1982 by Learning Technology Incorporated.)

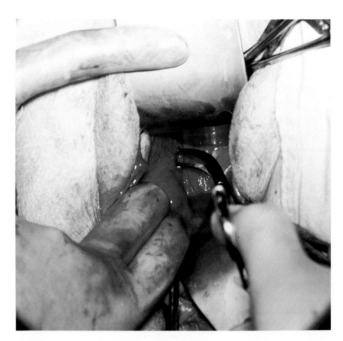

**Color Figure 16.3.** The right rectal pillar has been penetrated at a spot overlying the right ischial spine. The penetration is here being enlarged by opening the tips of a long, pointed forceps. (Photograph by Lester V Bergman, courtesy LTI Medica and The Upjohn Company. Copyright 1982 by Learning Technology Incorporated.)

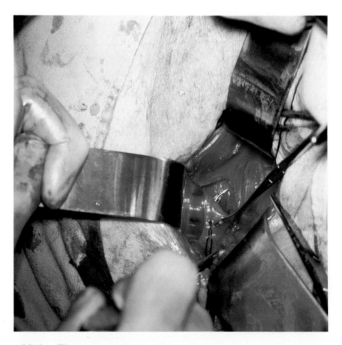

**Color Figure 16.4.** The sacrospinous ligament within the coccygeus muscle has been grasped in a long Babcock clamp, about 4 cm medial to the ischial spine. At a point about 3 cm medial to the spine, the sacrospinous ligament and coccygeus muscle have been pentrated by the tip of a Deschamps ligature carrier into which has been inserted a suture of No. 2 Dexon. (Photograph by Lester V Bergman, courtesy LTI Medica and The Upjohn Company. Copyright 1982 by Learning Technology Incorporated.)

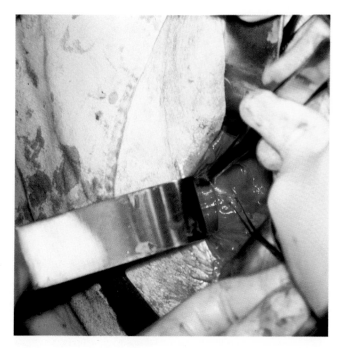

**Color Figure 16.5.** The Deschamps ligature carrier has been removed. This shows placement of the Dexon suture through the sacrospinous ligament and coccygeus muscle. Traction to the suture will move the patient on the table. The location of the ischial spine is indicated by the tip of the forceps in the upper part of the picture. One can readily see that the ligament has been penetrated 2.5 to 3 cm medial to the spine. (Photograph by Lester V Bergman, courtesy LTI Medica and The Upjohn Company. Copyright 1982 by Learning Technology Incorporated.)

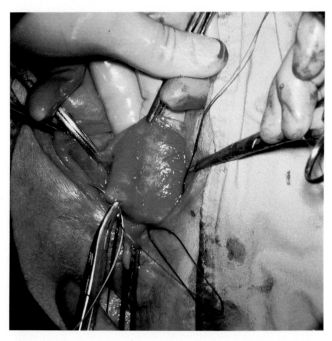

**Color Figure 16.6.** A free end of the Dexon suture is sewn through the undersurface of the full thickness of the fibromuscular wall. (Photograph by Lester V Bergman, courtesy LTI Medica and The Upjohn Company. Copyright 1982 by Learning technology Incorporated.)

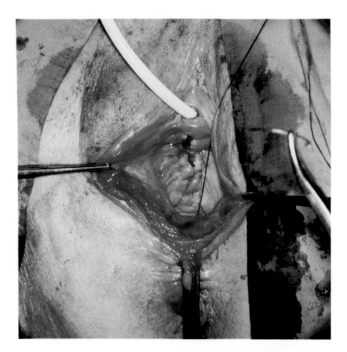

**Color Figure 16.7.** The remainder of the posterior vaginal wall is closed from side-to-side with a running subcuticular stitch, and the perineal body reconstructed. (Photograph by Lester V Bergman, courtesy LTI Medica and The Upjohn Company. Copyright 1982 by Learning Technology Incorporated.)

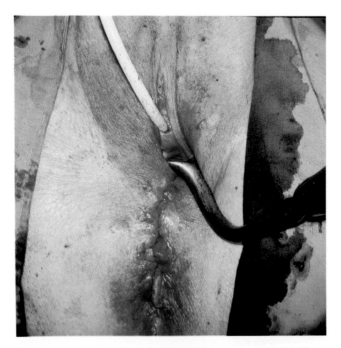

**Color Figure 16.8.** The vagina now has a relatively normal depth and axis, as shown by insertion of the Breisky-Navratil retractor. Digital examination confirms the integrity of the rectum. (Photograph by Lester V Bergman, courtesy of LTI Medica and The Upjohn Company. Copyright 1982 by Learning Technology Incorporated.)

patient may be reasonably comfortable for a while, the cause of the prolapse has not been relieved and, given enough time, continued progression of the prolapse will become evident. Although the uterine fundus may remain fixed to the abdominal wall, the uterus and cervix often will elongate until, ultimately, the vagina and those organs to which it is attached will come down again. The patient, meanwhile, has often forgotten the nature of her surgery many years before, and her operative records may have been lost and the surgeon may no longer be in practice. One may begin what appears to be a routine vaginal hysterectomy and repair only to find upon opening the peritoneal cavity that the fundus of the uterus extends all the way to the anterior abdominal wall (Fig. 16.19). A confirmatory tug on the cervix at that point will produce visible dimpling in the anterior abdominal wall. A drawback of the procedure of ventral fixation of either uterine fundus or posthysterectomy vaginal vault is the now exposed cul-de-sac. By having changed the axis of the vagina, the cul-de-sac has become even more vulnerable to increases in intra-abdominal pressure (Fig. 16.20). When Burch (4) presented his excellent results in treating incontinence by fixation of the vagina to Cooper's ligament, it was pointed out that the incidence of subsequent enterocele was between 11 and 15%. The probable explanation is that the change in vaginal axis caused the now unprotected cul-de-sac to become more directly vulnerable to increases in intra-abdominal pressure. The cul-de-sac should be clearly obliterated as a separate step with any abdominal surgery that changes the normal horizontal axis of the vagina.

### Sacropexy

Arthur and Savage (2) and Falk (6) attached the fundus of the uterus to the periosteum of the sacrum. Better still, one can remove the uterus and attach the vagina to the sacrum by a retroperitoneal bridge of Mersilene mesh, Gore-Tex, or fascia lata (10). This re-establishes a more or less horizontal vaginal axis.

The transabdominal method of retroperitoneal sacropexy is a satisfactory but complex procedure. This method is particularly attractive when the abdomen

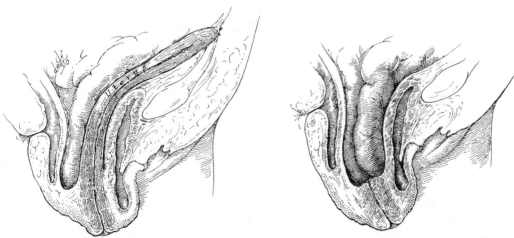

**Figure 16.19.** The failure of ventral fixation of the uterus to retard progression of genital prolapse is illustrated in the drawing to the left. The enterocele developing from the now unprotected cul-de-sac is noted. Eversion of the vagina after subtotal hysterectomy is illustrated in the drawing to the *right*. Although on superficial external examination the two conditions resemble one another, the technical details of subsequent surgical treatment are vastly different.

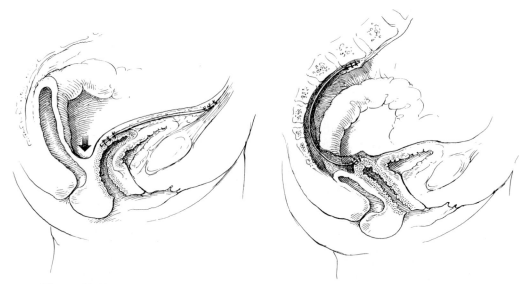

**Figure 16.20.** The unprotected cul-de-sac left after ventral fixation of the vagina is noted by the arrow in the drawing to the *left*. In the drawing to the *right*, the vagina has been fixed to the promontory of the sacrum by a retroperitoneal bridge of Mersilene mesh Gore-Tex or of fascia. The cul-de-sac is no longer vulnerable. (Reproduced with permission of JB Lippincott from Nichols DH: Repair of enterocele and prolapse of the vaginal vault. In Barber H (ed): *Goldsmith's Practice of Surgery*, 1981.)

must be opened for an unrelated reason, such as removal of an ovarian tumor or when the vagina is too short to be brought to the ischial spine. Coexistent intestinal diverticulosis risks future perforation of a diverticulum at the site of the mesh, and is a relative contraindication to the abdominal approach. If the mesh bridge becomes infected, it must be removed. A risk with this approach occurs when cystocele and rectocele are present. To attempt a vaginal repair and simultaneous transabdominal sacral fixation of the vagina appreciably increases the risk of infection at the site of the nonabsorbable sutures and Mersilene mesh, and it is not recommended. The repair of the cystocele and rectocele should be done at another time. Transabdominal sacropexy will correct eversion of the vaginal vault but not eversion of the lower vagina.

A transabdominal approach should be considered if massive vaginal eversion is secondary to a ventral fixation of the vagina or uterus, as it is difficult to return this type of vaginal axis to normal without freeing the vagina or uterus from its attachment to the anterior abdominal wall.

Massive eversion of the vagina is by no means uncommon after even a single pregnancy in a patient with a history of exstrophy of the bladder, even if the patient had been delivered by Cesarean section. The obvious anatomic weakness of the anterior vaginal wall is no comfort at all to the surgeon in providing an anatomic basis for suitable surgical support, because so many of these patients previously have had a cystectomy. One possibility, should there be an enormous appearance of a "cystocele" (namely, a massive relaxation of the anterior wall of the vagina with bulging and a feeling of falling out and fullness) but the patient has no uterine descent, is an operation involving modification of the Watkins-Wertheim transposition in which the fundus of the uterus is sewn to the periosteum of the pubic rami. To this may be added the Ocejo modification described by Gallo, in which the cervix is amputated and the uterus is opened before the transposition. The entire endometrial cavity is excised. The limits of the endometrial cavity to be removed may be defined by the intrauterine installation of an ampoule of indigo-carmine staining all the tissue a deep violet color. The uterine wall is reunited and the transposition finished.

When a procidentia accompanies a prolapse in this sort of situation, there often is no cardinal or uterosacral ligament strength to which to attach the vault of the vagina with confidence that it will stay there. An operation of Howard Jones has been employed successfully in which by a transabdominal approach the cul-de-sac of Douglas is obliterated and the vagina attached by an intermediate Mersilene strip to the periosteum of the pubis. Because there is no bladder to get in the way in this circumstance, this permits minimal displacement of the ureteral sigmoidostomy that may have been accomplished at the time of the preceding cystectomy, often in the patient's youth.

### Transabdominal Sacropexy

Anticipating some possible contamination of the operative field from the vagina, a single dose of an appropriate "prophylactic" antibiotic should be given preoperatively. The vagina is carefully packed with iodoform gauze and a Foley catheter is inserted into the bladder. The lower abdomen is opened through a midline lower incision and the abdomen is explored. The vaginal vault filled with packing is easily identified. A transverse incision is made in the peritoneum over the uppermost portion of the vagina, and the peritoneum is reflected both anteriorly and posteriorly for a distance of 2 to 3 cm. This line of cleavage should denude the musculoconnective tissue wall of the vagina. The bladder will be identified with its attachment to the anterior peritoneal reflection. Any appreciable enterocele sac should be identified and excised. A Dexon or Vicryl 2-0 guide suture is placed on each side of the vaginal apex, and three pairs of 2-0 coated *nonabsorbable* braided synthetic sutures are placed transversely 1 cm apart in the central portion of the vaginal vault through the full subepithelial fibromuscular thickness of the vaginal wall but not into the vaginal lumen. The vaginal pack is then removed, that the surgeon may be certain that no stitches have fixed it to the vagina.

A longitudinal incision is made through the peritoneum over the sacral promontory, extended caudally for 5 to 6 cm below and posteriorly to the promontory. The peritoneal flaps on either side are caught in retraction sutures left long enough to permit an adequate exposure of the bifurcation of the aorta and the vena cava. The midsacral artery and any nearby vein probably will need to be ligated to provide access to a 6- to 8-cm area of clean periosteum over the promontory of the sacrum between the common iliac veins. The exposed area of periosteum must be freed of all connective tissue, and hemostasis must assure a dry field where a segment of fascia lata, Gore-Tex, or plastic gauze is to be sutured to the periosteum.

A subperitoneal tunnel is established by dissection with a long, curved intestinal clamp or kidney stone forceps extending from the inferior edge of the incision over the sacral promontory beneath the peritoneum by blunt dissection across the posterolateral aspect of the right side of the cul-de-sac to the cut edge of the peritoneum overlying the vaginal apex. Alternatively, the peritoneum of the cul-de-sac may be incised longitudinally and reflected.

Small blood vessels may be electrocoagulated to assure a dry operative field. Three pairs of 2-0 braided nonabsorbable sutures are placed in the sacral periosteum, using a strong but small half-circle needle with a trochar point. The midpoint of a 2- to 8-inch piece of Mersilene mesh folded longitudinally (alternatively, a large strip of Gore-Tex on fascia) is brought to the vaginal apex. The braided plastic sutures are threaded through it and tied securely. The curved intestinal clamp running through the tunnel grasps the free end of the mesh or fascia now attached to the apex of the vagina and draws it to the promontory of the sacrum as the clamp is withdrawn. A little slack is left in the strip; it is not pulled so tightly as to elevate the cul-de-sac of the peritoneum appreciably. The nonabsorbable sutures previously placed in the periosteum over the sacral promontory are now passed through the appropriate points of the intermediate bridge; when all have been satisfactorily placed, they are tied, fixing the bridge to the sacral periosteum. Excess ends of the bridge are excised and the peritoneum closed with fine absorbable suture, obliterating any cul-de-sac, and the peritoneum closed. Unless one is planning an anterior colporrhaphy, a suprapubic pinup of the vesicourethral junction will lessen the chance of an unwanted postoperative urinary stress incontinence (Fig. 16.18). The vagina is redistended for 1 or 2 days with a splinting iodoform or gauze pack. The patient is permitted out of bed on the first postoperative day, and the urinary catheter is removed. It is our view that treatment of rectocele and cystocele are best managed at another time by a transvaginal approach directed at the sites of damage.

## CONCLUSION

Vaginal hysterectomy and repair, although usually successful, will not serve all patients with massive eversion of the vagina equally well. There are various causes, tissue strengths, and damages that should be identified and correlated with a choice of different surgical procedures. For those patients with vaginal vault prolapse but without usable cardinal-uterosacral ligament support, supplemental techniques for support of the vault must be added. The ultimate goal is to relieve symptoms and restore the natural depth and position of the vagina while at the same time effectively treating any coexistent pelvic disease, including cystocele, enterocele, and rectocele. This can be accomplished using techniques that will restore or preserve coital function.

It is usually unnecessary and often a distinct disservice to an active patient with prolapse to leave her with a short vagina or to perform partial or total colpectomy.

When colpectomy is performed, however, the results are better when any coexistent enterocele has been identified and the sac excised. Accurate perception and an adequate procedure cannot help but improve the long-term result of the surgery employed.

**References**

1. Amreich J: Aëtiologie und Operation des Scheidenstumpf prolapses. *Wien Klin Wochenschr* 63:74–77, 1951.
2. Arthur HGE, Savage D: Uterine prolapse and prolapse of the vaginal vault treated by sacral hysteropexy. *J Obstet Gynecol Br Emp* 64:355, 1957.
3. Baden WF, Walker TA: Physical diagnosis in the evaluation of vaginal relaxation. *Clin Obstet Gynecol* 15:1060, 1972.
4. Burch JC: Urethrovaginal fixation to Cooper's ligament for stress incontinence. *Am J Obstet Gynecol* 81:2, 1961.
5. Cox OC: Hystero-culpectomy. *Sibley Mem Hosp Alumni Assoc Bull* 1:9–16, 1958.
6. Falk HC: Uterine prolapse and prolapse of the vaginal vault treated by sacropexy. *Obstet Gynecol* 18:113–115, 1961.
7. Inmon WB: Pelvic relaxation and repair including prolapse of vagina following hysterectomy. *South Med J* 56577–582, 1963.
8. Nichols DH, Milley PS, Randall CL: Significance of restoration of normal vaginal depth and axis. *Obstet Gynecol* 36:241–246, 1970.
9. Nichols DH: Sacrospinous fixation for massive eversion of the vagina. *Am J Obstet Gynecol* 142:901, 1982.
10. Parsons L, Ulfelder H: *An Atlas of Pelvic Operations.* Philadelphia, WB Saunders, ed 2 pp 280–283, 1968.
11. Percy NM, Perl JI: Total colpectomy. *Surg Gynecol Obstet* 113:174–184, 1961.
12. Richter K: Die operative Behandlung des prolabierten Scheidengrundes nach Uterusextirpation Beitrag zur Vaginaefixatio

Sacrotuberalis nach Amereich. *Geburtshilfe Frauenheilkd* 27:941–954, 1967.

13. Richter K, Albrich W: Long term results following fixation of the vagina on the sacrospinal ligament by the vaginal route (vaginaefixatio sacrospinalis vaginalis). *Am J Obstet Gynecol* 141:811, 1981.

14. Sederl J: Zur Operation des Prolapses der blind endigenden Scheide. *Geburtshilfe Frauenheilkd* 18:824–828, 1958.

15. Symmonds R, Williams TJ, Lee RA, et al: Posthysterectomy enterocele and vaginal vault prolapse. *Am J Obstet Gynecol* 140:852, 1981.

16. Thompson HG, Murphy CJ, Picot H: Hystero-colpectomy for treatment of uterine procidentia. *Am J Obstet Gynecol* 82:743–753, 1961.

17. White R: An anatomical operation for the cure of cystocele. *JAMA* 53:1707–1710, 1909.

18. Zweifel P: *Vorlesungen über klinische gynakologie*. Berlin, Hirschwald p. 407, 1892.

# CHAPTER 17

# Urethral Diverticulum and Fistula

## URETHRAL DIVERTICULUM

Suburethral diverticula are not as uncommon as is widely believed, and the number found will be proportional to the diligence of the gynecologist in searching for them.

There is no need to repair an asymptomatic urethral diverticulum. Dribbling, dysuria, or dyspareunia, however, are symptoms that suggest indications for surgery.

Those symptomatic diverticula found in the distal urethra are prone to be associated with postmicturition dribbling, as Asmussen and Miller (1) have said: "The leakage can lead to a suspicion of stress incontinence because of the effect of straining and movement. Leakage, however, occurs soon after micturition, while in stress incontinence this is the one time when a patient can be almost certain that she will not leak, simply because the bladder is empty. After leakage has occurred from the diverticulum there is a tendency for the patient to be dry until after the next micturition. In stress incontinence the reverse is the case-she leaks more when the bladder is full." Significant urinary leaking is less common in patients in whom there is a diverticulum of the proximal urethra, but dysuria and dyspareunia are of greater intensity, proportional to the degree of diverticular infection (1). Intradiverticular stones may be found in those present for a long period of time, and are secondary to chronic urinary stasis. The stones may precipitate hematuria and may contribute to the cause of urethral malignancy, which must be thoughtfully diagnosed.

Urethral diverticula are most frequently found in the middle third and outside the posterior or posterolateral wall of the upper urethra, and their walls are adherent to all nearby structures with which they are in contact including the wall of the vagina. The sac of a diverticulum may occasionally extend ventrally alongside the urethra on one or both sides.

The origin of urethral diverticula is not clear, but when the wall includes only fibrous tissue and is without an epithelial lining, it is believed that the condition is one acquired from infection and obstruction of a paraurethral duct (6, 7). When muscle is present in the diverticular wall, as is true of bladder diverticula, a possibly congenital origin is suggested. It should be differentiated from a Gartner's duct cyst, that contains mucus, has a distinct epithelial lining, and does not communicate with the urethral lumen.

The condition should be suspected when there is a history of dysuria, dribbling, and dyspareunia, but positive findings are not always obvious on physical examination, as the contents of some urethral diverticula may be easily discharged into the urethral lumen producing temporary collapse of the sac. Urine exudate obtained from stripping the urethra is suspicious, and the diagnosis may be confirmed by radiography (in which the sac may be filled with

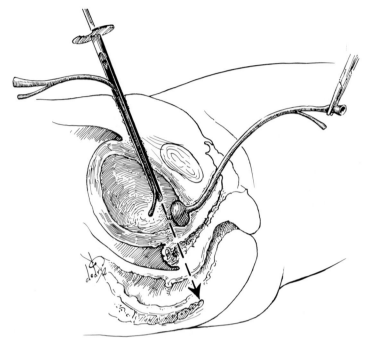

**Figure 17.4.** The bladder has been distended by 400 ml of sterile saline solution instilled through a transurethral Foley catheter, shown in place and clamped. At a midline point two fingerbreadths above the superior border of the pubis, a No. 22 spinal needle was introduced through the anterior abdominal and bladder wall and pointed toward the coccyx. When a free flow of clear urine has been observed, the needle is immediately removed and a 1.5-cm transverse incision through the skin only is made using a No. 12 scalpel blade at the site of the needle puncture. The operator, having noted the approximate depth at which the spinal needle entered the bladder, bluntly introduces the Campbell trochar in the same direction until the characteristic "give" is noted. The sharply pointed obturator of the trochar is withdrawn about an inch, the blunt end of the sleeve is inserted an additional inch or two, and the obturator is removed. There is prompt escape of urine and saline, and immediately a No. 16 Foley catheter is inserted through the trochar into the bladder as shown. The 5-ml bulb is inflated, the trochar is removed, and a brief tug on the catheter until resistance is encountered brings the now inflated bulb to the undersurface of the fresh cystostomy. (Reproduced with permission from Nichols DH, Milley PS: A simplified technique for suprapubic cystostomy. *Ob/Gyn Digest* 12:30–35, 1970.

## URETHROVAGINAL FISTULAE

Urethrovaginal fistulae present special problems in repair that Keettel et al. (4) have identified:

1. The extent of urethral damage;
2. The involvement of the vesicourethral junction;
3. The extensive scarring;
4. Often there is insufficient tissue for a second layer closure.

A fistula involving the middle or lower third of the urethra may not produce incontinence, but the fistulous opening permits urine to be discharged into the vagina at the time of urination. There will likely be an unpleasant uriniferous

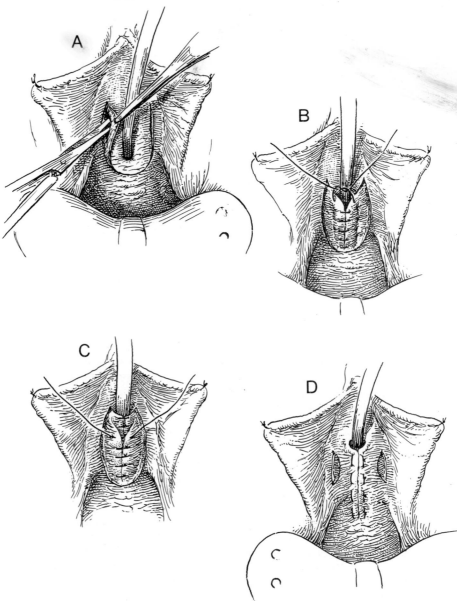

**Figure 17.5.** Construction of a neourethra is depicted. The labia minora have been stitched out of the way to improve the operative exposure, and a Foley catheter has been inserted into the bladder. The tissues to be mobilized may be infiltrated by epinephrine-lidocaine solution to reduce blood loss, and a U-shaped incision is made as shown in *A*. The flap is undermined medially so that the medial margins of the incision may be joined together in the midline surrounding the catheter as shown in *B*. A second layer approximates the subepithelial connective tissue as shown in C, and the lateral incisional margins are brought together by a series of interrupted mattress stitches as shown in *D*). Any tension on the suture line is relieved by lateral relaxing incisions as shown. Placement of a fascia lata vesicourethral sling as a future procedure may be required to establish continence. In a sense, the operation is a miniaturized counterpart of the Williams vulvovagino-plasty (Figs. 21.2 and 21.3).

odor in the vagina, and the postmicturition dribbling from the vagina is certain to have been noticed. Openings that develop in the upper third of the urethra, closer to the vesical neck, are likely to be associated with either intermittent or, at times, total urinary incontinence, mainly dependent upon the extent to which a functionally sphincter-like tone has or has not been maintained (5).

Asymptomatic urethrovaginal fistula may occasionally be found on routine pelvic examination, perhaps to the surprise of the examining physician as well as the patient. Such a fistula may have been accounting for no discernible or troublesome complaint, and it need not be repaired if unassociated with chronic urinary infection, not responsible for an unpredictable stream when voiding, and unaccompanied by evidence of neoplasia. When the history suggests, or there is record of a previous operation for excision or drainage of a urethral diverticulum or suburethral abscess, the site and origin of a urethral fistula are immediately suspect. When the fistula is associated with a chronic bloody vaginal discharge or hematuria, however, the possibility of malignant disease must be the first considered, and appropriate biopsy must be taken before consideration of surgical reconstruction. Urethroscopy and cystoscopy should be included in the investigation, and, during surgery, areas of hard tissue found not to represent calculus formation should be promptly biopsied and submitted for immediate tissue diagnosis.

When biopsy of the urethra or adjacent tissue is reported to indicate invasive malignant disease, treatment should be that appropriate for the malignancy and will usually involve radiation and/or surgery, the details of which are beyond the scope of this discussion.

When a fistula indicates surgical reconstruction of the urethra, the choice of operative procedure should be determined by need for restoration or improvement in function, in which consideration of involuntary urinary incontinence, whether continual or intermittent, is of paramount importance. When incontinence is not a consideration, the surgeon should first mobilize the urethra, undercutting the wall of the vagina to the extent necessary to permit excision of the fistulous track and closure of the defect without tension. Alternately, the fistulous opening may be inverted into the urethral lumen without excision of the track as long as the subepithelial connective tissues of the urethra can be approximated without tension, using interrupted fine absorbable sutures. Such a defect should usually be closed transversely to avoid or minimize the postoperative urethral stricture. Repair should be accomplished with a catheter in the urethra. The site of repair may be insulated from the vaginal incision by the vaginal flap technique (3), as described in Chapter 18.

The repair of a fistula at or near the vesical neck often requires a special technique. After preliminary infiltration with dilute lidocaine-epinephrine solution and insertion of a transurethral Foley catheter, an inverted U-shaped incision is made through the full thickness of the anterior vaginal wall. The vaginal wall is carefully reflected by sharp dissection exposing the full length of the fistulous track, and the dissection is carried around and cranial to the fistula (Fig. 17.6A). The track is excised from the wall of the urethra or bladder neck, as well as the vagina (Fig. 17.6B), and the urinary defect is closed by a deep layer of running mattress suture of fine absorbable suture (3-0 polyglycolic or chromic) and a superficial layer of interrupted mattress sutures of the same material (Fig. 17.6C inset). A bulbocavernosus fat pad may be transplanted to insulate the bladder or urethral repair from the vagina (Fig. 17.6D). The incision in the anterior vaginal wall closed by interrupted sutures and the vagina packed overnight with iodoform gauze. The transurethral Foley catheter is removed in favor of postoperative suprapubic catheter drainage to keep the catheter away from the site of the repair.

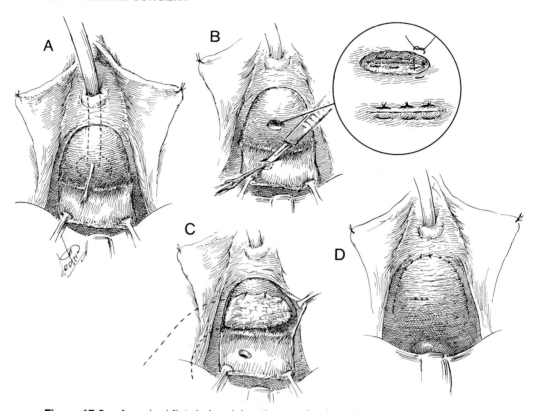

**Figure 17.6.** A vaginal fistula involving the proximal urethra at the bladder neck is shown. Bladder drainage may have been conveniently obtained by suprapubic cystos and a separate transurethral Foley catheter insertion. An inverted U-shaped incision is made in the anterior wall at the hymenal margin from the eight-o'clock position on the patient's right to the four-o'clock position on the patient's left, and the cut edges of the vagina are grasped with Allis forceps (A). By sharp and blunt dissection, the full thickness of the anterior vaginal wall is separated from the underlying connective tissue and displaced posteriorly. This mobilization continues around the fistula until the neck has been mobilized 1.5 to 2 cm in all directions, after which only the track is excised (B). If located at the vesical neck, the surrounding bladder muscle will retract to some extent, and the vesicourethral opening of the fistula will appear even larger than the original vaginal opening. No sutures penetrate the bladder lining, and no knots are tied within the bladder. The submucosal connective tissue around the fistula is closed transversely with a running horizontal mattress stitch of 3-0 absorbable suture material reinforced by a second layer of interrupted mattress stitches. Transverse closure in this area reunites the vesical and urethral portions of the trigone and, by its direction, lessens the chance of postoperative stricture. It is often desirable to reinforce this repair with an additional layer of living tissue by either pubococcygeus muscle transplant or bulbocavernosus fat pad transplant (C) as described in Chapter 11. The inverted U-shaped incision in the anterior and lateral vaginal wall is closed with interrupted sutures (D), any episiotomy or Schuchardt incision is repaired, and the vagina is lightly packed for 24 hours. If the bladder is to be drained by suprapubic cystostomy, the transurethral catheter may be removed, avoiding subsequent contact between the catheter and the vesicourethral side of the fistula repair.

## MARTIUS BULBOCAVERNOSUS FAT PAD TRANSPLANT

This tissue has been employed as a means of bolstering the vesicourethral junction, but, because it contains a large amount of fat, the tissues are physiologically inert. We have elected to use this technique principally to reinforce a fistula repair (Fig. 17.7) by interposing a layer of living tissue and its new blood supply between the sites of repair in adjacent organs.

When incontinence due to vesical neck incompetence coincident with fistula repair is expected, some additional supplementation or reinforcement of the tissues beneath the vesicourethral unction should be considered, either simultaneous with the primary repair or as a future secondary procedure. The pubococcygeus muscle transplant (see Chapter 11, Figs. 11.21 and 11.22) will provide the security of intermittent striated muscle contraction, which seems to offer an advantage over the Martius bulbocavernosus fat pad translocation in this situation because although the latter brings additional blood supply into the area and bolsters the suburethral connective tissue, it does not provide for any eventual contribution to sphincteric contraction. Lateral vaginal relaxing

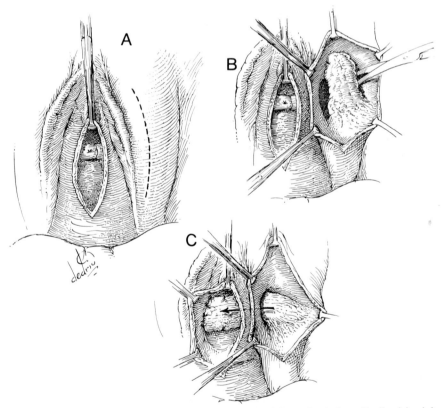

**Figure 17.7.** The bulbocavernosus fat pad transplant. In *A*, longitudinal incision has been made to the central position of the left labia majora. By sharp dissection a thumb-thick pedicle of fat and bulbocavernosus muscle has been freed from all but its inferior attachment *(B)*. A tunnel has been established beneath the vulvar and vaginal skin, and the freed margin of the pedicle has been brought through the tunnel without constriction and has been sewn to the undersurface of the vaginal flap of the opposite side, as shown in *C*.

incisions in a sagittal plane (see Fig. 20.2) may be necessary to avoid tension in a new suburethral suture line. Either local or systemic estrogen therapy, preferably started before surgery, may be helpful in the healing of the vaginal wound of a postmenopausal patient.

## References

1. Asmussen M, Miller A: *Clinical Gynaeco-logical Urology*. Oxford, Blackwell Scientific Publications, pp 172–175, 1983.
2. Bhatia NN, McCarthy TA, Ostergard D: Urethral Diverticula: Urethral Closure Pressure Profile. In Zinner NRn Sterling AM (eds): *Female Incontinence*. New York, Alan R Liss, Inc, pp 239–242, 1981.
3. Judd GE, Marshall JR: Repair of urethral diverticulum or vesicovaginal fistula by vaginal flap technique. *Obstet Gynecol* 47:627–629, 1976.
4. Keettel WC, Sehring FG, deProsse CA, et al: Surgical management of urethrovaginal and vesicovaginal fistulas. *Am J Obstet Gynecol* 131:425–431, 1978.
5. Kunz J: *Urological Complications in Gynecological Surgery and Radiotherapy*. Basel, S. Karger AG, pp 73–74, 1984.
6. Spence HM, Duckett Jr JW: Diverticulum of the female urethra: clinical aspects and presentation of a simple operative technique for cure. *J Urol* 104:432–437, 1970.
7. Spraitz AF, Welch JS: Diverticulum of the urethra. In *1964–1965 Collected Papers in Surgery from the Mayo Clinic and the Mayo Foundation*. Philadelphia, WB Saunders, vol 56, pp 195–198, 1965.
8. Symmonds RE, Hill M: Loss of the urethra: a report on 50 patients. *Am J Obstet Gynecol* 130:130, 1978.
9. Tancer ML, Hyman R: Suburethral diverticulitis in the female. *Am J Obstet Gynecol* 84:1853–1858, 1962.

# CHAPTER 18

# Vesicovaginal Fistulae

## REPAIR OF VESICOVAGINAL FISTULAE

Fistulae involving the female genitalia may be the result of trauma, necrosis secondary to invasion by neoplastic growth, or rarely, the reaction to certain types of necrotizing inflammation. Genital tract trauma is by far the most common cause.

Unrecognized or unrepaired full-thickness trauma involving the urinary or the intestinal system will usually result in fistula formation, which explains the necessity of immediately recognizing unexpected penetration of a neighboring viscus at the time of any gynecologic operation or obstetric procedure. The presence of a *small* amount of urine in the bladder is desirable at the time of vaginal hysterectomy or anterior colporrhaphy, as its appearance in the operative field will usually alert the surgeon to the likelihood of a penetrating injury. When such an injury is even suspected, the question must be answered and an appropriate repair accomplished without delay. The incidence of accidental penetration is small and becomes smaller as the experience of the operator increases. Nevertheless, accidental injuries due to unexpected relationships will occur occasionally with every surgeon, whether he operates occasionally or frequently. The techniques of repairing fresh injury and the postoperative management of such repair are considered in detail in Chapter 22.

## VESICOVAGINAL FISTULA

This type of urinary fistula is likely to develop as a result of unrecognized or inadequately repaired sites of trauma. A history of previous low cervical cesarean section is a predisposing factor during hysterectomy due to altered tissue relationships between the bladder and cervix. It is important to remember that a history of previous cesarean section will be present in about 20% of the present generation of parous patients requiring hysterectomy in the future. Preoperative intravesical instillation of 60 ml of indigo carmine or methylene blue solution is especially helpful when operating on the patient with a history of previous cesarean section. Not only can the violet-stained bladder mucosa be sometimes seen *before* it might be opened, but violet stained urine in the operative field is a priori evidence of unwanted penetration.

When vesicovaginal fistula follows hysterectomy, it is likely to be located at the very apex of the vagina if the vaginal cuff was not closed, or just anterior to the suture line if it was. Vesicovaginal fistula in the lower vagina is more likely to follow previous colporrhaphy.

A fistula first recognized after hysterectomy is usually the result of an unrecognized penetration or laceration at the time of the primary operative procedure, the result of trauma recognized but inadequately repaired, or perhaps the result of postoperative necrosis of a small area of bladder epithelium secondary to an infected hematoma or to devascularization by a suture placed into or immediately adjacent to the lumen of the bladder. Carelessly placed hemostatic matress sutures in the bladder wall near the cut edge of the vagina may devitalize the spot of tissue in which they have been placed. Incomplete surgical separation of the bladder from the vaginal cuff during hysterectomy will place it at risk.

The presence of unsuspected postoperative hematuria after the initial operative procedure should alert the operator to the possibility of a later fistula, particularly when bloody urine persists longer than the first 48 postoperative hours. Inspection by cystoscopy is then desirable, and catheter drainage should usually be prolonged for a number of days beyond the usual period. When a fistulous track, even though small, is relatively short, incontinence is the rule. When the track is longer, and particularly when tortuous, incontinence is likely to be intermittent because the flow of urine through the track may be inversely proportional to the amount of urine within the bladder. This type of intermittent incontinence seems especially prone to infection and calculus formation along the track.

The presence of an intermittent spontaneous bloody urethral or urinary discharge is particularly ominous, and when present, the coexistence of malignant disease relating to the fistulous track must be evaluated by adequate study and biopsy, followed when indicated by treatment appropriate to the malignant disease.

The possibility of multiple fistulae must always be considered during investigation of any patient with a recognized fistula. Should an additional track escape recognition, an apparently successful surgical correction of the one recognized fistula will in no way eliminate a continued incontinence resulting from an unrepaired coexistent fistula, leading both operator and patient to suspect a treatment failure when, in fact, the failure may not have been due to the treatment but rather to the inadequacy of the preoperative study and appraisal. Careful review of the history and circumstances preceding recognition of a fistula is always indicated.

The differentiation between a vesicovaginal or ureterovaginal fistula is of prime importance. In making this distinction the tampon test (9) is helpful and may be performed as follows:

The test is to inject 6 to 8 ounces of strongly colored methylene blue or indigo carmine solution into the bladder and then to insert a rather long menstrual tampon in the vagina. The patient is instructed to walk about for 10 or 15 minutes, after which the tampon is examined. If the lowest part alone is wet and blue, the patient presumably suffers from stress incontinence of urine or detrusor instability. If the upper thirds are wet and blue, the indication is a vesicovaginal fistula; if the upper third is wet but not blue, the diagnosis is of a damaged ureter.

There are several excellent techniques of repair, adaptable to a variety of clinical circumstances, but we will consider those that seem most applicable to the women seen in urban communities and in whom coexistent neoplastic disease of the pelvis has been excluded. In younger patients with a history of urinary loss, particularly when there is evidence of congential malformation in the genitalia, thorough inspection of the urinary as well as the genital tract is indicated. Intravenous pyelography may be the only way an aberrant or third ureter opening into the vagina will be demonstrated. It is equally important to know whether the patient with a urinary fistula has bilateral ureteral patency, two normally placed ureters or perhaps only a single kidney and ureter, this latter situation should certainly be known to the operator before the repair of a urinary fistula is planned or undertaken. The relationship of a fistula to the ureteral orifices, bladder neck, and trigone should be studied by preoperative cystoscopy. The operative preparation of the patient should, therefore, include a pyelogram as well as cystoscopic investigation.

Electrosurgical or chemical cautery of a very small fistulous opening has been recommended by others (3) from time to time on the basis and with the hope that coagulation will destroy the epithelial lining of the track and may be effective in permitting spontaneous healing in a small percentage of cases of tiny fistula. It is followed by immediate decompression of the bladder by constant drainage for 2 to 3 weeks, and is most likely to succeed when the fistula is only 1 or 2 mm in diameter, follows an oblique course, and exists with a thick, healthy bladder around the fistulous tract, as may be seen after an inadvertent stitch through the bladder wall.

If the injury follows an obstetric laceration, a repair should be accomplished within 24 hours of the injury. If a fistula develops after hysterectomy or failure of a previous fistula repair, a usual interval of between 3 and 6 months, preferably the latter, should pass to permit adequate lymphatic drainage to return to the tissue and the infection, swelling, and edema of surgery to subside. If the fistula appears after necrosis from irradiation, the vagina should be given effective estrogen supplementation and the repair postponed at least a year to permit the causative endarteritis obliterans to have ceased to progress (13). When active malignancy has been excluded by biopsy of any suspicious area in the margin of the fistula, successful repair generally requires not only delicate handling and approximation of tissue, but introduction of a new layer of tissue bringing with it a new blood supply between the repair of the organs involved. If the labia are fleshy, one may use for this new layer a bulbocavernosus fat pad transplant. If the labial tissues are atrophic, a nonirradiated graft of omentum, blood supply intact, may be brought down and sutured in place to provide the new blood supply and the necessary insulation.

While awaiting repair, some temporary but socially welcome relief can be obtained by wearing the intravaginal Tassett cup (Vagicup) modified for the collection of body fluids by tubing from the bottom of the cup to a leg bag. The resulting improvement will relieve the physician of some of the burden so often imposed by the patient anxious for a quick repair at a time when the condition of the tissues is not favorable or optimal for surgical repair. We have had no experience with cortisone treatment to accelerate tissue preparation for surgery and prefer to wait the necessary time required for inflammation and edema to subside.

It is desirable to examine both sides of the fistulous tract in choosing the appropriate surgical procedure for the repair of a genital fistula. This will reveal information about the size of each aperture and will afford better opportunity to appraise scarring, fibrosis, and the possibility of multiple openings.

Principles of urinary fistula repair include the following:

1. Postpone the repair until infection and inflammation have subsided and there may be healthy granulation tissue present.
2. Dissect, mobilize, and excise the epithelialized track and adjacent scar tissue until healthy, normal tissue is reached, converting the lesion to a fresh wound. It will be recalled that it is the rule for a fresh wound of bladder or rectum to heal promptly and primarily if initial repair is adequate and appropriate. It should be closed without tension.
3. One should try to interrupt the continuity of the fistulous track so that the orifice of repair in one viscus no longer overlies or underlies its counterpart.
4. Approximate anatomically strong layers or flaps and, when available, interpose between the previous fistulous orifices of a strong tissue layer having an independent blood supply.
5. When infection or abscess formation is likely, provision should be made for adequate drainage of the low pressure side of the previous track.
6. Decompression of the bladder postoperatively.
7. If the ureter is adjacent to or incorporated in the fistula, it should be catheterized at the time of the repair to avoid unintentional operative

ureteral stricture; if it appears likely that it will be compromised by the repair, a ureteroneocystostomy may be desirable.

8. Supplement or replace estrogen pre- and postoperatively if the patient is postmenopausal.

9. Lateral vaginal relaxing incisions should be used if the repair has been closed under tension.

A few special instruments can be very helpful at the time of fistula repair, such as a pair of fine dissecting scissors, right-angled scissors, Sims hooks, and Sims or Breisky retractors. A small suction tip is desirable.

A variety of scalpel blades and handles should be available to the operator, particularly including the Nos. 11 and 15 type blades and the no. 7 type scalpel handle. Knowledgeable interested assistance at surgery can also be of great help, as will a flexible operative time schedule that permits the operator to employ as much surgical time as necessary for the particular reconstruction, because the length of an adequate operation is not always predictable.

Adequate exposure of the fistula is of paramount importance; and if for any reason this cannot be obtained with the exaggerated lithotomy position, an alternate would be the knee chest position or even the jackknife or Kraske position in which the patient is face down and the hips well flexed, the table being bent at this point with extra padding under the hips. This will enable the operator to look down on the fistula. Adequate, well-focused lighting is equally important, and at times the operator may find it advantageous to wear a forehead fiberoptic light to concentrate illumination and reduce annoying shadows.

Mobilization of a fistulous tract can be improved by insertion of a small or pediatric-sized Foley catheter (no. 8, 9, or 10) into the bladder through the fistula itself. When the bulb on the Foley is inflated, the catheter that serves as an identifying handle permits traction of the fistula in all directions (6). If the fistulous opening is too small to permit the entry of a small Foley catheter, the opening can be enlarged gently by spreading the tips of a small hemostat or inserting a small Hegar dilator. Infiltration of the area by dilute epinephrine-lidocaine solution offers hemostatic effect, and, by the local hemostatic effect, small sponges (wisps, pushers, or "peanuts") soaked in the solution of epinephrine often improve the surgeon's visibility, especially when the healthy mucosal tissue is being dissected and mobilized. There may be considerable oozing but few vessels are large enough to clamp and tie.

Most experienced gynecologic surgeons will repair vesicovaginal fistulae using a transvaginal approach, reserving the transabdominal route (10) for very unusual situations in which mobility is limited, the ureter is involved, there have been repeated previous failures, or sometimes when the fistula has developed in tissues previously irradiated.

If the patient has a deep vagina and there is a posthysterectomy fistula located at the very apex of the vagina, the simplest and most effective operative repair will often involve utilization of the Latzko colpocleisis (8, 11, 12). This technique can be useful also for a small residual vault fistula remaining after previous closure of a larger fistula. If any problem in exposure of the fistula is encountered, a preliminary episiotomy or Schuchardt type incision (see Chapter 10) is strongly recommended in order to improve accessibility and assure visibility of the fistula. Adequate exposure is an essential ingredient of a successful operative closure.

## Latzko Technique

In this technique (Fig. 18.1), a 1.5- to 2-cm disk comprising the vaginal epithelium only is excised from around the fistulous opening. When approxi-

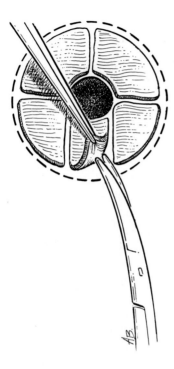

**Figure 18.4.** Ueda's (14) alternate method of closing a large fistula is shown. The vaginal wall around the fistula is divided into five sections as shown. Four are removed, but the fifth, the width of the fistula, is developed as a flap.

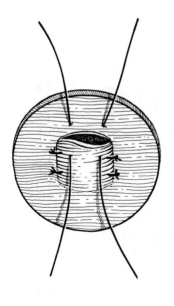
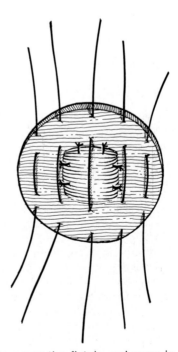

**Figure 18.5.** The vaginal flap has been turned to cover the fistula and sewn in place by several interrupted sutures, as shown to the *left,* sufficient to make the closure watertight. A second layer of sutures approximates the exposed tissues, as shown to the *right,* and when these have been tied the cut edges of the vagina are approximated by interrupted through-and-through sutures.

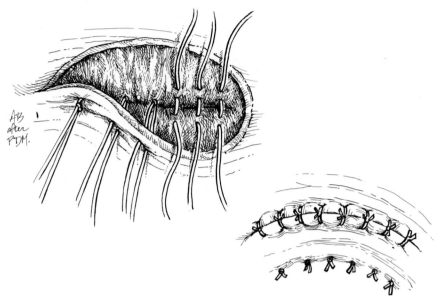

**Figure 18.6.** Hurd's alternate method of closing the vault (5), useful for a recurrent fistula, is shown. The posterior vaginal wall margin has been undermined for 1 ½ cm and the ends of the final reinforcing layer of stitches approximating the bladder wall have been tied, reinserted through the full thickness of the vaginal wall as shown, and tied again to avoid overlapping of the closure of the bladder with that of the vagina. The vaginal incision is closed by a separate layer.

The operation does not shorten the vagina and has proved popular for many years. He was once asked why he preferred a transvaginal to a transabdominal exposure and replied, "If you were going to have your tonsils taken out, would you prefer they be removed through your mouth or through an incision in the side of your neck?"

### Modern Sims Technique

After suitable exposure has been obtained, the margins of the fistulous track, often quite vascular, should be injected or infiltrated by a few cubic centimeters of 0.5% lidocaine in 1:200,000 epinephrine solution.

A small Foley catheter is inserted through the fistula (enlarged if necessary by the tip of a small hemostat) into the bladder, and the bulb is inflated. Traction on the catheter will stabilize the position of the fistula and bring it closer to the operator (Fig. 18.7).

The circumference of the fistula is circumscribed by the point of the scalpel blade 1/2 to 1 cm from the edge of the fistula. A sagittal incision is made completely through the vaginal wall (but not into the bladder muscularis or cavity) for a distance of 1 cm superior and inferior to the fistula using the No. 11 taper-pointed Bard-Parker blade (Fig. 18.8). The vaginal wall is undercut about 1 cm along each side of the fistulous track (Fig. 18.9A). Undercutting is continued until the bladder adjacent to the fistulous track is mobilized sufficiently to facilitate closure without tension.

A circular incision is made through the full thickness of the bladder wall (Fig. 18.9, *B* and *C*), and the fistulous track and Foley catheter are removed. Any remaining fibrous tissue is carefully excised to a point where normal tissue vascularity is apparent, because it is desirable to remove as much scar and fibrous tissue as possible in order to convert the edges of the defect to a state

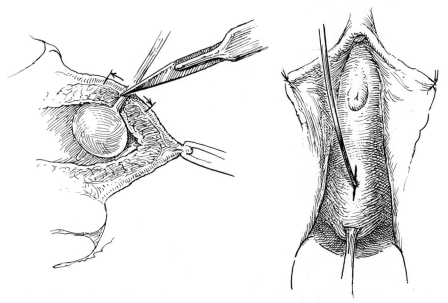

**Figure 18.7.** A pediatric-sized Foley catheter has been inserted through the fistula and a linear incision made in the anterior vaginal wall.

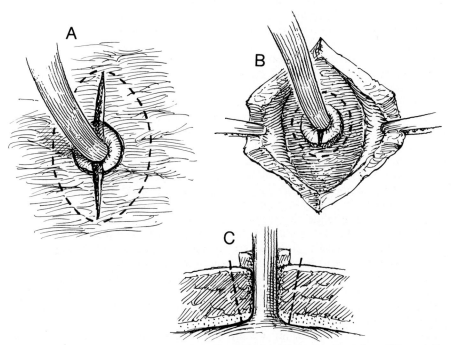

**Figure 18.8.** The fistulous track is circumscribed by an incision *(A)* and the anterior vaginal wall undermined by sharp dissection to the limits indicated by the *broken line*. The flaps are mobilized *(B)* and the round segment containing the fistula and surrounding cicatrix excised along the pathway indicated by the *broken line* in *B* and *C*, leaving a circular defect in the bladder wall.

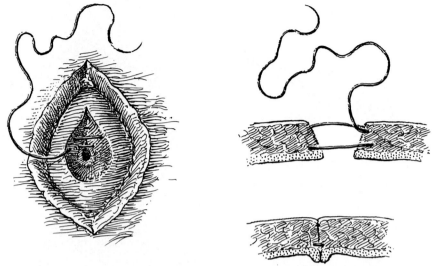

**Figure 18.9.** The muscularis of the bladder wall is reunited by a suture line of running or fine mattress sutures, with no knots protruding into the lumen of the bladder. If there has been sufficient mobilization and the bladder wall edges can be brought together without tension, the axis of bladder closure may be at right angles to that planned for the vagina. A second layer may be placed to insure watertightness.

resembling a fresh operative wound. If necessary for hemostasis, the bladder mucosa is closed with a layer of running 3-0 polyglycolic or chromic suture, using a subcuticular stitch that inverts any exposed bladder mucosa into the lumen of the bladder (Fig. 18.10). The watertightness of the closure may be tested by the instillation of sterile milk or infant formula into the bladder and additional sutures are inserted if necessary. If the cut edge of the vaginal incision appears ragged, or torn, or suspiciously thin, it may be trimmed and the full thickness of the vaginal membrane closed from side to side with vertical mattress sutures of 2-0 monofilament nylon (Fig. 18.9). This second layer of closure takes much of the tension from the stitches of the first layer. All of these interrupted stitches are best placed and held before they are tied, and when tied, the operator should be certain to incorporate a double turn on the first cast of each knot followed by four additional casts of the suture to obviate postoperative slipping. Moir has correctly emphasized that these sutures should be tied only tightly enough to approximate the tissue securely, but not so tight as to strangulate the tissue. The ends of any nonabsorbable sutures should be left long to facilitate their removal about the 21st postoperative day.

Full-thickness lateral vaginal relaxing incisions, as noted in Chapter 20, may be made to relieve any tension on the suture line, after which the vagina should be loosely packed with iodoform gauze for 24 hours. An indwelling catheter is inserted to assure bladder contraction for 10 days. If the patient is postmenopausal, both local and systemic estrogen should be administered through the postoperative period.

For the larger vesicovaginal fistula, it is particularly important to assure mobilization of vaginal wall from bladder wall by a more extensive dissection, in order to assure the interposition of a significant layer of subcutaneous tissue between the sutures closing the bladder and those closing the defect in the vagina. When the vaginal wall is suitably redundant, a vaginal lapping technique emphasized by Aldridge (1) and Judd and Marshall (8) may provide a

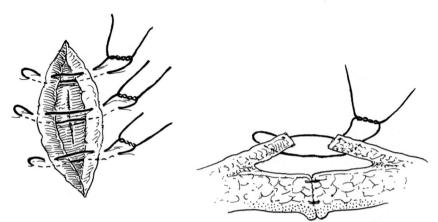

**Figure 18.10.** The vaginal wall is closed by interrupted vertical mattress sutures.

useful means of insulation and reinforcement as a result of the interposition of an additional layer of supporting tissue between closure of the bladder wall and closure of the vaginal incision (Fig. 18.11).

### Technique of Vaginal Lapping

If a hysterectomy has been performed immediately preceding the operation to be described, the anterior vaginal vault has been opened. The full thickness of the anterior vaginal wall may then be incised in the midline, resulting in an inverted T-shaped incision of the anterior half of the vaginal membrane. If no hysterectomy has been performed, and none is to be performed, this incision

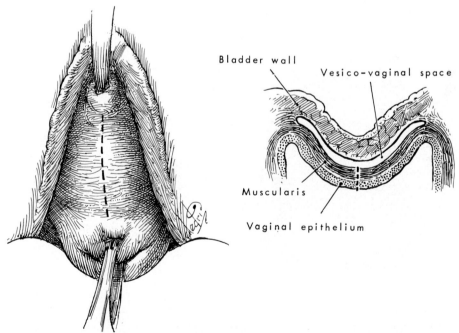

**Figure 18.11.** The vaginal lapping technique. An incision is made through the full length and full thickness of the anterior vaginal wall into the vesicovaginal space, as shown by the *dotted line*.

(Fig. 18.12) is made through the full thickness of the anterior vaginal wall in the midline, entering the vesicovaginal space (see Chapter 11).

This incision should be deep enough to leave all vaginal fibromuscular connective tissue attached to the vaginal flap. Equivalent full-thickness vaginal flaps are developed by opening laterally into lines of cleavage, identifying the vesicovaginal space on each side, and this mobilization is extended almost to the pubic ramus on each side.

The urogenital diaphragm containing the pubourethral "ligaments" is now identified and plicated beneath the vesicourethral junction (Chapter 11), but this suture should be tied and held long, rather than cut, to facilitate identification later in the procedure.

The connective tissue "capsule" of the bladder is then plicated to the degree that seems advisable, using 2-0 polyglycolic suture (Fig. 18.13). Care must be taken to avoid tying these sutures too tightly thus avoiding tissue strangulation at the points of approximation. A satisfactory degree of plication should reduce the transverse diameter of the bladder wall that had been sagging into the vesicovaginal space and at the same time thicken the bladder capsule and somewhat decrease future tension on the flap by limitation of potential bladder expansion in this area.

The underlying fibromuscular layer of the right vaginal flap is then split from the vaginal epithelium (Fig. 18.14) to the lateral margins of the vesicovaginal space. This line of cleavage should separate the musculoelastic layer of the vaginal wall from the overlying layer of vaginal epithelium. The vaginal flap of the left side is not similarly split, however, and all connective tissue should remain attached to the epithelial layer of the left flap of the vagina in order to preserve as much of its blood supply as possible.

The medial edge of the right inner vaginal or fibromuscular flap is sewn to the undersurface of the unsplit full-thickness flap of left vaginal wall, along the

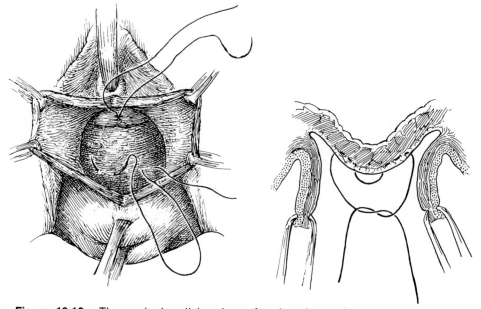

**Figure 18.12.** The vaginal wall has been freed and retracted laterally, the pubourethral plication stitches have been placed and tied, and the bladder capsule is being plicated with interrupted sutures to reduce the transverse diameter of the vesicovaginal space and thus thicken the bladder capsule.

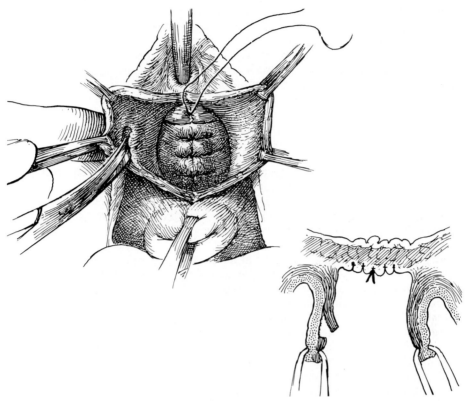

**Figure 18.13.**  The fibromuscular layer of the right vaginal flap is dissected from the superficial vaginal skin as shown.

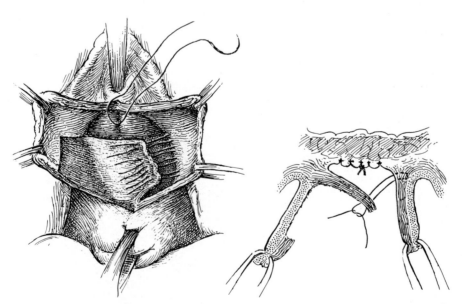

**Figure 18.14.**  The fibromuscular layer of the right vaginal flap is sewn to the undersurface of the unsplit left vaginal wall.

lateral extent of the vesicovaginal space, by a series of interrupted sutures of 2-0 polyglycolic suture (Fig. 18.15). Each untied suture is held loosely until all have been placed, and then all are tied.

The ends of the suture previously placed to shorten the pubourethral ligaments are brought through the vaginal flap and again tied, but not too tightly, on the vaginal side of the suture line (Fig. 18.16).

An appropriate amount of the right epithelial covering layer of vaginal flap is then trimmed along the left lateral margin of the vesicovaginal space (Fig. 18.17), at which point the edges of the vaginal membrane again become adjacent and roughly parallel, overlying the now doubled fibromuscular tissue layers. Finally, the full thickness of the unsplit left vaginal flap should be attached along the cut edge of the right flap by a series of interrupted sutures of 2-0 polyglycolic suture (Fig. 18.18).

Leaving the vaginal muscularis attached to the epithelium on one side assures preservation of its blood supply, and the procedure as described effectively doubles the thickness of the connective tissue layer supporting the anterior vaginal wall.

Any significant damage or relaxation of the posterior vaginal wall and perineum should also be repaired. Postoperatively, it might be advisable to place postmenopausal patients on estrogen with the intent of improving the vascularity and wound healing in these estrogen-sensitive tissues.

Under rare circumstances if unusual thinness of the anterior vaginal wall and preservation of full vaginal depth and width is strongly desired, the Ocejo modification of the Watkins-Wertheim interposition operation may be useful in patients in whom the uterus is still present. The modification championed by Gallo (4) in which the cervix is amputated and the endometrium is excised (Fig. 18.19) through a longitudinal incision in the anterior wall of the uterus, safely removes this future source of potential endometrial trouble or symptoms.

## VESICOUTERINE FISTULAE

Vesicouterine or vesicocervical fistula with its accompanying incontinence is almost invariably the aftermath of a cesarean section at which the integrity of

**Figure 18.15.** The pubourethral "ligament" stitch is sewn to the undersurface of the vagina.

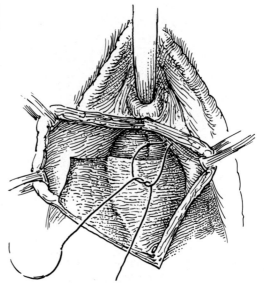

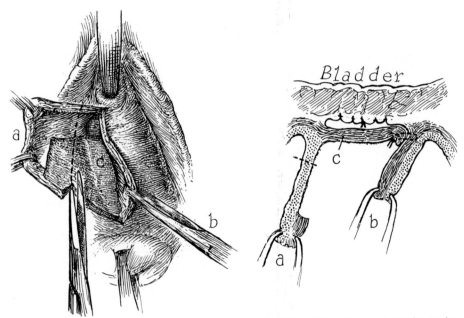

**Figure 18.16.** The excess of the split right vaginal flap *(A)* is trimmed, as shown by the *broken line*. The fibromuscular layer of the right flap *(C)* has been sewn to the undersurface of the unsplit left flap *(B)*.

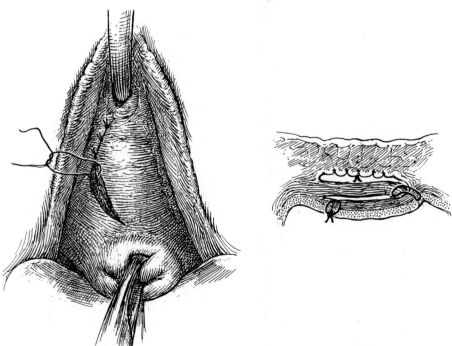

**Figure 18.17.** The full thickness of the left flap is sewn to the right.

**Figure 18.18.** The uterine corpus may be transposed between the bladder and the vagina in certain cases of vesicovaginal fistula when the blood supply is poor. In Acejo's (4) modification, the endometrium has been removed by sharp dissection and the cavity obliterated by sutures, as shown. An elongated cervix will have been amputated.

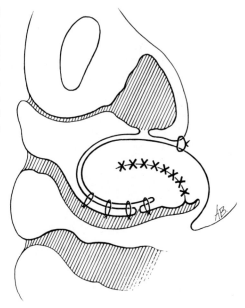

the bladder was compromised by a suture used in the repair of the uterine incision. It occasionally follows uterine rupture with precipitate labor (2). Surgery requires the anatomic dissection and separation of the bladder from the uterus at the site of the fistula, with freshening of the edges and separate repair of each organ using absorbable suture. A period of not less than 10 days of postoperative catheter decompression of the bladder is desirable.

## VESICOCERVICAL FISTULAE

Urinary incontinence may not always be evident with vesicocervical fistula; and occasionally, the sole symptom will be menstrual hematuria, erroneously suggesting endometriosis of the bladder. In such istances, some valve-like arrangement due to a flap effect within a fistulous track permits fluid to pass from the uterus to the bladder but not in the reverse direction.

### Additional Postoperative Care

Although the bladder that has been totally incontinent as a result of a vesicovaginal fistula for a number of years is usually capable of physiologic regeneration and restoration of function within a few weeks as the result of its long period of rest, after repair the patient should be expected at first to demonstrate relatively small bladder capacity and should have been warned to expect a certain amount of urgency and need to empty her bladder frequently for the first few postoperative weeks, even during the night. It might be suggested that she set an alarm clock to arouse her for this purpose in order to avoid noctural distention. Because primary healing is so very important, such a patient should be maintained on urinary antisepsis for several weeks from the time of surgery.

## URETEROVAGINAL FISTULAE

Although freshly damaged or transected ureters may be transvaginally reimplanted into the bladder at the time of the initial injury if the operator is familiar with the technique of repair, the postoperative ureterovaginal fistula is most often approached through a transabdominal route, either for reconstruction or reimplantation. The related techniques are not included within the scope of this text.

## References

1. Aldridge AH: Modern treatment for vesicovaginal fistula. *J Obstet Gynecol Br Emp* 60:1, 1953.
2. Al-Juburi A, Aloosi I, Khundra S: Unusual vesicocervical fistulas. *J Obstet Gynaecol* 4:264, 1984.
3. Falk HC, Orkin LA: Nonsurgical closure of vesicovaginal fistulas. *Obstet Gynecol* 9:538–541, 1957.
4. Gallo D: Ocejo modification of interposition operation. In *"Urologica Ginecologica"*. Guadalajara, Gallo, 1969.
5: Hurd JK: Vaginal repair of vesicovaginal fistula. In Libertino JA, Zinman L (eds): *Reconstructive Urologic Surgery*. Baltimore, Williams & Wilkins, 1977.
6. Janisch H, Palmrich AH, Pecherstorfer M: *Selected Urologic Operations in Gynecology*. Berlin, Walter de Gruyter, 1979.
7. Judd GE, Marshall JR: Repair of urethral diverticulum or vesicovaginal fistula by vaginal flap technique. Am J Obstet Gynecol 47:627–629, 1976.
8. Latzko W: Postoperative vesicovaginal fistulas. Am J Surg 58:211–228, 1942.
9. Moir JC: *The Vesicovaginal Fistula*. London, Balliere, Tindall & Cassell, 1967.
10. O'Connor VJ Jr: Repair of vesicovaginal fistula with associated urethral loss. *Surg Gynecol Obstet* 146:251–253, 1978.
11. Robertson JR: Vesicovaginal fistulas. In Slate WG (ed): *Disorders of the Female Urethra and Urinary Incontinence*. Baltimore, Williams & Wilkins, 1982.
12. Tancer L: Personal communication.
13. Turner-Warwick R: The use of pedicle grafts in the repair of urinary tract fistulae. *Br J Urol* 44:644, 1972.
14. Ueda T, Iwatsubo E, Osada Y, et al: Closure of a vesicovaginal fistula using a vaginal flap. *J Urol* 119:742-743, 1978.

# CHAPTER 19

# Rectovaginal Fistulae

A rectovaginal fistula may occur at any level within the vagina but is most common in the lower third. Most of these have resulted from obstetric trauma, most often at the apex of an improperly healed repair of a fourth degree perineal laceration. The patient may give a history of much difficulty expelling the fecal bolus with her first bowel movement and after much straining probably compromises the repair. Although the tissue may have been properly approximated during the initial repair, a breakdown occurs cranial to the perineum, often between the fifth and tenth day after repair. In many instances of fistula it is likely that prophylaxis, including the liberal use of stool softeners and a low residue diet, might have prevented the complication (6). By these means it may be better for the patient to keep her bowel movements on the soft side for a few weeks postoperatively.

Other causes of rectovaginal fistula are from other trauma, suture penetration during episiotomy repair or perineorrhaphy, Crohn's disease, infection and necrosis of a vaginal hematoma from hysterectomy, perineorrhaphy, or posterior colporrhaphy and postpelvic radiation, particularly after trauma to the vagina in the presence of endarteritis obliterans, and the growth of residual or recurrent cancer.

The possibility that a gastrointestinal-vaginal fistula in the upper vagina arises from small bowel should be considered if the patient passes liquid stool through the fistula while passing solid stool through the rectum, or if the vagina and vulva are excoriated as might result from digestion of the skin with small intestinal digestive enzymes.

Although occasionally congenital in origin (11), the rectovaginal fistula seen today in the civilized or developed countries of the world is usually the aftermath of trauma either unrecognized or unrepaired, or inadequately and unsuccessfully repaired during the initial attempt. Fistulae may be single or multiple, or a single fistula may have several connecting tracks that communicate within the subepithelial tissues with one another, occasionally originating from several openings into the rectal lumen. Less commonly, a single opening in the rectal mucosa may communicate with several fistulous openings in the vagina and perineal skin. The relationship of a fistulous track or tracks to the external anal sphincter is of paramount importance in planning surgical repair.

Before repair, a relative degree of constipation will permit reasonable fecal continence, but success is not usually achieved in the control of flatus. It is, in fact, the inability to avoid involuntary loss of flatus that usually first makes a fistula known to the patient and equally often accounts for a patient's decision to seek surgical repair. During a period awaiting surgery, there are several things the patient can do to lessen the quantity of flatus, much of which is related to unabsorbed nitrogen from swallowed air. The patient can be advised not to talk while there is food in her mouth, to chew her food well, eating slowly without gulping, and to finish and swallow one mouthful before adding to the food being chewed. Such simple measures will often reduce considerably the amount of air being swallowed and, as a result, the amount of gas that is likely to be expelled.

When repair of coexistent rectovaginal and vesicovaginal fistulae is being considered, the vesicovaginal fistula should be repaired first, lest postoperative scarring from the rectovaginal fistula repair compromise the operative exposure should re-repair be required.

If the vesicorectovaginal fistula followed pelvic irradiation, usually one should require a preliminary diverting transverse colostomy, followed in 2 or 3 months by repair of the vesicovaginal fistula in the usual manner, then repair of the rectovaginal fistula, which may at times involve a colpocleisis, followed finally, after 2 or 3 additional months, by closure of the colostomy.

It is important to emphasize principles in the management of rectovaginal fistula that, if observed, will increase the probability of successful surgical treatment. These are:

1. A time for fistula repair should be chosen when granulation tissue, infection, and edema are minimal.
2. The repair must interrupt the continuity of the fistula.
3. The repair need not necessarily involve levator plication with its resultant risk of dyspareunia, but a layer of tissue should be interposed between the rectal wall sutures and those in the vaginal wall, if possible.
4. Excise the epithelialized fistulous track.
5. Closure of the tissues in more than one layer is recommended. (A second layer takes much of the tension from the suture line of the first layer.)
6. Interpose a layer of fresh tissue with an independent blood supply between the layers of repair if necessary, as with postirradiation fistulae.
7. The vaginal side of the fistula may be left open for drainage. When a rubber drain is used, it should be left in place for 2 to 7 days. The time for removal will depend upon the size of the fistula, the amount of drainage present, and whether an abscess was encountered during the procedure.

## BOWEL PREPARATION

The standard antibiotic erythromycin-neomycin bowel preparation (1 gm of each by mouth at 1:00, 2:00, and 11:00 PM the day before the operation) is associated with a high incidence of troublesome and annoying gastrointestinal side effects, so we now employ cefoxitin sodium (Mefoxin), which is given 2 gm intravenously on call to the operating room and 2 hours later during surgery if necessary, or 2 gm in the recovery room if surgery is completed in less than 2 hours from the initial dose and 2 gm the evening of surgery.

As Menaker (10) has stated, ". . . systemic antibiotics administered preoperatively and for a short perioperative interval . . . has little effect on intestinal colonization . . . antibiotics are not indicated merely to cover breaks in the operative technique." Only clear liquids by mouth are taken for the 2 days before admission to the hospital, and a half bottle of citrate of magnesia or two bisacodyl (Dulcolax) tablets are given the afternoon before admission. There should be two Fleet's enemas an hour apart the day before surgery, and the morning of surgery plain water or saline enemas until the return is clear. The use of GoLYTELY, consumed after a 3- or 4-hour fast the evening before surgery, seems to an effective substitute.

The choice of a number of surgical procedures from which one might choose in determining the surgical therapy for a rectovaginal fistula is predicated on many things. Foremost among these is the location of the fistula: high, mid, or low vagina: Second is the etiology of the fistula: trauma, postradiation, postoperative, postepisiotomy, Crohn's disease, active malignant disease, etc. An additional consideration is the need for preserving or restoring coital function of the vagina. Another factor is the age of the patient, whether it be at any point in the full life spectrum from the congenital or traumatic problems of infancy to the effects and influences of advanced years.

The gynecologic surgeon should be familiar with a number of techniques for surgical treatment of a rectovaginal fistula, that the one chosen be likely to best fit the specific needs of a particular patient.

## RECTOVAGINAL SEPTAL DEFECTS

The choice of procedure for repair of rectovaginal septal defects is determined by the etiology and the age of the patient (from infancy to the advanced years) but for the most part by the location of a rectovaginal fistula (low, mid, or high within the vagina), the presence or absence of a perineal body, and the integrity of the exterior anal sphincter (12). The goals of surgery are as for all reconstructive surgery, to relieve the symptoms and to restore the anatomy and function to normal. The effective combination must be thoughtfully planned and carefully executed for each patient.

It must be remembered that for genital fistulae there is a high pressure side and a low pressure side, as noted by Corman (4). In the presence of a symptomatic fistula the flow of material from a hollow viscus is always from the high pressure side to the low pressure side. With rectovaginal fistula, the rectum is the high pressure side, the vagina the low. Material flows from the rectum into the vagina, not from the vagina into the rectum. (With vesicovaginal fistula, the bladder is the high pressure side.) Primary attention must be given the closure of the high pressure side that must be closed securely and effectively. Even if unattended the low pressure (i.e., the vagina) will generally close spontaneously once the continuity of the fistula has been interrupted and the high pressure side effectively closed. However, the vaginal continuity over the rectum is made stronger by excision of the epithelium lining the vaginal opening and loosely approximating the sides of the vaginal defect, but with the stitches far enough apart to permit postoperative drainage, if there is any.

Repair should be considered when fistulae have caused troublesome symptoms and when local edema and inflammation have subsided (usually coincident with relief or pain) and should embrace the following technical considerations:

1. The epithelial track should be excised and the edges inverted into the lumen when possible.
2. The fistula should be closed securely in two layers, usually in a transverse axis, and without tension.
3. Meticulous hemostasis should be accomplished.

Because of the high vascularity of the pelvis, hemostasis in the area of fistula repair is essential to improve wound healing and lessen the chances of hematoma and abscess formation. Infiltration by up to 50 ml of a "liquid tourniquet" such as 0.5% lidocaine in 1:200,000 epinephrine solution is helpful, although neosynephrine solution or saline may be substituted when indicated by the presence of severe hypertension or of coronary heart disease.

Nine basic operative procedures with which the surgeon might wish to become familiar are:

1. closure in layers without disrupting perineum;
2. closure in layers following episioproctotomy;
3. transperineal mucosal flap transplant dorsal to an intact external sphincter;

4. transperineal mucosal layers and closure ventral to an intact external sphincter;
5. the transrectal anterior rectal mucosal flap transplant;
6. the Noble-Mengert-Fish anterior rectal flap operation (Chapter 14);
7. the Warren-Miller vaginal flap operation (Chapter 14);
8. transabdominal procedures for fistula located in the vault of an immobile vagina that, when following radiation, might include temporary transverse colostomy;
9. colpocleisis or colpectomy (Chapter 16).

All of these should be included within the armamentarium of the gynecologist so that a choice can be made on the basis of the patient's needs rather than a particular technique of operation with which the surgeon is comfortable but which may not be universally applicable or suitable to the clinical circumstances of a particular patient.

## DIAGNOSIS

Although some rectovaginal fistulae are asymptomatic, the majority are not. The presence of fistulae can be suspected from incontinence of rectal gas or of liquid or solid stool even in the presence of an intact perineum and functional external anal sphincter. When these contaminants are passed through the vagina, the bacterial concentration may precipitate a chronic, recurrent vaginitis. There may be dyspareunia when infection and fibrosis are present.

Most cases of rectovaginal or rectoperineal fistula repair should be preceded and accompanied by suitable proctoscopy. Occasionally, the rectal opening of the fistula will be difficult to demonstrate except by gentle probing under anesthesia. When it is still not demonstrable with certainty, traction by an Allis clamp on the external secondary opening, as described by Bacon and Ross (1), will usually produce dimpling at the primary opening, which will often be found in an anal crypt. If visualization is still unclear, the surgeon may inject the fistulous tract with methylene blue using a Nos. 18, 19, or 20 needle that has been cut off about 1 cm from its hub. Through an anoscope look for the blue dye coming through the rectum, and look also for branches of the fistula (13).

The most common postpartum rectal vaginal fistulae are those located in the lower third of the vagina. For these fistulae a sliding rectal flap procedure, such as that described with the Noble-Mengert-Fish operation, mobilizes then excises a portion of the anterior rectal wall including the fistula and, if the external anal sphincter has been lacerated, permits reunification of its severed ends and construction of a perineal body (see Chapter 14). Corman's modification using a cruciate perineal incision is useful when there is ample perineal skin (4), and it is desired to narrow the introitus and restore or build up a defective perineum (Figs. 19.1-19.3).

If abundant perineal skin is lacking, which is quite common, and it is desired to narrow a gaping introitus, the Warren-Miller flap operation is a useful alternate, permitting narrowing of the introitus with coincident reconstitution of the integrity of an interrupted external anal sphincter and perineum (see Chapter 14).

When the fistula is in the midvagina and the external anal sphincter and perineal body are intact, a layered closure is useful. The full thickness of the vaginal wall is incised into the rectovaginal space and the rectum and vagina carefully separated from one another. The fistulous track is transected and the rectal track excised in its entirety. The rectal wall is closed by two layers of submucosal interrupted size 3-0 polyglycolic acid-type mattress sutures placed

**Figure 19.1.** When the vagina is wide and the perineum is thin, the cruciate incision of Corman is useful. Incisions are made in the full thickness of the skin as shown by the *dotted line* and two skin flaps, A and B, are noted.

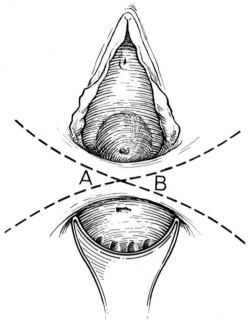

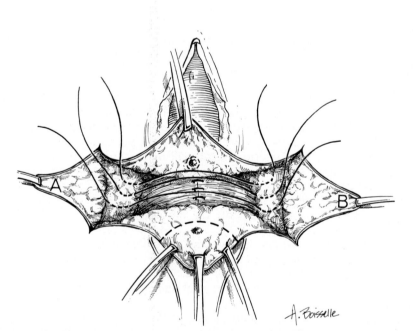

**Figure 19.2.** The flaps have been dissected widely and the fistulous track transected. Lateral subcutaneous tissues including external anal sphincter reinforcement are being brought together in the midline. Excess anal wall containing the rectal side of the fistula will be excised along the path of the *dotted line*. The vaginal side of the track will be excised as shown.

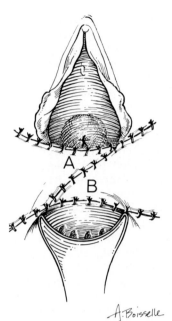

**Figure 19.3.**    Flaps *A and B* are sewn to each other as shown, narrowing the vagina and thickening the perineum. The vaginal wound is closed with a single interrupted stitch.

2 or 3 mm apart in the rectal wall. These may be placed transversely in the muscular wall of the rectum or longitudinally (9) depending upon available exposure, if the latter will not compromise the rectal lumen. A second layer not only reinforces the first, but takes some of the tension from the first layer of closure. The epithelialized track through the wall of the vagina is excised and the opening loosely approximated in a longitudinal direction by interrupted sutures of polyglycolic acid placed no more closely than 1 cm apart, to allow for adequate possible postoperative drainage. Alternately, and after irrigation of the wound, the posterior vaginal vault may be split and a layer of rectovaginal septum interposed from side to side. The edges of the vaginal incision are freshened and made symmetrical, and the vagina is closed with interrupted sutures.

When the operator has determined to use a layered closure after re-creation of a fresh third degree laceration with excision of epithelialized fistulous track, and there is little available other tissue to use, the interposition of some "levator" stitches between the rectum and vagina, placed without palpable ridges, will increase the thickness of the perineum and insulate the site of the rectal repair from that of the vaginal side of the fistula.

Rectovaginal fistulae in the pregnant patient resulting from obstetric trauma of a previous delivery may be closed at the time of delivery by episioproctorrhaphy-the excellent blood supply and laxity of the perineal muscles during pregnancy favor good healing. By a fresh incision an episioproctotomy is performed, "re-creating" a fourth degree laceration. The fistulous track and scar tissue are excised and the wound repaired as if it were a fresh fourth degree laceration. Our objection to episioproctorrhaphy in the treatment of rectovaginal fistulae in the non-pregnant patient is that in the event of postoperative infection with abscess formation, the perineal body and external anal sphincter integrity may be destroyed. Infection in this area even without tissue destruction in abscess formation may initiate chronic painful inflammation, edema, and spasm of the pubococcygeal portion of the levator ani muscle, giving rise to the "levator syndrome" that is so resistant to effective treatment.

For the patient with an intact perineum and intact external anal sphincter in whom the fistula is in the lower third of the vagina, the transperineal rectal flap-sliding operation of Inmon is our choice, as it does not disturb the perineal body but does permit plication of an intact but lax external anal sphincter, if desired (Fig. 19.4).

When the fistula is located in the midvagina and the perineal body and external anal sphincter are intact, the operation of Thompson (13) using a transverse perineal incision is useful. In this operation (Fig. 19.5) a perineal incision is made beneath the posterior vaginal wall ventral or anterior to the external anal sphincter, and the rectovaginal space is entered. Identification of the fistula during dissection of the vaginal wall is aided by passage of a malleable probe. After the rectum and vagina have been separated from one another, first laterally, then cranially to the fistula, the fistula is transected at its central portion as noted in Figure 19.5F. The fistula is transected and the epithelialized track excised from both rectal and vaginal wall (Fig. 19.5). The rectal defect is closed transversely with two layers, one of interrupted submucosal and the other of intramural sutures, and the vaginal wall closed longitudinally. Interrupted sutures for the vagina may be placed in a single layer, rather widely apart to permit possible postoperative drainage. The perineal skin may be closed transversely, but if it is desired to lengthen the perineal body, the skin and subcutaneous tissue may be approximated in the midline (Fig. 19.5K). However, when considerable fibrosis of the perineum is apparent and such a repair as described would result in a reduction in vaginal caliber and size of the perineum and be certain to cause dyspareunia, an alternate and preferable approach would involve a surgical technique that would preserve the vaginal diameter and the integrity of the external anal sphincter. One such operation is the transrectal sliding mucosal flap operation (5, 7, 8).

## Transrectal Mucosal Flap Transplant Technique

The patient is face down in a jacknife position, with small sandbags elevating the hips. The fistula may then be evident and explored from the rectal side using a small malleable blunt probe until the probe is palpable within the vagina.

With the Smith self-retaining retractor in place, and aided by a Sims retractor providing exposure in the vagina, the rectal circumference of the fistula may be infiltrated by 0.5% lidocaine in 1:200,000 epinephrine solution, and the rectal ostium circumscribed by an incision placed 0.5 to 1 cm from the margins of the track (Fig. 19.6). This incision is extended distally onto the perineum, where removal of an inverted V-shaped wedge of skin and subcutaneous tissue exposes the anal sphincter. The incision is deepened to identify both internal and external anal sphincters, that may be partially divided sufficiently to remove any tendency toward a ridge or shelf-like effect. The rectovaginal septum is identified close to the posterior wall of the vagina, and the rectovaginal space and anterior rectal wall are mobilized for about 3 cm above the site of the fistula.

A figure-of-8 suture is then placed through the rectal opening of the fistula and tied to the needle eye of the blunt probe. By traction upon the probe from the vaginal side, the fistulous track is inverted into the vagina and cut off flush with the vaginal skin. A series of interrupted 2-0 absorbable polyglycolic sutures fix the rectal muscularis to the cranial edge of the external anal sphincter, and another layer of sutures sews the mucosal edge of the anterior rectal wall to the posterior surface of the external anal sphincter. A small Malecot or Penrose drain may be placed through the vaginal opening at the site

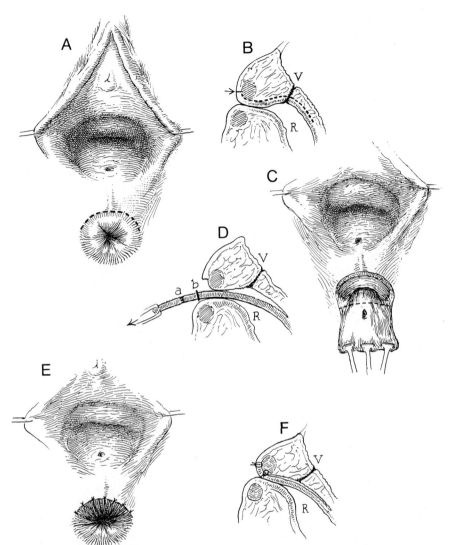

**Figure 19.4.** A transperineal rectal flap operation is depicted. A rectovaginal fistula proximal to an intact external anal sphincter is noted. Preliminary infiltration by lidocaine 0.5% in epinephrine 1:200,000 of all tissue to be dissected will diminish blood loss. The site for an incision is identified by the *broken line (A)*. This is seen in sagittal section *(B)* where *V* indicates vagina and *R* the rectum. The dissection beneath the perineal body proceeds to, opens and develops the rectovaginal space. Traction to the anterior rectal wall stretches it until the fistulous opening in the rectum is exteriorized *(C)*. This is seen in sagittal section *(D)* in which the fistula *(a)* has been exteriorized. The underside of the perineal body and the external anal sphincter can be reinforced by interrupted sutures. The rectal flap is excised along the *broken line* that corresponds to *b* in the sagittal view. The remaining anterior rectal wall *(b)* is tacked to the capsule of the external anal sphincter and the edge sewn to the perineal skin *(E)* completing the operation. The sagittal view *(F)* shows the interruption of the continuity of the fistula. There is no longer communication between the rectum *(R)* and the vagina *(V)*. The vaginal side of the track will granulate in and rapidly disappear. Because it is epithelialized, it too may be readily excised during the operation.

of the previous fistulous tract where it is sewn in place with a single absorbable suture and the anal canal is lightly packed with a plug of Vaseline gauze. An indwelling Foley catheter is inserted into the bladder.

Postoperatively, the preliminary antibiotic can be continued for a short time unless a significant diarrhea develops, in which case the antibiotic should be promptly terminated and the diarrhea brought under control. The patient should be kept on a clear liquid diet for 3 days and when she is passing gas, she is gradually changed to a low-roughage or bland diet for 3 weeks. Stool softeners should be given, and if there has been no bowel movement by the

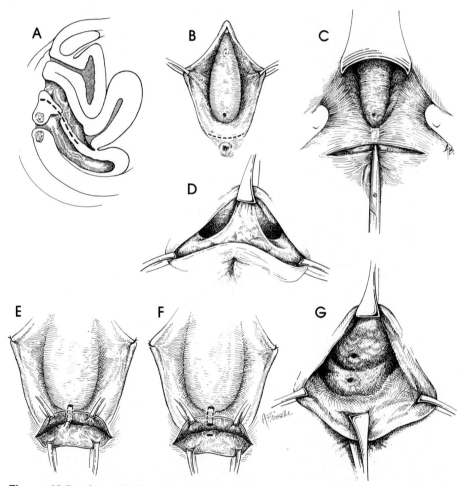

**Figure 19.5.** A sagittal section of the pelvis showing a rectovaginal fistula is shown in *A*. The fistula is independent of the intact external anal sphincter, which will be spared by an incision made along the path of the *dashed line*. Notice that the dissection between rectum and vagina extends well above the area of the fistula, in order that it may be closed without tension. The transverse incision in the perineum is shown by the *dotted line* in *B,* anterior to the external anal sphincter. The dissection between rectum and vagina is begun as shown in *C*. Tunnels into the rectovaginal space lateral to the fistula are established as shown in *D*. The rectovaginal fistula is identified in *E* and transected in *F*. The dissection into the rectovaginal space is carried cranial to the fistula as in *G*.  (*continued*)

seventh day, a gentle laxative should be added. The vaginal drain should be removed between the fifth and seventh postoperative days, depending upon the amount of drainage and the stability of the patient's temperature. Sitz baths may improve comfort and be given twice daily after the drain has been removed. Coitus is neither advised nor permitted until the end of the third postoperative month.

The Warren flap operation and the Noble-Mengert-Fish operation are useful when there is no functional anal sphincter, as they are often used as very successful surgical procedures to remedy an old fourth degree laceration (Chapter 14) and may be employed when a bridge of tissue not containing significant or functional sphincter muscle connects one side with the other. In the latter condition, the bridge that consists primarily of scar tissue is cut across at the beginning of the operation, and the procedure is essentially the same as that used for reconstructing the vagina after an old healed fourth degree laceration. They require approximation of the anal sphincter anterior to the anterior rectal wall. If, rarely, the reconstructed anal sphincter is smaller

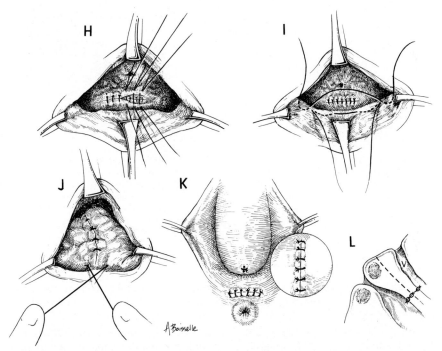

The rectal side of the fistula is closed transversly using two layers of interrupted mattress sutures of 3-0 polyglycolic acid sutures as shown in *H*. A layer of tissue between the rectum and the vagina is brought together in a longitudinal direction with suture placement as shown in *I*. Any necessary perineorrhaphy is accomplished, and when these sutures have been tied the longitudinal orientation is clear as shown in *J*, whose axis is at right angles to the transverse closure in the anterior wall of the rectum. The epithelialized vaginal track is excised, and the vaginal wall may be lightly closed with a single stitch, if desired, or left open for drainage. The incision in the perineum is closed with interrupted sutures, as shown in *K*. If it is desired to thicken the perineum, it may be closed longitudinally as shown in the *inset* within the circle. The sagittal section showing the end result is noted in *L*. The integrity of an intact external anal sphincter has been spared.

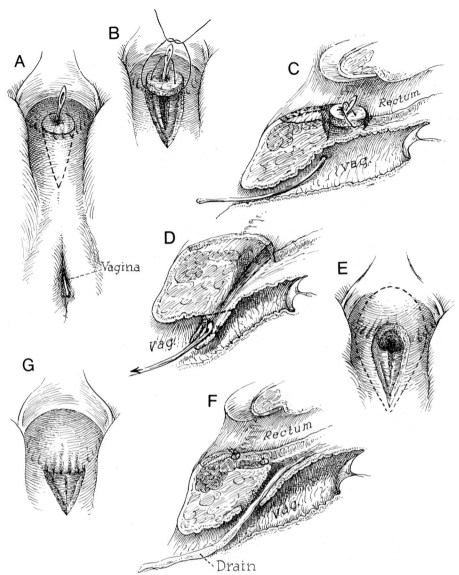

**Figure 19.6.** The transrectal mucosal flap transplant is depicted. With the patient face down and in a jackknife position, the posterior rectal wall is displaced by a retractor, and the fistula is explored from the rectal side by a small malleable probe *(A)*. The rectal circumference of the fistula is infiltrated by 0.5% lidocaine in 1:200,000 epinephrine solution and the opening circumscribed by an incision placed 1 cm from the margin. This incision is extended distally onto the perineum, and a V-shaped wedge of epithelium is excised as indicated by the *dotted line*. Sufficient superficial fibers of the rectal side of the anal sphincter are incised as to remove this as an obstruction postoperatively to the passage of stool and gas *(B)*, and the mobilized rectal opening of the fistula is sewn to the eye of the malleable probe *(B)*. This is shown in sagittal section in *C*. Traction on the vaginal end of the probe is made as shown in *D*, inverting the fistulous tract into the vagina where it is excised as indicated by the *dotted line*. The anterior rectal wall is separated from the vagina for about 2 cm *(E)*. A series of interrupted sutures fixes the rectal wall to the internal anal sphincter *(F)*, and another layer of sutures sews the mucosal edge of the anterior rectal wall to the posterior surface of the external sphincter *(G)*. A small drain may be placed through the vaginal opening at the site of the previous fistula and fixed in place with a single absorbable stitch.

than one fingerbreadth, a complementary paradoxical external anal sphincter transection at the five-o'clock position may be beneficial.

For fresh and unepithelialized fistulae involving the upper third of the vagina, usually after hysterectomy with postoperative pelvic abscess, many such fistulae will close spontaneously if the patient is placed on a no-residue all elemental diet with clear liquids for several weeks inactivating the lower bowel. Several weeks of local estrogen therapy will be beneficial even preoperatively and postoperatively if the patient is postmenopausal. For those vault fistulae that do not close spontaneously, the smaller may be closed transvaginally by a Latzko partial colpocleisis, but laparotomy should be considered for those that are large, and after inflammation and edema have subsided. After bowel preparation, the rectum and upper vagina are separated from each other by sharp dissection. After excision of the epithelialized margins, the rectal opening is closed transversely in two layers and the vaginal opening longitudinally in one layer, interposing or covering each with a layer of mobilized peritoneum. Complementary defunctioning temporary colostomy is usually not necessary unless there has been a history of prior therapeutic pelvic irradiation.

For those fistulae that occur after therapeutic doses of pelvic radiation, usually years later consequent to the reduction in blood flow that occurs with endarteritis obliterans, one should first confirm that no active malignant disease exists by biopsy of viable tissue from the fistula margin. Having determined this, nightly application of intravaginal estrogen cream is prescribed, so as to improve the local blood supply and thicken the genital epithelium. Repair should be delayed for about 1 year from the time this fistula is first noticed, so as to permit adequate stabilization of the blood supply and further confirmation of the absence of recurrent malignancy in this area. Premature repair of this type of fistula, although morphologically correct at the conclusion of the operation but before restabilization or arrest of the vascular obliteration, is prone toward recurrence of the fistula the size of which may be greater than that of the original and more difficult ro repair. For the meticulous and technically precise surgeon, Boronow's operation of partial colpocleisis of the upper vagina is appropriate (3). The somewhat fibrotic vaginal vault fistula is surgically exposed using a Schuchardt incision, and the vagina is carefully dissected from the anterior rectal wall for 1 to 2 cm in all directions at the site of the fistula. Meticulous hemostasis is achieved to prevent postoperative hematome formation, and the defect in the anterior rectal wall is closed transversely without tension by a two-layered interrupted fine polyglycolic acid suture technique, thus closing the high pressure side of the fistula. A bulbocavernosus fat pad is mobilized, swung beneath the anterior vaginal wall and sewn in place covering the site of the fistula repair, and the vagina is closed. A no-residue oral elemental diet is maintained for several weeks, followed by a low-residue diet and stool softeners. Nightly instillation of intravaginal estrogen cream is continued for many weeks until healing, followed by long-term weekly dosage.

Because fistulae resulting from Crohn's disease do not characteristically respond to standard surgical technique, it is essential to recognize this disorder before a surgical approach can be recommended. Suspicion occurs when there is no known mechanical trauma to explain the origin of the fistula, and the patient may give a history of weight loss and frequent loose bowel movements, often accompanied by intestinal cramping. The fistula is invariably quite painful to touch (especially during the active phases of the disease) even when such a fistula has been present for a considerable length of time. Its edge has the roughened red appearance of granulation tissue. Confirmation of this suspicion may be obtained from biopsy, endoscopy, and study of the films of upper and lower gastrointestinal radiography. Repair of the Crohn's induced rectovaginal fistula in the lower vagina may be considered during a phase of temporary remission of the disease, and use of a rectal flap-sliding operation permits excision of bowel wall containing the fistula, but the patient must be made aware of the high risk of surgical failure or of exacerbation of the disease. Preoperative preparation may include 1 month's administration of metronidazole (Flagyl) (2), 1000 mg daily along with 20 mg of prednisone daily.

Sigmoid-vaginal fistula is usually the result of perforation of a sigmoid diverticulum coincident with abscess formation from diverticulitis in a usually older patient with diverticulosis. A transabdominal operation often combined with partial colectomy is the proper approach for surgery for this type of fistula.

Colpocleisis is reserved primarily for the large fistula that is sometimes seen after radiation, in which the viability of the adjacent tissue is so poor that good wound healing cannot be optimistically predicted. It, of course, destroys function of most or all of the vagina, and this must be thoroughly explained to, understood, and agreed upon by the patient.

Transabdominal closure of the fistula is generally reserved for those in the vault of the vagina in which accessibility from below may be limited and repair of the bowel more difficult due to decreased visibility once the two organs have been separated. This is more often seen in the longstanding epithelialized rectovaginal fistula after hysterectomy and pelvic abscess that may limit vaginal mobility. When it follows pelvic irradiation, successful closure may require temporary transverse colostomy and bringing into the repair an interposing layer of fresh tissue with an independent blood supply, such as the omentum or the bulbocavernosus fat pad. This is because postradiation fibrosis includes coincident obliteration of local blood vessels with development of "endarteritis obliterans," which effectively reduces the blood supply to the irradiated tissues.

Late recurrence of rectovaginal fistula, even 10 or 15 years after the time of an original repair, will occasionally be seen; and for this reason it is desirable for the operator periodically to examine the patient over a long period of time.

A rectoperineal fistula not communicating with the anal sphincter is treated by simple excision of a wide area of surrounding skin, at least 1 cm lateral to each side of the fistula. A probe is placed into the fistulous track that is then incised through the full thickness of the overlying skin and subcutaneous tissue. The surrounding skin margin is widely excised, removing the fistulous track. Any bleeding vessels are tied, and the wound is packed open, to granulate in from the bottom. It is desirable that the skin margins be the last portion of the wound to close. Healing requires a 4- to 6-week period, but the patient remains surprisingly comfortable and there is little disability.

## Postoperative Care of the Patient After Fistula Repair

The following recommendations are made regarding postoperative care of the patient after fistula repair:

1. Stool softeners such as docusate sodium (Colace) should be given for 5 weeks. One may give tincture of opium, 10 drops in water 3 times a day for 5 days if cramps are troublesome.
2. A clear liquid diet is advised postoperatively for 3 days, then low residue for 3 weeks.
3. There should be a bowel movement between the 5th and 7th day postoperatively while the patient is still in the hospital. Small doses of GoLYTELY are preferable to an enema at this time. No coitus is permitted for 2 or 3 months postoperatively.

### Abscess Formation

The timing of a fistula repair should be such as not to involve an abscess, because the presence of an infection will seriously impede the quality of wound healing. When, at surgery, an unexpected abscess is encountered in the tissues between the rectum and the vagina, the intended procedure must be modified and simply becomes an unroofing operation in which the full thickness of the vaginal wall overlying the abscess is widely excised (Fig. 19.8). This will permit immediate and adequate drainage. Such a wound will also granulate in from the bottom up, and in some instances the communication with the rectum will be closed by the granulation of the base of the wound and no further surgery will be necessary. These principles are demonstrated in Figure 19.7.

## RECTOUTERINE FISTULA

Unless associated with an invasive neoplasm, rectouterine fistulae are almost invariably the result of coexistent diverticulosis that became adherent to the posterior wall of the uterus, after which an abscess formed and ultimately eroded into the uterine cavity. The condition produces a profuse, cloudy, watery discharge from the cervix that is usually sufficient in amount to require the patient to wear sanitary protection. Early in its course of development the discharge may be intermittent, coinciding with flare-ups of activity within the abscess cavity, and between spells of watery leukorrhea the patient may be relatively comfortable. The diagnosis is readily confirmed by a barium enema and sigmoidoscopy. Treatment is surgical, sometimes requiring a preliminary

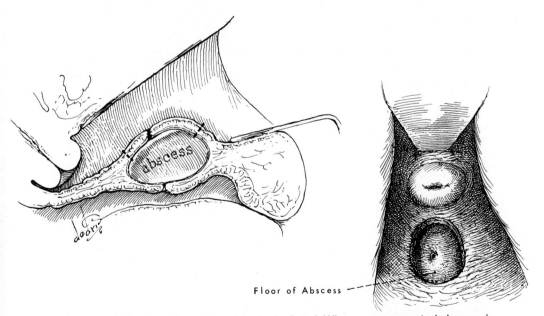

Floor of Abscess

**Figure 19.7.** An unroofing procedure is depicted. When an unexpected abscess is encountered in the course of the fistulous track, the cavity is widely exposed by cutting away a generous circumference of posterior vaginal wall as indicated by the *dotted line* in the drawing at the *left*. This exposes the floor of the abscess, as seen at the *right* of the illustration, with the visible central dimple indicating the communication to the rectum. The cavity should be packed and allowed to granulate in.

colostomy, then a bowel resection and hysterectomy 2 or 3 months later, and closure of the colostomy as a tertiary procedure 2 or 3 months after hysterectomy.

## VESICORECTAL FISTULA

This is a rare late complication after hysterectomy and, because of its location high within the vault of the vagina, will usually require a transabdominal approach with dissection followed by separate repair of each organ system. Depending upon the size of the fistula and any previous irradiation, a preliminary diverting colostomy may be desirable.

### References

1. Bacon HE, Ross ST: *Atlas of Operative Technique: Anus, Rectum, and Colon.* St Louis, CV Mosby, p 110, 1954.
2. Bernstein LH, et al.: Healing of Perineal Crohn's Disease with Metronidazole. *Gastroenterology* 79:357–365, 1980.
3. Boronow RC: Management of radiation-induced vaginal fistulas. *Am J Obstet Gynecol* 1:1–8, 1971.
4. Corman ML: *Colon and Rectal Surgery.* Philadelphia, JB Lippincott, pp 108–110, 1984.
5. Gallagher DM, Scarborough RA: Repair of low rectovaginal fistula. *Dis Colon Rectum* 5:193, 1962.
6. Hauth JC, et al.: Early Repair of an External Sphincter Ani Muscle and Rectal Mucosal Dehiscence. *Obstet Gynecol* 67:806–809, 1986.
7. Jackman RJ: Rectovaginal and anovaginal fistulas: A surgical procedure for treatment of certain types. *J Iowa State Med Soc* 42:435–440, 1952.
8. Laird DR: Procedures used in the treatment of complicated fistulas. *Am J Surg* 76:701, 1948.
9. Leacher TC, Pratt JH: Vaginal repair of the simple rectovaginal fistula. *Surg Gynecol Obstet* 124:1317–1321, 1967.
10. Menaker GH: The use of antibiotics in surgical treatment of the colon. *Surg Gynecol Obstet* 164:581–586, 1987.
11. Rock JA, Woodruff JD: Surgical correction of a rectovaginal fistula. *Int J Gynaecol Obstet* 20:413–416, 1982.
12. Rosenshein NB, Genadry RR, Woodruff JD: An anatomic classification of rectovaginal septal defects. *Am J Obstet Gynecol* 137:439–442, 1980.
13. Thompson JD: *Transperineal Repair of a Rectovaginal Fistula.* Ob-Gyn Illustrated, New Scotland, NY, Learning Technology Incorporated, 1985.

# CHAPTER 20

# The Small Vagina

When the mature vagina cannot admit nor contain one's sexual partner with comfort, there is a major threat to conjugal harmony. Disproportion in size is a frequent cause of pain and discomfort.

The etiology is varied, including such congenital deformities as absence of the vagina and uterus, absence of the lower half of the vagina, and obstructive transverse septa at any level, including an imperforate hymen. A longitudinal vaginal septum may exist with duplication of the birth canal and the presence of a rudimentary uterine horn may produce dyspareunia as well as dysmenorrhea. Thick lateral bands connecting the external urethral meatus to the hymenal margin may be a source not only of dyspareunia but, by dragging upon the meatus during coitus, may invite recurrent postcoital cystitis (1).

Menopausal change may be a factor, especially when there has been pelvic irradiation or when the aging process has been accompanied by an unusual degree of progressive atrophy and shrinkage. The coital problem may be compounded by some relative flaccidity of the sexual organ of the marital partner, making vaginal penetration difficult.

Iatrogenic causes are significant and range from postepisiotomy scarring and discomfort to the posthysterectomy vagina that is too short, especially after radical surgery with partial vaginectomy. The vaginal diameter may be too narrow as a consequence of excessive subepithelial plication or excision of a more than adequate amount of vaginal membrane with colporrhaphy. Subepithelial ridges that have been produced become more tender as the fibrosis of postoperative scarring progresses.

Contributing psychosomatic factors must be added to the above, including fear of being hurt, the psychologic scarring after rape, the fear of becoming pregnant, fear based on lack of knowledge concerning sexual practices, and, to some, an unconscious or conscious desire to inflict punishment upon oneself or one's marital partner.

These factors may be etiologically grouped in any combination and successful treatment requires identification and proper attention to each contributing factor.

## TREATMENT

A hallmark of treatment is prevention. If the patient is postmenopausal, and particularly if there is sign of mucosal or vulvar atrophy, more or less permanent estrogen replacement will strengthen, restore, and preserve vaginal elasticity in estrogen-sensitive pelvic tissues.

Proper techniques of either vaginal or abdominal hysterectomy, particularly when some degree of genital prolapse is present, require shortening of elongated cardinal and uterosacral ligaments that should be firmly attached to the vault of the vagina. When these ligaments are hypertrophic, the technique of cul-de-plasty (see Chapter 10) is useful in preserving or restoring vaginal length. In principle, this fixes the vaginal vault to the undersurface of strong uterosacral ligaments, which have been brought together in front of the vagina, lessening any tendency toward enterocele formation. This technique can be used successfully with either vaginal or abdominal hysterectomy, but with the latter, the surgeon must be especially careful not to produce ureteral obstruction.

Effort should be made to identify actual or potential enterocele and any excess peritoneum should be excised before high peritonealization. The vaginal vault can be strengthened by excision of any excess width.

Preservation of vaginal depth by fixing the vault above the levator plate will lessen any tendency for telescoping, as increases in intra-abdominal pressure compress the vagina against the levator plate. If strong and surgically useful cardinal-uterosacral ligaments are lacking, alternative methods of colpopexy to support the vault must be used even at the time of hysterectomy (see Chapter 16). As Amreich has pointed out, a short vagina ending anterior to the levator plate will tend with time to become even shorter, as intra-abdominal pressure may be transmitted in the axis of the vagina.

It is essential that the surgeon carefully calculate the amount of the vagina to be excised with colporrhaphy, to permit an acceptable postoperative vaginal width. There should be suitable allowance for any anticipated shrinkage with ageing and hormone withdrawal (i.e., all other things being equal, one would excise less vaginal membrane from a premenopausal patient in whom postoperative vaginal shrinkage has yet to occur). Allowance should be made for the age and genital size of the patient's marital consort. In the temporary absence of sexual activity, periodic insertion of a vaginal obturator will be of value if there is any tendency toward stricture or stenosis.

With lower vaginal agenesis, a tunnel is dissected through the vestibular area toward the upper vagina. If a functional uterus is present, a hematocolpos will have been confirmed by rectal examination. The upper vaginal canal can be mobilized, opened, stretched, and sewn to the skin of the vestibule, to cover the raw lower area. It should not be necessary to perform a graft.

The uterus may be present in a patient with a transverse vaginal septum at any level. Interestingly, there is no associated urinary track anomaly suggesting a significant difference from the Rokitansky-Kuster-Hauser syndrome. A vaginal septum or imperforate hymen is treated by appropriate excision.

When the vagina is short, as from previous radical pelvic surgery that has included partial vaginectomy, the distal vulvovaginoplasty of Williams (8) may add 1 to 3 inches to the length. For those requiring still more depth, construction of a new upper vagina by a partial McIndoe procedure may be accomplished (see Chapter 21). Additional depth may be created as well as maintained by the use of appropriate vaginal obturators (2, 4).

When the vagina is narrow or constricted at a specific point, additional width can be obtained by surgery at an appropriate level, the technique and procedure depending upon the site of the constriction.

Most commonly, this occurs at the perineum, often after overenthusiastic perineorrhaphy or hurried inadequate reapproximation of an episiotomy. This is particularly true when the pubococcygei have been approximated anterior to the rectum (see Chapter 12). A midline perineotomy with a suture of the wound in the direction at a right angle to the incision may be all that is required, although this will shorten the vagina a small bit. If atrophy is present, a bilateral episiotomy with sliding of the skin margins (8) (Fig. 20.1) will widen the introitus.

## CORRECTION OF A MIDVAGINAL STRICTURE OR STENOSIS

Stricture of the midportion of the vagina may be overcome by the use of lateral relaxing incisions made through the full thickness of the vagina (Fig.

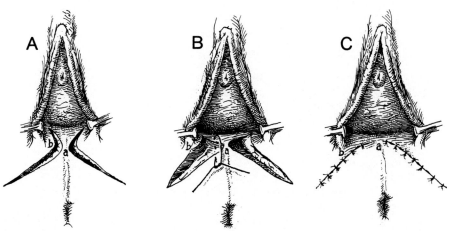

**Figure 20.1.** Bilateral episiotomy is performed *(A)*. Repair is begun at the medial edge *(b)* in such a fashion that *(b)* is no longer adjacent to *(a)* but is in fact moved laterally on each side a distance sufficient to enlarge the introitus as much as is necessary. The end-result *(C)* shows the now widened introitus.

20.2). The margins of the incision are undercut, and the vaginal caliber is maintained by a suitable obturator during epithelialization and healing. If the freshly excised vaginal wall is still on the scrub nurse's table, a patch may be cut of a size sufficient to fill the defect in the lateral vaginal wall and sewn in place as a full-thickness graft (Fig. 20.3).

Lateral vaginal relaxing incisions can be made in a constricted vagina at any time, even years later, although a brief rehospitalization and anesthetic is required. The technique and aftercare are precisely the same as when done in the fresh surgical patient.

With moderate constriction of the lower vagina, as seen for example in the patient with congenital adrenal hyperplasia, a fasciocutaneous flap from the labia may be developed and swung into place bridging the defect created by a fresh episiotomy (6). This is illustrated in Figure 20.4.

Extensive constriction of the lower half of the vagina from either congenital underdevelopment or postoperative stricture consequent to the surgical excision of too much tissue may be relieved by the use of full-thickness skin flaps (5) from the inner thigh, a modification of the Graves operation (3) for construction of a neovagina. Convalescence requires several weeks of relative rest and several months' use of a vaginal obturator.

## GRAVES PROCEDURE

The Graves procedure (3) was described as a method of treating congenital absence of the vagina, in which a tunnel between the bladder and rectum was established and lined by four full-thickness flaps of skin. Two were raised from the medial surface of the thighs, and two were raised from the full-thickness of the skin medial to the labia majora, and including the labia minora, which were spatulated. These were all sewn together, inverted into the tunnel of the neovagina, and held there by a glass obturator until fixed to the walls of the cavity.

When a major stricture or atresia of the lower half of the vagina is encountered that is more extensive than can be relieved by simple midline perineotomy closed transversely, a modification of the Graves procedure is useful, in which two full-thickness flaps of an appropriate size are mobilized

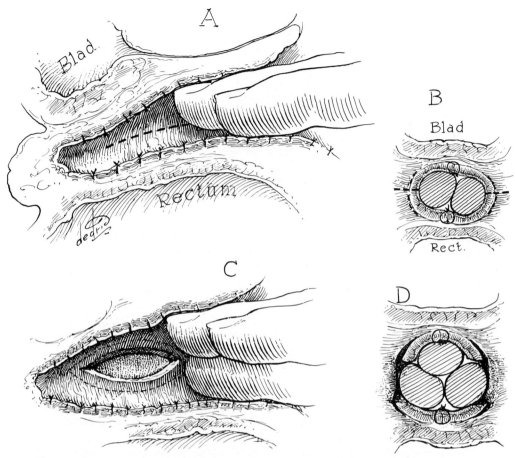

**Figure 20.2.** Digital examination of the vagina immediately after colporrhaphy discloses an unexpected stenosis in the upper half that will admit but two fingerbreadths *(A)*. The sites of the lateral relaxing incisions are indicated by the *dotted lines (B)*. These incisions are made through the lateral wall of the vagina to a depth sufficient for the vagina to comfortably admit three fingerbreadths *(C)*. The vaginal wall is undercut for a centimeter in each direction *(D)*. Any obvious bleeding vessels are clamped and tied, and a firm vaginal packing is inserted. This may be replaced within a day or so by a large vaginal obturator or mold, to keep the cut edges of the relaxing incisions apart until healing and epithelialization are well under way, usually by the 5th postoperative day, after which the obturator or dilator may be worn at night for an additional 2 or 3 weeks. Thus, the integrity of the colporrhaphy incisions in the anterior and posterior vaginal walls is not compromised.

from the medial surface of each thigh and swung into the vagina to cover the site of a fresh midline episiotomy (Figs. 20.5 to 20.11). Polyglycolic acid-type suture is used throughout.

## TECHNIQUE OF VULVOVAGINAL SKIN FLAP ROTATION (MODIFIED GRAVES OPERATION)

1. The perineum and the medial skin of each thigh are thoroughly infiltrated by subcuticular 0.5% lidocaine in 1:200,000 epinephrine solution. Approximately 100 ml are used.

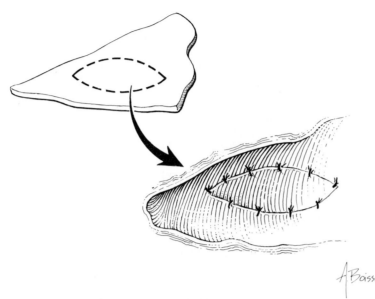

**Figure 20.3.** A full-thickness graft may be cut from the vaginal membrane previously excised with the colporrhaphy. The proper size of the graft is that which will fit the defect in the lateral vaginal wall created by the relaxing incisions. It is held in place by a few interrupted stitches, as shown.

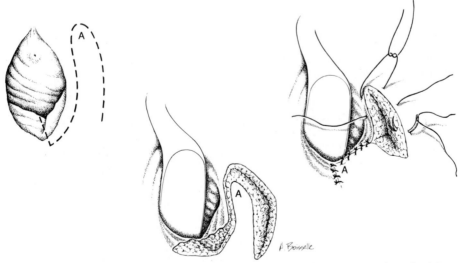

**Figure 20.4.** Labial cutaneous flap. The site of a perineotomy and an incision through the full-thickness of the labia skin and subcutaneous fat is made as shown by the *broken line* in the drawing to the *left*. The base of the flap is wider than the apex as seen in the *center* drawing. The flap has been freed from the underlying fascia and swung into the defect created by the perineotomy, and fixed in place by a few interrupted stitches as shown. The labial defect is closed. Note the change in location of the tissue marked with the *asterisk*. Transplanted hair growth is minimal.

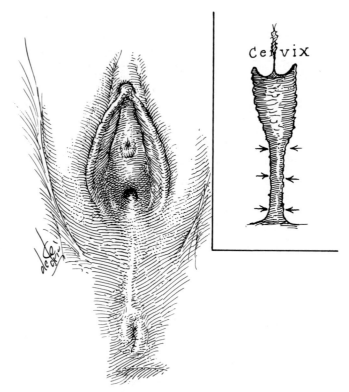

**Figure 20.5.** The vulvovaginal skin flap rotation is shown. The vulva is illustrated. The small opening into the vagina illustrates the vaginal diameter for the lower half of the vagina. A cross-section of the vagina *(right)* shows the extent of the stricture (marked by the *arrows*).

**Figure 20.6.** The perineum and skin of the medial thighs have been infiltrated with lidocaine-epinephrine solution. A large midline episiotomy will be made as shown by the *broken line*. It extends halfway up the posterior vaginal wall to above the stricture. The lower vagina must accommodate three fingerbreadths in diameter.

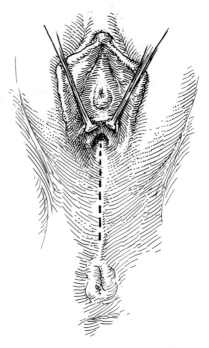

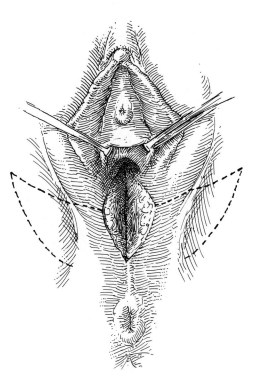

**Figure 20.7.** The large midline episiotomy has been made. Skin flaps are marked out of such a length and width so that when united, they will fill the raw area of the episiotomy.

2. A deep midline episiotomy is made with the skin edges separated widely enough to establish the desired vaginal diameter.
3. Skin flaps are marked off with indelible stain to a size sufficient for each to fill half of the space created by the unrepaired episiotomy.
4. Full-thickness flaps are cut, all the way to the underlying fascia, leaving the subcutaneous fat attached to the undersurface of the flap.

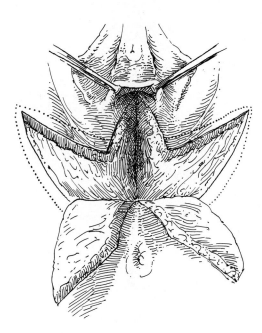

**Figure 20.8.** The full-thickness flaps are cut, including the fat and subcutaneous tissue down to the fascia. The residual skin of the thigh is undermined as shown by the *dotted lines*.

**Figure 20.9.** The medial margins of the flaps are sewn together in the midline. The apex of the now united flaps is held by a single stitch which will be sewn to the apex of the episiotomy. Excess subcutaneous fat beneath the flaps is trimmed.

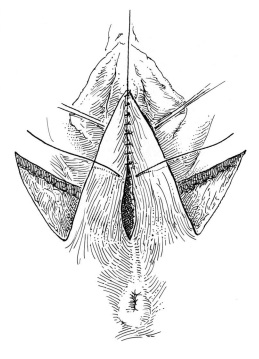

**Figure 20.10.** The lateral edges are sewn to the sides of the episiotomy, and the skin of the thigh is approximated as shown. Penrose drains have been placed beneath the skin flaps on the thigh, a Foley catheter placed in the bladder, and a plastic obturator inserted into the vagina.

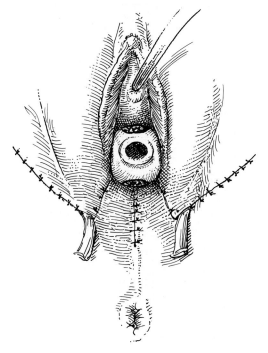

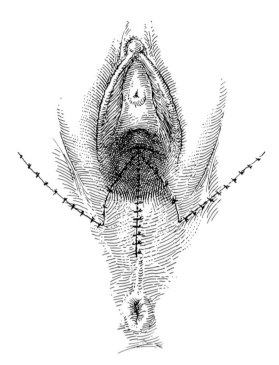

**Figure 20.11.** The end result is shown after removal of the drains and the obturator.

5. The residual skin of the thigh is undermined preparatory to its approximation.
6. The flaps are swung medially to meet in the midline, where their medial edges are approximated with interrupted sutures.
7. Incisions in the thigh are closed from side to side, and the apex of the now united flaps is sewn to the apex of the episiotomy. Any excess adipose tissue is trimmed from the underside of the flap.
8. The lateral margins of the flap are fixed to the edges of the episiotomy with a few interrupted sutures.
9. A Penrose drain is inserted beneath the skin of each thigh, a Foley catheter is inserted in the bladder, and a splinting obturator is inserted into the vagina.
10. The obturator and the Foley catheter are removed on the 4th postoperative day, and the flaps and vagina are thoroughly inspected to determine healing. The obturator is replaced, to be removed each time the patient voids. After 2 or 3 weeks, the mold is worn for several months only at night until healing has been completed.

When the vagina is both too short and too narrow and generally inelastic consequent to fibrosis and scarring from previous surgery, the vulvovaginoplasty of Williams (8) may be of use if the labia are thick and well developed; but if atrophic and thin, vaginectomy followed at the same operation by construction of an Abbe-McIndoe-type neovagina is useful (see Chapter 21).

Long-term postoperative estrogen replacement is of value when indicated and frequent wearing of a suitable obturator is often desirable in order to maintain both vaginal depth and width.

# EVERTED SHORTENED VAGINA

One will occasionally encounter the multioperated patient with total eversion of a shortened vagina-too short, in fact, to reach the sacrospinous ligament. There are several surgical treatment alternatives from which to choose.

1. Ingram-Frank dilators (4) lubricated with estrogen creme may be used to lengthen the vagina until it will reach the sacrospinous ligament at which time sacrospinous colpopexy may be performed.
2. Transabdominal sacrocolpopexy may be performed using an intermediate bridge of fascia lata or of a synthetic plastic material.
3. Sacrospinous colpopexy may be performed using deliberate suture bridges of nonabsorbable synthetic monofilament material, such as Prolene, Surgilene, or Gore-Tex. If the labia are of sufficient size, a Williams vulvovaginoplasty may be added to provide a supplemental depth of an additional 1 ½ or 2 inches of vaginal length.

### References

1. Cummings KG, Gibbons RP, Correa RJ, et al: Scientific Exhibit, American College of Obstetricians and Gynecologists, 1976.
2. Frank RT: The formation of an artificial vagina without operation. *Am J Obstet Gynecol* 35:1053, 1938.
3. Graves WP: Operative treatment of atresia of the vagina. *Boston Med Surg J* 163:753, 1910.
4. Ingram JM: The bicycle seat stool in the treatment of vaginal agenesis and stenosis. *Am J Obstet Gynecol* 140:807, 1981.
5. Martin LW, Sutorius DS: An improved method for vaginoplasty. *Arch Surg* 98:716, 1969.
6. Morton KE, Davies D, Dewhurst J: The use of the fasciocutaneous flap in vaginal reconstruction. *Br J Obstet Gynecol* 93:970–973, 1986.
7. West JT, Ketcham AS, Smith RR: Vaginal reconstruction following pelvic exenteration for cancer or postirradiation necrosis. *Surg Gynecol Obstet* 118:788, 1965.
8. Williams EA: Congenital absence of the vagina: A simple operation for its relief. *J Obstet Gynecol Br Commonw* 71:511, 1964.

# CHAPTER 21

# Creation of a Neovagina

A neovagina may be developed through the use of a number of techniques, a particular one chosen according to the circumstances, needs, and motivations of the individual patient. Although the most common etiologic factor is vaginal agenesis with the Mayer-Rokitansky-Küster-Hauser syndrome, which occurs in one of about five thousand female births, replacement of the vagina may also be considered after vaginectomy, as from cancer, or after extensive scarring from trauma or infection. Surgery may range from construction of the entire length of a vagina or only a portion of vagina depending on the circumstances.

## TIMING OF TREATMENT

Development of a neovagina need not wait until the time of anticipated marriage or coitus, as several months may be required for the postoperative swelling, edema, pain, and tenderness to subside, precluding comfortable coitus until this has eventuated. Because the length of postoperative convalescence is unpredictable, an ideal time for this construction is at the beginning of the patient's summer vacation. Because the entire treatment concept is weighted with psychologic overtones, the need for emotional maturity on the part of the patient is great. Her understanding of the necessary aftercare and its critical importance in determining the success of the procedure requires coincident strong patient motivation after a realistic description of the entire procedure and process and the alternative methods of treatment have been presented. Some positive assessment of her personal commitment, willingness, and motivation must be appropriately developed for there to be a probable long term success of her treatment. The patient must be given ample time to consider the treatment alternatives, her personal commitment to the success of the venture, and to develop a realistic appraisal of her personal long-term goals concerning the operation. There must be opportunity for her to develop and ask relevant questions and to obtain appropriate answers before a final decision is implemented.

Empathy, understanding, patience, and kindness on the part of the surgeon are part of a friendly and effective doctor-patient relationship. If emotional maturity is lacking, a surgical plan to implement the goals should be postponed and the patient referred for psychologic and social counseling. Treatment usually should not be started until these qualities have been assured, attained or developed.

There are many effective treatment options from which to choose depending upon many variable factors. These include:

1. the perceived wishes and plans of the patient;
2. the motivation of the patient and her degree of emotional maturity;
3. an accurate estimate of the patient's ability to participate effectively in the necessary follow-up program;

4. the familiarity and experience of her surgeon with each of the surgical treatment techniques;
5. the support of the patient's family.

At times, various combinations of treatment may be advised for a particular patient depending upon her various specific needs.

## CHOICE OF PROCEDURE FOR CONSTRUCTION OF THE NEOVAGINA

There are at least 11 different surgical procedures currently in use to create a neovagina and fulfill a variety of clinical indications and circumstances. There are specific indications for each, and the responsible gynecologic surgeon owes it to the patient to be familiar with a number of these techniques in order to choose one that will be likely to be of greatest benefit to a specific patient.

For some persons, a full-length neovagina will be required; for others, a supplemental or additional length is needed. Occasionally, partial or complete vaginectomy followed by creation of a neovagina is indicated, i.e., total vaginal stenosis, or after extirpation for malignant disease (5, 15).

When the possible need for construction of a neovagina has been determined, it is time to introduce the patient and her companion or family to the mechanics of surgery and postoperative care for the various solutions, with a thoughtful and detailed discussion of the techniques of aftercare and probable length of time involved. Some various options of interest to a particular patient may be described, a broad range of questions solicited to which practical answers are provided, and the patient's views concerning herself, her problem, and her attitude toward a particular treatment strategy should be determined, as best as she can predict. This broad-ranged discussion should be realistic in its appraisal and assurances, empathetic, and unhurried. It will likely involve more than one discussion. Meanwhile, a necessary work-up, if not already accomplished, is undertaken consisting of a thorough physical examination including appraisal of secondary sex characteristics and any possible endocrinopathy, rectal-abdominal examination and deep abdominal palpation, karyotyping, and evaluation of any pelvic masses. Ultrasound or intravenous pyelography is required to locate conclusively the number, size, and placement of the patient's kidneys, and to determine the possibility of a pelvic kidney or of a hematometria. The patient's understanding of the problem and its solution should lead to objective interpretation of its personal and psychosocial significance as might be applied to her own social environment or plans for personal sexual intimacy. Her willingness and determination to become involved in a realistic sequence of postoperative planning must be confirmed.

The surgeon must evaluate the patient's motivation and psychologic maturity as would relate to her aftercare and follow-through. The surgeon must describe to the patient how this might differ with each of the treatment options offered.

It is now commonly agreed that timing of reconstructive surgery because of congenital absence of the vagina, previously assigned to the premarital state, now be offered at the time of endocrine maturity irrespective of the current social status. It presumes that the patient has the maturity to comprehend the social, economic, convalescent, and psychologic dimensions consequent to *her* decision concerning treatment.

Whatever method is selected, it is helpful for the gynecologist to maintain a list of previous surgical successes of patients who might be willing to discuss with the new patient their experience concerning neovaginal reconstruction.

A choice of procedure can be made from among the following current operations. Under various circumstances, a combination of two or more may be of advantage to a particular patient.

When a strongly motivated patient with a recognized perineal indentation or shortened vagina is anxious to pursue a nonsurgical development of a neovagina, the Frank pressure-by-obturator method can be remarkably effective (9). The simplest of the surgical approaches is the William's vulvovaginoplasty (22). This creates a pouch-like vagina by sewing together vulvar skin incisions overlying the labia majora.

In Western Europe and Asia, the Vecchietti (20) transabdominal procedure is sometimes used. The elasticity of the pseudohymenal tissues are stretched to create a neovagina using traction from *above*. A retroperitoneal loop of suture is introduced from the abdomen to the vulva, where it is threaded through a 2 cm plastic olive. The abdominal ends of the suture are attached to adjustable tension springs in a metal frame that lies on the patient's abdomen and make constant traction to the perineal olive. It stretches the elastic skin with which it migrates upward over a period of several days, creating a vaginal cavity of the desired depth. This seems to create effectively a vagina of sexually usable depth in a period of about 7 or 8 hospital-based days, but persistent frequent sexual activity or wearing of an obturator is required to maintain vaginal depth and patency.

Of the transperineal surgical procedures that may be considered, that of Wharton (21) is probably the least complicated. The cavity of a neovagina is created by surgical dissection, bleeding is carefully controlled, and an obturator is inserted to be worn most of the time until the cavity has been thoroughly epithelialized, which requires a space of several months, and postoperative use of an obturator for a long time is essential to maintain adequate width. The inconvenience of a chronic bloody discharge during most of this period of time is a disadvantage and inconvenience, and there may be more abundant scar tissue formation around the neovagina as time goes on tending toward vaginal stricture if it is not kept open by an obturator.

For many years, this has been often replaced by the Abbe-McIndoe operation (1, 12, 19) in which the cavity described above has been lined by a split-thickness skin graft. This requires postoperative attention to the donor site, as well as the wearing of an obturator for many months, taking it out only for a bowel movement or to empty the bladder, and wearing it nightly during sleep for and additional 6 to 12 months, the frequency depending upon the stability of the vaginal size.

Much the same effect appears to be achieved by lining the cavity with human amnion (18), usually obtained from a cesarean section delivery, and amnion, mesenchymal side out, is placed around the intravaginal obturator and left in place for 5 postoperative days, at which time the obturator is removed. It is covered with a new layer of amnion, and reinserted. After 5 more days, the obturator is taken out only for voiding and passage of stool, and replaced for most of the time. Granulation tissue is minimal, as there are areas effectively covered by amnion, and epithelialization gradually develops beneath the amniotic membrane. Failure to wear the obturator long enough can result in a rapid contraction of the neovagina during this healing phase.

In years past, a loop of small intestine has been used to line a newly created neovagina, the Baldwin procedure, but the amount of mucous discharge has been so great as to be uncomfortable and inconvenient for the majority of patients and the method is no longer used.

In the Schubert operation, the rectum was transplanted to the site of the neovagina, and the large intestine brought down to form a new rectum. Better results have been obtained by the Ober-Meinrenken operation (10, 13, 14) in which a loop of sigmoid colon is mobilized by a transabdominal approach, and brought down to line a fresh neovaginal cavity that has been made to open into the peritoneal cavity. A major advantage of this procedure is that it does not appear to require postoperative stretching and wearing of an obturator as is necessary with the McIndoe operation, but the procedure has an obvious disadvantage in that it requires assumption of the operative risks and convalescence coincident with a large bowel resection and anastomosis. It is particularly helpful when the surgeon wishes to replace the upper vagina that had been removed by cancer surgery or after radiation therapy. It provides a supplement to the vaginal size.

It is possible to line the vagina with a transplant of skin made by bivalving pedicles from the labia minora and inner surfaces of the thigh-modifications of the Graves operation (see Chapter 20). This does provide some sensory coital perception within the neovagina (17). It is important that these pedicles be held in place by a suitable obturator and that the length of the pedicle be no greater than three times the width, lest the vascular supply of the pedicle be disturbed.

In some centers, a combined abdominal-perineal approach is employed in which the undersurface of a cylinder of peritoneum is dissected from within the pelvis, brought down into a fresh neo-vagina and attached to the vulvovaginal skin by a circumferential placement of sutures (4). The "vaginal vault" of peritoneum is closed by a transabdominally placed purse-string stitch, and over a period of months, epithelialization develops beneath the peritoneum.

It is thus clear that in various parts of the world surgical community a number of operative approaches to the construction of the neovagina are currently being performed. There are advantages and disadvantages to each, and the selection of an appropriate procedure must take into account the patient's willingness to participate in the necessary postoperative follow-up program, the depth of her maturity, and of her perception of herself. The timing of the operation seems best when the patient can afford adequate postoperative convalescence and develop obturator use experience, in the majority of techniques. Therefore, the most popular time for surgery with the school-aged girl is early in the spring or summer vacation.

## NONSURGICAL TREATMENT

If the patient has a dimple at the site of the absent vagina, about one-third of them can use the Frank dilator method. It takes about 9 months of daily dedicated and concentrated use to achieve a satisfactory vagina.

This re-establishment of vaginal depth and width by a program of continued pressure using progressively longer and wider firm obturators has been advocated by Frank (9) and, more recently, by Ingram (11) for the cooperative patient. Success requires daily applications of significant pressure by the obturator to the site of vaginal obstruction. It requires significant perineal pressure totalling about 2 hours per day using graduated sized dilators (first, to achieve depth, then width). The patient should be seen for examination, reassurance, and reinforcement at the relatively frequent intervals of from 2 to 4 weeks between visits, and the size of the obturator exchanged for the next larger size as vaginal deepening develops. If she should decide later that she is unwilling to continue this approach, an alternate surgical plan can be offered at any time. Given an enthusiastic patient and therapist, successful results may be achieved over a period of 6 to 9 months. Ingram (11) has developed a unique program in which obturator pressure to the site of the neovagina is maintained for a total of 2 hours each day by the act of sitting on a specially designed bicycle seat (Fig. 21.1) freeing the patient's hands. The obturator length is

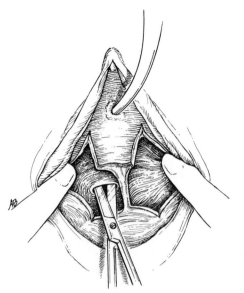

**Figure 21.6.** Lateral tunnels are made by both sharp and blunt dissection between the urethra-bladder and rectum.

(21) procedure. Epithelialization of the neovagina occurs from the edges of both isograft and vaginal orifice. The technique is illustrated in Figure 21.10. At the conclusion of the operation a vaginal form made of a condom tightly packed with foam fubber is inserted into the neovagina, the labia majora loosely stitched together, a transurethral or suprapubic catheter placed in the bladder, and the patient given a nonresidue diet. The mold is removed on the 14th day and the patient given a solid obturator to be lubricated with estrogen cream and worn most of the time with pressure to the point of discomfort for 3 months, at which time coitus may be initiated. Once fully epithelialized, this neovagina is not as vulnerable to postoperative contraction as is that lined by a split-thickness skin graft, though its size should be tested frequently by the use of

**Figure 21.7.** A midline "raphe" is developed.

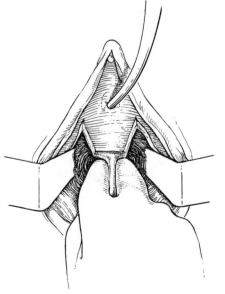

**Figure 21.8.**    The raphe is cut, completing the separation between bladder and rectum.

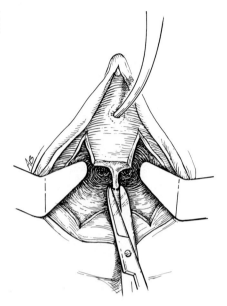

the solid obturator, the use of which may be reintroduced from time to time as necessary.

A massively scarred and nonfunctional vagina may be removed by vaginectomy (Fig. 21.11) and replaced by a neovagina using a full-thickness skin graft (2, 5, 15). Indigo-carmine solution is instilled into the bladder through a Foley catheter and dissection proceeds. A protective finger is inserted into the rectum. Tunnels are established by sharp dissection along the sides of the vagina and these are connected by sharp dissection beneath the anterior and posterior walls of the vagina, removing the full-thickness of the vaginal wall and the surrounding scar tissue.

Human amnion, usually freshly obtained from someone's cesarean section, may be used to line the freshly developed neovaginal canal instead of a split-thickness skin graft (7, 18). It is bacteriostatic and is placed over the obturator smooth side in and inserted into the neovagina. The obturator is removed in 5 or 6 days, recovered with fresh amnion, and reinserted for an additional week. A firm obturator is inserted and vulvar squamous epithelium will gradually grow in beneath the adherent amnion. The smooth surface of the

**Figure 21.9.**    The tunnel of the neovagina is shown in sagittal section, the operator's fingers demonstrating its depth and axis. An obturator covered by split-thickness skin can now be inserted.

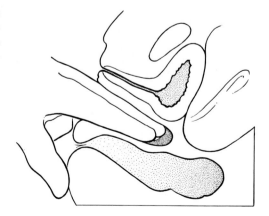

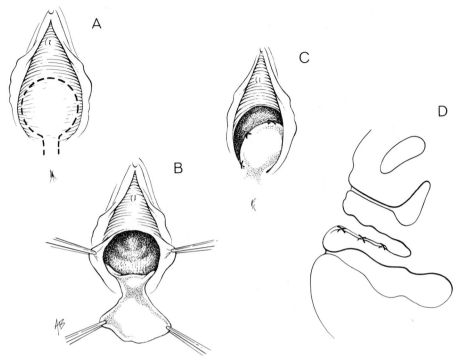

**Figure 21.10.** A racquet-shaped full-thickness incision is made inside the labia minora as shown (A). The skin flap is dissected from the underlying tissues, preserving its attachment at the base of the "handle" (B). The flap is displaced posteriorly and the tunnels for the neovagina are created by both blunt and sharp lateral dissection. They are united by incision of the raphe between them, separating the bladder from the rectum. The flap isograft is unfolded into the new tunnel so as to cover its lower and posterior surface and fixed in place, underside down by some interrupted sutures (C). This is shown in sagittal section (D). An obturator or form is inserted and held in place by suture together of the labia majora.

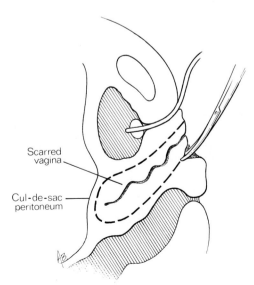

**Figure 21.11.** A massively scarred vagina is shown in sagittal section. A Foley catheter is in the bladder. The entire vagina is excised by sharp dissection along the plane indicated by the *broken line* (1), starting laterally, then posteriorly, and finally anteriorly, beneath the urethra and bladder. An obturator, suitably covered with a split-thickness skin graft, will be placed in the tunnel.

Scarred vagina

Cul-de-sac peritoneum

neovagina 1 month postoperatively is deceptively smooth and shiny. It must be remembered that this covering is essentially a temporary mesenchyme, and is not as yet mature squamous epithelium. Therefore, it retains a great capacity for accelerated shrinkage, and the patient must use the obturator, dilator, or stent adequately postoperatively. In most instances, this will require wearing it constantly for 12 months, removing it only to void or for a bowel movement, until the neo-vagina is well-covered by mature squamous epithelium and subepithelial cicatrization has been stabilized.

There is a place for the Ober-Meinrenken operation (13) (sometimes popularly called the "Schubert-Schmidt" operation) using a loop of transplanted colon for the neovagina of the patient whose vagina is shortened after a cancer operation such as exenteration, in which circumstance it may be added as part of the original exenterative procedure. It is also of value in the patient neither psychologically nor socially able or likely to use dilators of the neovagina regularly in the postoperative period and who is not sexually active (10, 13, 14).

## COMPLICATIONS OF THE NEOVAGINA

Eversion of the vault or stricture of the neovagina are uncommonly seen, but must be addressed promptly if the vagina is to be salvaged. Eversion may be a consequence of the natural absence of strong natural tissues supporting the vault of the neovagina. This weakness is made greater if the underside of too much peritoneal cul-de-sac is exposed during creation of the tunnel.

In making the Abbe-McIndoe cavity, the tip of the cavity should come to a point as it nears the abdominal peritoneum to lessen the chance of postoperative enterocele and eversion of the neovagina. If a wide area of cul-de-sac peritoneum is exposed through the neovagina, the risk of postoperative eversion of the neovagina with enterocele is considerable, which then might require a separate future secondary operation for support. An everted vault must be supported surgically by reoperation.

In the patient with eversion of a neovagina, the surgeon should carefully evaluate the patient for the presence of a pelvic kidney, as this will determine whether or not there is operative room for a transabdominal sacral colpopexy. When room is lacking a transvaginal surgical remedy can be offered. For the transvaginal surgical colpopexy the neovagina may be sewn to the sacrospinous ligament or to the "white line" (arcus tendineus) just anterior to the site of the ischial spine.

Stricture of a neovagina develops after infection and scarring and when the patient has been remiss in wearing the postoperative mold during the required time. It may develop literally overnight. In the instance of a postoperative shrinking neovagina, which is too uncomfortable to permit progressive stretching as by an obturator, the condition may be remedied surgically by lateral incisions in the three- and nine-o'clock position that meet at the top of the vagina and extend across the vault. This is followed by the wearing of an obturator postoperatively until epithelialization and healing have taken place, and until the patient becomes sexually active. During the healing interval, the patient must wear an obturator as instructed.

### References

1. Abbe R: New method of creating a vagina in a case of congenital absence. *Med Rec* 54:836–838, 1898.
2. Berek JS, Hacker NF, Lagasse LD, et al: Delayed vaginal reconstruction in the fibrotic pelvis following radiation or previous reconstruction. *Obstet Gynecol* 61:743–748, 1983.
3. Counseller VS, Davis CE: Atresia of the vagina. *Obstet Gynecol* 32:538, 1968.
4. Davydov SN: Modifizierte Kolpopoese aus Peritoneum der Excauatio Rectouterina.

*Obstet Gynecol* 12:55, 1969. Quoted in Käser O, Iklé FA, Hirsch HA: *Atlas der Gynäkologischen Operationen*, 4 Auflage, Stuttgart, Georg Thieme Verlag, 1983.

5. DiSaia PJ, Rettenmaier MA: Vaginectomy. In Sanz LE (ed): *Gynecologic Surgery*. Oradell, NJ, Med Economics Co Inc, pp 151–157, 1988.

6. Evans TN, Poland ML, Boving RL: Vaginal malformations. *Am J Obstet Gynecol* 141:910, 1981.

7. Feroze RM, Dewhurst CJ, Welply G: Vaginoplasty at the Chelsea Hospital for Women: A comparison of two techniques. *Br J Obstet Gynaecol* 82:536, 1975.

8. Fleigner JR: Congenital atresia of the vagina. *Surg Gynecol Obstet* 165:387–391, 1987.

9. Frank RT: The formation of an artifical vagina without operation. *Am J Obstet Gynecol* 35:1053, 1938.

10. Goligher JC: The use of pedicled transplants of sigmoid or other parts of the intestinal tract for vaginal construction. *Ann Roy Coll Surg Engl* 65:353–355, 1983.

11. Ingram JM: The bicycle seat in the treatment of vaginal agenesis and stenosis: A preliminary report. *Am J Obstet Gynecol* 1:867, 1981.

12. McIndoe AH, Banister JB: An operation for the cure of congenital absence of the vagina. *J Obstet Gynaecol Br Commonw* 45:490, 1938.

13. Ober KG, Meinrenken GH: Allgemeine und spezielle chirurgische operationslehre. In Kirschner M: *Gynäkologische Operationen*. Berlin, Springer 1964. Quoted in

Käser O, Iklé FA, Hirsch HA: *Atlas of Gynecological Surgery,* ed 2, New York, Georg Thieme Verlag, 1985.

14. Pratt JH: Use of the colon in gynecologic surgery. In Sturgis SH, Taymor ML (eds): *Meigs and Sturgis, Progress in Gynecology,* Vol. V, New York, Grune & Stratton, pp 435–446, 1970.

15. Rettenmaier MA, DiSaia P: Understanding current vaginectomy techniques. *Contemp Obstet Gynecol* 30:109–117, 1987.

16. Sheares BH: Congenital atresia of the vagina-a new technique for tunnelling the space between the bladder and rectum and construction of a new vagina by a modified Wharton technique. *J Obstet Gynecol Br Emp* 67:24–31, 1960.

17. Song R, Wang X, Zhou G: Reconstruction of the vagina with sensory function. *Clin Plast Surg* 9:105–108, 1982.

18. Tancer ML, Katz M, Veridiano NP: Vaginal epithelialization with human amnion. *Obstet Gynecol* 54:345–349, 1979.

19. Thompson JD, Wharton LR, TeLinde RW: Congenital absence of the vagina. *Am J Obstet Gynecol* 74:397, 1957.

20. Vecchietti G: Le neo-vagin dams le syndrome de Rokitansky-Kuster-Hauser. *Rev Med Suisse Romande* 99:593–601, 1979.

21. Wharton LR: A simplified method of constructing a vagina. *Ann Surg* 107:842–847, 1938.

22. Williams EA: Congenital absence of the vagina: A simple operation for its relief. *J Obstet Gynaecol Br Commonw* 71:511, 1964.

# CHAPTER 22

# Complications and Sequelae of Vaginal Surgery

## PREOPERATIVE DIAGNOSIS AND PREVENTION

Every surgeon must recognize the obligation to acknowledge personal weaknesses and to review them from time to time so as to improve continually and to prevent less than satisfactory results. The surgeon should review the patient's hospital record immediately before surgery to refresh one's memory of significant points in the patient's history and preoperative laboratory findings and the recommendations of consultants. This review should include the findings of medical students, house officers, fellows, and referring physicians. When specific changes in the usual preoperative preparation of the patient are indicated, it is important to be sure they have been performed.

The surgeon's thinking should also have been organized in regard to the whole spectrum of postoperative complications. Such contemplation will not only provide better preparation for the management of such complications as they may occur occasionally in the management of his or her own patients, but the busy surgeon also will be called upon increasingly for advice, or to assume the management of complications developed from the patients of fellow practitioners.

Complications can be grouped conveniently into three general categories: intraoperative, early, and late postoperative complications.

## INTRAOPERATIVE COMPLICATIONS

Aside from the immediate problems associated with the administration of anesthesia, complications that occur during surgery are principally related to hemorrhage or accidental injury of adjacent organs or tissues.

In the evaluation and control of hemorrhage it is important to differentiate first between venous and arterial bleeding. Venous bleeding can be usually controlled by extrinsic pressure, whereas arterial bleeding requires prompt and accurate ligation or electrocoagulation. It is essential to be familiar with the details of circulatory anatomy of the region, including the collaterals. When ligation at the point of bleeding is not possible, ligation should be performed at a site proximal to the site of bleeding. The anesthesiologist should be notified regarding the possible need for transfusion when blood loss becomes excessive. Because blood loss tends to be directly proportional to the duration of the operative procedure, time-saving surgical efficiency is obviously important. The occurrence of postoperative infection is also directly proportional to the length of the operative procedure, tending to increase when the duration of surgery exceeds 2 hours. Accidental trauma also includes undesirable laceration, avulsion, or unwanted incision of nearby pelvic organs, and it is essential that any suspected injury be evaluated and treated promptly. A problem that is neglected intraoperatively eventually may require one or more secondary surgical procedures, which can be as damaging to the surgeon's reputation as they may be to the patient's health. There is no room for procrastination while hoping that suspected damage did not occur, or that by ignoring the possibility, the problem will go away.

All sites of possible trauma should be considered preoperatively. It is useful to maintain a file of literature references on the management of obscure and uncommon complications, such as trauma, avulsion, incision, or transection of the ureter (16), bladder, small intestine, large intestine, and rectum, as well as the pelvic musculature.

Laceration or incision into a pelvic viscus should be repaired as soon as it is recognized. The tissues must be adequately mobilized and the repair accomplished under direct vision. The remainder of the operation should proceed as planned. To manage such problems effectively requires candor, scientific objectivity, and confident surgical technique.

For the repair of visceral injury we favor two or three layers of fine absorbable suture (3-0 polydiaxanone, polygluconate, polyglycolic-acid type, or chromic). An important principle when a mucosal stitch is required is to place the knots within the lumen of intestine or rectum where they may fall away readily when the required support has been developed through healing. In the repair of injuries to the bladder or ureter, knots should be extralumenal in order to lessen the chance of calculus formation at the site of the suture (Fig. 22.1). The major contribution to support must come as a result of accurate approximation of the submucosal muscular layers. Although mucosal sutures are hemostatic, they supply minimal support. A layer of watertight running horizontal mattress sutures in the muscular layer inverts the previous stitches, and another layer of interrupted reinforcing mattress stitches may be added, if desired, to lessen the tension on the deeper layer. Care must always be taken to avoid tying mattress sutures so tightly as to strangulate the tissues involved. The manner of suture placement is identified in Figures 22.2 and 22.3. If the

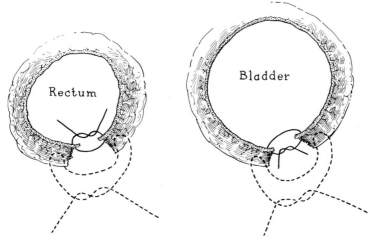

**Figure 21.1.** Suture placement for a traumatic laceration of a viscus is shown. The knot of a mucosal stitch is tied within the lumen of the rectum, as shown to the *left,* but outside the lumen of the bladder, as shown on the *right.* The muscularis is approximated by one or more layers of inverting mattress sutures, as shown by the *dotted lines.*

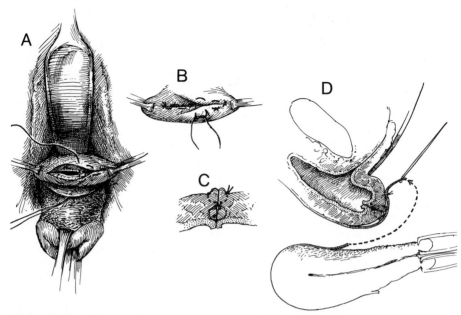

**Figure 22.2.** Closure of accidental cystotomy is depicted. The defect has been identified and widely mobilized. A suture tagging the peritoneum is noted on the left side of *A* and on the right side of *D*. If no mucosal stitch is used, a running mattress suture in the muscularis, starting and finishing lateral to the defect, may be placed as shown in *A*. This may be covered by a second layer of interrupted mattress sutures *(B)*, establishing full-thickness reapproximation of the muscularis as seen in cross-section *(C)*. An anterior peritoneal flap is excised from the anterior surface of the uterus as shown *(D)* and tacked in place over the operative repair, providing the security of an additional fresh tissue layer.

ureteral orifices are near or part of the laceration, ureteral catheters should be inserted. Ureteroneocystostomy should be performed if ureteral integrity cannot be assured. In the case of traumatic penetration of the wall of bladder near its attachment to the cervix, the adjacent peritoneum can be mobilized and sewn over the site of the repair after the defect in the musculature has been repaired (8), to provide support and added blood supply (Figs. 22.2*D* and 22.3). If there is a question of penetration of the mucosa or wall of the rectum, the operator's finger should be inserted immediately in the rectum for confirmation. Any demonstrable defect should then be repaired. A finger in the rectum is often quite helpful as a guide.

When there is a recognizable escape of a urine-like fluid into the vagina during the course of surgery, the possibility of bladder injury should be suspected. It is for this reason that it is desirable to have some urine in the bladder during surgery. We request patients who will undergo vaginal surgery to void shortly before coming to the operating suite and then to be catheterized at the beginning of surgery only if bladder distention is evident on bimanual examination. After repair of a recognized penetration in the wall of the bladder, watertightness may be tested by the instillation of a methylene blue, indigo carmine solution, or sterile milk (evaporated milk, sterile condensed canned milk, or sterile infant formula milk from the nursery). Sterile milk has the obvious advantage over dyes, in that prolonged staining of adjacent tissues does not occur if leakage is demonstrated. After additional reinforcing sutures have been placed, the repair should again be tested for leakage. If the ureter is

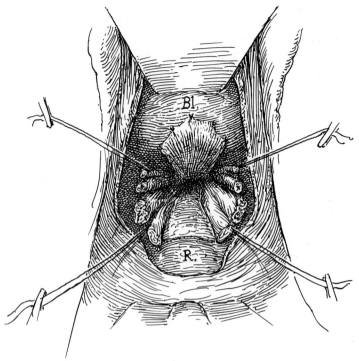

**Figure 22.3.** Frontal view of the tongue of anterior peritoneum covering the site of cystotomy repair. Vaginal hysterectomy has been completed, and the peritoneal cavity will now be closed in the usual fashion. The positions of the bladder *(B1)* and rectum *(R)* are noted.

transected, as may occur quite inadvertently when the patient has an undiagnosed duplication of the ureter on one or both sides, the severed ureter can be successfully reimplanted under direct vision. Two weeks of postoperative splinting by both ureteral and urethral catheters is desirable.

When grossly bloody urine is found postoperatively, and no injury of the bladder wall has been recognized, the bladder should be decompressed by catheter drainage. Generally speaking, in the absence of significant damage to the bladder wall, hematuria should clear grossly within 48 hours, and microscopically within 72 hours. If it is not clear after 72 hours, the patient should be examined cystoscopically to evaluate and treat the possibility of bladder trauma, such as an unexpected stitch through the bladder wall. The most likely cause is trauma from suture penetration. Even after unrepaired cystotomy, an empty bladder has a remarkable capacity to heal itself. In those instances where adequate surgical exposure is not feasible, 2 weeks of continuous catheter drainage will usually permit a fresh wound to heal spontaneously. But if the traumatized bladder is permitted to distend, a pinpoint opening may fail to close or may even enlarge and, when epithelialized, is likely to give rise to a fistula.

After repair of a laceration of the rectum, 3 days of clear liquid postoperative diet followed by a low-residue diet may be desirable during the first postoperative week, with a rectal tube gently inserted if gas pains or distention develop. A stool softener and gentle laxative should be taken for several weeks postoperatively. In all instances, the patient should be informed of the unexpected trauma and its repair so that she understands the important details of her operation and the need for special postoperative care, perhaps making her convalescence different from others thought by the patient to have had "the same operation."

Uncontrolled genital hemorrhage can be treated by tamponade and packing and, in rare circumstances, by the umbrella pack (2) may be lifesaving (Figs. 22.4 to 22.6). The ring and clamp are removed in 12 hours. The surface veil of the pack may be left in place for several days, although gradual removal of its interior packing is usually desirable beginning 24 hours after insertion of the pack. Often the removal of remaining packing or "veil" by traction after several days can be accomplished best by employing a twisting motion.

## EARLY POSTOPERATIVE COMPLICATIONS

A gentle bimanual examination is necessary at the completion of every vaginal operation, not only to detect swelling or hematoma but also to determine if the reconstruction has been successful. If there is an undesirable ridge in the posterior vaginal wall it should be corrected immediately, even if it is necessary to reopen the posterior vaginal incision. Such a ridge is likely to be a source of future discomfort or dyspareunia and is likely to become more fibrotic and more tender as time goes on. Similarly, any undesirable vaginal stricture or stenosis should be approached aggressively and immediately. These complications result either from the excision of too much vaginal

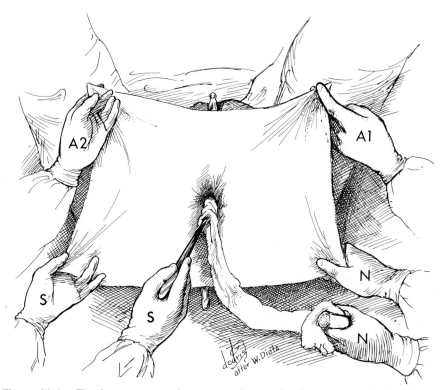

**Figure 22.4.** The four corners of a gauze veil or umbrella are supported as shown. A hand of the assistants *(A1, A2)* is shown. There is an anterior intraperitoneal retractor in place behind the veil. The nurse *(N)* feeds the gauze packing to the forceps of the surgeon *(S)*, who pushes the packing, now covered by the veil, well within the peritoneal cavity taking the central portion of the veil along with it.

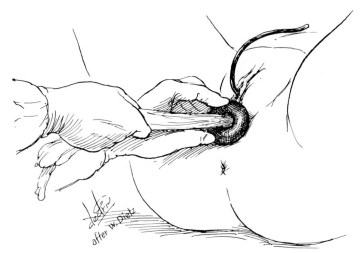

**Figure 22.5.** When the pelvis has been thoroughly packed, the four corners of the veil are led through the center of a rubber ring or doughnut pessary, and traction is applied which will compress the packing against the source of the bleeding. (After Werner P, Sederl J: *Abdominal Operations by the Vaginal Route.* Philadelphia, JB Lippincott, 1958)

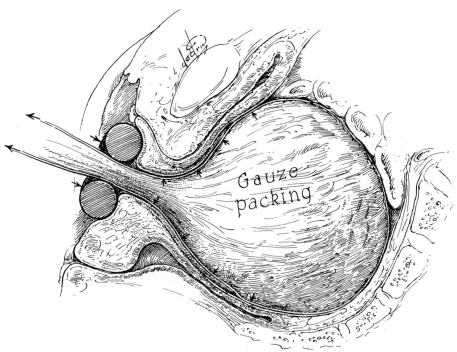

**Figure 22.6.** Sagittal view showing the effect of compression by the intra-abdominal gauze packing. *Small arrows* denote the areas to which pressure is applied.

membrane at the time of surgery or excessive plication of slack in the subepithelial fibromuscular connective tissues. Since the anterior and posterior walls of the vagina have received the principal attention during repair, they are also the most vulnerable for future or subsequent trauma.

Correction of individual stenosis should be carried out with relaxing incisions in the lateral walls of the vagina on one or both sides as described in Chapter 20. The vaginal wall may be undermined for a distance of 1 cm along the margins of each incision to enhance the relaxation. The epithelium need not be closed, but it is desirable to place a secure intravaginal pack that should be left in place for 2 days; then followed by the regular insertion of a vaginal obturator until healing is satisfactory.

If the defect created in the lateral walls of the vagina by relaxing incisions appears excessive, a full-thickness graft using a portion of the patient's own vaginal wall may be used to fill the defect (see Fig. 20.3). At the time of colporrhaphy, the excised pieces or strips of vaginal membrane can be wrapped in sterile sponges soaked with saline and retained on the nurse's instrument stand for possible grafting later in the procedure.

Adequate inspection should be followed by accurate hemostasis if excessive blood loss persists at the conclusion of a vaginal operation. If significant venous oozing is noted during the first 24 postoperative hours, a gauze packing of the vagina should be inserted. It will act not only as a wick in soaking up blood or serum that would otherwise accumulate and will also gently tamponade the operative site and compress the connective tissue spaces. When appreciable bleeding occurs through a pack, however, it usually indicates unsecured hemostasis of some significance, which should be investigated by examination of the patient in the lithotomy position with good lighting and suitable relaxation. When the bleeding point is found, it should be promptly ligated.

When a vaginal pack is in place, the patient will usually experience difficulty in voiding and will need an indwelling Foley catheter. In the absence of bladder trauma or surgical repair, the catheter should be removed at the same time as the intravaginal packing. Bathroom privileges may be permitted then, but daily palpation of the lower abdomen and careful recording of the patient's voiding pattern should be continued during the early postoperative period.

As a last step after conclusion of a vaginal operation, a gentle rectal examination should be performed before the patient is fully awake and before she has left the operating table, so that any unsuspected damage may be identified and repaired. Careful search should be made for any stitches that might have penetrated the rectal mucosa. A penetrating stitch should be exposed with adequate retraction and cut on the lumenal side so that the loose ends will retract into the wall of the rectum. Postoperative difficulty is then unlikely.

Finally, an accurate description of the surgical procedure should be dictated promptly before the details that may later assume considerable importance become less clear or are simply forgotten.

## Postoperative Ileus

Significant intestinal paralysis is less common after vaginal surgery than abdominal surgery. Patients usually resume an adequate fluid intake and regular diet soon after postoperative nausea subsides following pelvic repairs. Moving about, both in and out of bed, is good prophylaxis; and although the patient is usually not hungry, frequent sips of tap water and occasional small amounts of solid food will usually initiate peristalsis. If postoperative distention and ileus develop, additional days will be required for a return to normal. Intravenous feedings should be continued so long as the abdomen is tympanitic, distended, and relatively silent to auscultation. Peristalsis will eventually return coincident with the expulsion of flatus. If gastric dilation with nausea and vomiting develops, nasogastric decompression should be instituted with appropriate increase in intravenous fluids.

## Intestinal Obstruction

Obstruction of small bowel is usually due to pathologic fixation and kinking of a loop of small intestine, occasionally from a misplaced stitch, but more often the result of attachment to a devitalized tissue surface. It can also be produced by kinking from traction to an unfreed adhesion of bowel to adnexa. Obstruction is more common when there are extensive intraperitoneal manipulations or when the patient has sustained adhesions from previous intra-abdominal surgery.

Postoperative obstruction is usually partial at first, and the patient may complain only of anorexia and intermittent colicky pain. Patients who have had previous surgery should be watched with more concern during the first postoperative week, even after resumption of normal peristalsis and bowel function. Tachycardia may occur with only a mild temperature elevation, but peristalsis is usually hyperactive. A flat plate of the abdomen is desirable at this point, and intravenous feeding and intestinal decompression should be considered. Obviously, partial obstruction, when aggravated by postoperative edema, will respond to conservative management, and there will be a gradual return to normal bowel function. When such improvement is to occur it will become evident within 2 or 3 days in the majority of cases. When spontaneous improvement is not apparent, however, the condition of the patient soon changes with the appearance of projectile vomiting, more frequent and severe crampy abdominal pain, and waves of audible hyperperistalsis coincident with the height of the crampy pain. The patient appears acutely ill, becomes mildly shocky, and develops severe electrolyte disturbances. X-ray studies are now diagnostic, and laparotomy with surgical relief must be undertaken as soon as intravenous feeding and gastric decompression have improved electrolyte imbalance and dehydration. Clinical deterioration can occur in hours. Each postoperative patient should be observed by her own physician daily during her hospital stay, and more often when necessary. A 1- or 2-day delay in the diagnosis and treatment of complete intestinal obstruction may result in postoperative mortality.

At laparotomy, the site of the obstruction is usually readily apparent and blunt dissection by simple finger separation of the bowel from the point to which it has become adherent can be accomplished. The involved loop of bowel should be carefully inspected to ensure its viability and should be observed over a period of several minutes to be certain that both color and peristalsis return. If they do not, resection of the loop may be necessary. If the obstruction cannot be found with ease, a running inspection of the intestines should be performed, beginning with the distal segment of collapsed bowel. If the operative field is obscured by excessive balloon-like intestinal dilation, this may need to be decompressed by insertion of a large-bore hypodermic needle to which suction tubing has been attached. After decompression, the needle is removed, and the point of penetration is closed with a purse-string suture of fine chromic catgut or polyglycolic suture on an atraumatic or intestinal needle (6). When the patient's condition appears critical and will not permit the time necessary for adequate exploration and possible resection, an enterostomy proximal to the point of obstruction may be indicated and should be accomplished without extensive handling of the multiple loops of distended bowel.

## Postoperative Infections

Postoperative fever most often originates from problem areas called the "five W's": Wind (pulmonary), Water (urinary), Wound (abscess), Walk (phlebitis), and Wonder drugs (drug reactions). As has been noted in the review of postoperative complications by Cruse (3), major temperature elevation during the first 48 hours is usually the result of atelectasis, especially if the patient is a heavy smoker. Prompt physiotherapy emphasizing incentive spirometry and prolonged inspiration is the backbone of early treatment. Onset of fever during the 3rd postoperative day is usually from urinary infection. Fever beginning between the 3rd and 5th day is likely to be due to wound infection initiated at the time of surgery. Septic thrombophlebitis may be the explanation of fever originating between the 3rd and 7th postoperative day; between the 10th and 14th day, pulmonary embolism becomes a more likely possibility.

It is especially important that an evening temperature be recorded, because an elevation at this specific time may be the earliest objective evidence than an infection is developing. Costovertebral angles should be percussed daily beginning the evening of the day of surgery and unilateral discrepancy should be investigated promptly by infusion pyelography. In the absence of other findings, unexplained ileus should elicit suspicion of unilateral ureteral ligation, and an intravenous pyelogram ordered without delay. Infection involving the urinary system is more likely in the patient with a history of urinary tract infections.

Fever persisting beyond the 1st and 2nd postoperative days will often prove to be from infection within the pelvis, often within the site of an unsuspected pelvic hematoma. Prompt and gentle daily palpation of the abdomen for tenderness or masses and gentle bimanual examination of the pelvis are indicated. Abscess formation should be expected and the majority of such abscesses will point to and drain into the vaginal vault and be evidenced by a sudden seropurulent discharge followed by almost immediate clinical improvement. Suspected abscess formation may be investigated by rectal examination and gentle digital exploration of the vault of the vagina. While the natural tendency of this development is to drain spontaneously, this course may be aided easily by gentle digital probing of the suture lines in the vagina over a period of several days. A culture and sensitivity study of any appreciable exudate is desirable.

When the abscess cavity involves or is adjacent to the pelvic peritoneum, signs of pelvic peritonitis usually involve lower abdominal distention, lower abdominal pain, anorexia, and depressed peristalsis. Although adnexal abscess is uncommon after vaginal surgery, this possibility should be suspected when a unilateral pelvic mass is present in a patient in whom ovulation had been occurring regularly. Relatively late development is almost characteristic of this complication, and it may, therefore, not become evident for days or weeks following discharge from the hospital. Ledger et al. (11) emphasized that the "diagnostic possibility of an adnexal abscess should be considered in any febrile patient readmitted after a recent pelvic operation." Such adnexal abscesses localize relatively high in the pelvis and may not be palpated but may be identified by ultrasound or computerized axial tomography (CAT) scan (10). Spontaneous drainage through the vaginal vault is unlikely and transabdominal salpingo-oophorectomy is usually required. Various studies have demonstrated an increased probability of postoperative infection and morbidity among premenopausal as compared to postmenopausal women undergoing vaginal surgery, probably related to the increased vascularity of their tissues and the increased probability of a hematoma, which becomes a focus of infection.

Greater sexual activity increases vaginal bacterial contamination. A larger variety of organisms within the vaginal flora are ready for proliferation under the conditions present after vaginal surgery during the menstrual years and infection by virulent anaerobic vaginal bacteria may result.

Infection can be minimized by careful anatomic dissection (which minimizes trauma), adequate hemostasis, and provision for drainage when indicated. Also, the short-term use of an appropriate broad-spectrum antibiotic is helpful, given an hour before surgery, and repeated if the operation is longer than of 2 hours duration. It is given to those patients in whom it is expected that the peritoneal cavity will be entered during the course of the transvaginal operation, as well as in those less common instances in which the surgery will involve relatively inaccessible although extraperitoneal connective tissue spaces, such as the pararectal, prevesical, or retrorectal spaces that have no natural path of drainage to the outside.

Anaerobic bacterioid infections are characteristically foul-smelling and result in characteristic systemic reactions. Dangers are greater when a body temperature of 103 degrees or higher develops along with a white blood count higher than 15,000 or less than 4000/cmm. Under such circumstances, any purulent exudate should be cultured for both aerobic and anaerobic organisms, and serious consideration should be given to administration of antibiotics or antibacterials with anaerobic coverage. Antibiotics that will penetrate an abscess include:

1. clindamycin;
2. cefamandol;
3. cefoxitin;
4. metronidazole.

### Septic Shock

Septic shock should be considered when a shock-like state develops postoperatively without evidence of blood loss. Peripheral vascular collapse from endotoxins will often produce subnormal temperature, hypotension, metabolic acidosis, oliguria, and mental confusion. There will be no response to transfusion. Once the peripheral circulatory collapse has been overcome by intravenous fluids, ideally monitored by central venous pressure or pulmonary wedge pressure measurements, treatment may include norepinephrine and also dopamine and large doses of an appropriate antibiotic. Search should be made for an abscess cavity. Ultrasound or CAT scan studies may be helpful (10). When found, an abscess should be cultured and excised or drained.

### Necrotizing Fascitis

Necrotizing fascitis and synergistic bacterial gangrene are rare, serious virulent and toxic infections that can develop subcutaneously at any time. The overlying skin is dark, bullae may be present, and thrombosis of nearby blood vessels may precipitate edema of the skin rendering it anesthetic. Prompt recognition is essential, and the primary treatment is adequate surgical debridement, as extensive as necessary to excise the bacterial inoculum completely. Subcutaneous fascial damage is extensive, but muscle may be spared, as would not be the case were crepitant gas gangrene present as associated with clostridial infection.

### Hemorrhage

Careful observation of the patient's vital signs during the first 2 postoperative days will provide evidence of intraperitoneal bleeding. It is important to monitor the patient's hemoglobin and hematocrit. A coagulation defect should be suspected when the patient shows unexpected ecchymoses or when a sample of venous blood fails to form a firm clot. If external blood loss is insignificant and bleeding seems to be persistent, the patient who is unusually restless should be prepared for laparotomy. Bleeding points should be identified and ligated, any hematoma should be evacuated, and a search should be made for the source of bleeding.

If intra-abdominal hemorrhage has stabilized at the end of the first postoperative 24 hours, and there is no evidence of further bleeding, operative intervention is seldom necessary unless infection intrudes, at which time a presumed hematoma may become infected and require drainage. Under unusual circumstances where shock due to blood loss has intervened and massive postoperative hemorrhage is evident within the bases of the cardinal ligaments, aggressive surgery may be required, including bilateral ligation of the hypogastric and ovarian arteries (14). This procedure should not be time-consuming, and the response in arresting an alarming rate of hemorrhage will be dramatic. Experience with the technique of transperitoneal bilateral hypogastric artery ligation should be part of the surgical armamentarium of every gynecologic surgeon, particularly when the technique can be readily learned by isolation of the hypogastric arteries on fresh autopsy material. Once the arteries have been identified, the relevant surgical anatomy and the position of the ureter and the vein clearly distinguished, and these structures excluded from the operative field, sutures for ligation can be properly placed around the hypogastric artery and below the origin of the superior gluteal artery. The overlying peritoneum is closed with fine absorbable suture, care being taken to avoid the nearby ureter. Such practice provides a convenient and easy way to learn or to teach this procedure to one's self or to others, and when the occasion does arise that ligation must be performed as an emergency procedure, the operator can proceed knowledgeably and efficiently with a technique based on some previous personal experience.

Externally evident hemorrhage after vaginal surgery is usually of extraperitoneal origin. When this is mild in quantity and approximates that seen with the menstrual period, firm vaginal packing will usually provide sufficient tamponade to achieve control. If this is insufficient and blood loss appears either accelerated or sustained, surgical intervention may be indicated. When this development is seen during the 1st postoperative day, the rapidity of blood loss is a reliable indication of the size of the vessel accounting for the bleeding. Suspicion that sustained intraperitoneal bleeding from an unsecured uterine or ovarian artery is accounting for blood loss indicates the need for a prompt surgical approach. Persistent transvaginal bleeding after a vaginal repair will usually arise from a small artery in the edge of a vaginal incision.

Blood loss occurring from the 6th to perhaps the 14th postoperative day is most likely the result of local infection that has hastened suture absorption or has eroded into an adjacent vascular bed. At this stage, tissues are edematous and friable, and additional sutures will not be secure. Dissection will destroy tissue planes and break up established barriers of "inflammatory membrane," thereby resulting in dissemination as well as an increase in the clinical virulence of the infection. Undiagnosed diabetes should be excluded and, if found, appropriate measures employed. Tight vaginal packing may prove effective even in the presence of infection and broad-spectrum antibiotics should be administered. Local application of the microfibrillar collagen, Avitene, may be effective. It exerts its hemostatic effect by attracting functioning blood platelets that adhere to the microfibrils, triggering the formation of thrombi in the adjacent tissue. Because it can cause fibrosis with ureteral obstruction, Avitene should not be used near the ureter. The bladder should be put at rest by an indwelling catheter. If vaginal packing is not effective and a coagulopathy has been excluded, the patient should be returned to the operating room. If transvaginal control of excessive bleeding cannot be achieved, the possibility of bilateral hypogastric artery ligation should be considered. Should this fail, massive hemorrhage may be controlled by percutaneous transcatheter embolization, using the skills of a radiologist experienced in this technique (15 ).

Hematoma formation may be intraperitoneal or extraperitoneal, but occasionally when retroperitoneal it is ominous because it affords an excellent culture medium in proximity to the vaginal or rectal flora and is likely to account for postoperative abscess formation. When a hematoma is palpable and is increasing significantly in size, it should probably be evacuated. Again, it is important to note that a coagulopathy must be excluded.

Small hematomas in the vault of the vagina or beneath a reapproximated tissue plane will generally liquify, and although they may become infected, they usually drain spontaneously through the vaginal suture line. Because these hematomas are more common in the vault of the vagina, the surgeon may wish to leave a small opening in the very center of the vault for drainage at the time of hysterectomy.

### Thrombophlebitis

Elastic stockings that have been worn preoperatively and during the operative procedure should be continued for the initial 3 or 4 postoperative days until the patient is comfortably ambulatory. Daily rounds include palpation of the patient's calves and attention to complaint of leg pain, particularly if unilateral. Superficial thrombophlebitis may be treated with elastic stocking compression of the extremity, elevation, and external heat. Phenylbutazone (Butazolidin alka) three times daily for 7 to 10 days will often add to the patient's comfort. Anticoagulation is desirable only when there is evidence of upward expansion of the thrombophlebitis despite the use of the measures already described. The importance of prophylaxis cannot be overemphasized. All patients should be instructed on the importance of frequently moving their extremities and encouraged to move about in bed freely, starting from the time of recovery from anesthesia. The patient should be encouraged to be up in a chair 2 or 3 times daily beginning on the 1st postoperative day, being told clearly that moving her legs will aid her circulation. Oversedation should be avoided.

Of ominous significance is evidence of a thrombophlebitis in pelvic veins, an uncommon development manifested by lower abdominal pain and tenderness to deep palpation without change in hematocrit and without a palpable lower pelvic mass as might be seen with a hematoma. Often accompanied by a high spiking fever and coincident tachycardia, pelvic thrombophlebitis is surprisingly resistant to antibiotic therapy, but it does respond dramatically to anticoagulation with heparin.

When there is a predisposition to thrombophlebitis as indicated by obesity or a history of thrombophlebitis, the increased likelihood of this potentially dangerous development should be anticipated postoperatively. Preliminary preoperative determination of partial thromboplastin time to identify previous unsuspected bleeding disorders will help considerably to prevent its development. If partial heparinization is desired, 5000 units of heparin are given subcutaneously three times daily *beginning the day before the operation* and continued through the first 4 or 5 postoperative days. Because increased operative and postoperative bleeding can be expected, the importance of meticulous surgical hemostasis cannot be overemphasized. Defibrotide may prove to be a safer antithrombotic than heparin (see Chapter 23).

### Treatment of Acute Inflammatory Thrombophlebitis of the Leg

When massive thrombosis occludes practically all of the veins of the leg, the entire leg becomes deeply cyanotic and extremely painful. Total heparinization should be accomplished promptly and thrombectomy should be considered.

### Treatment of Deep Vein Thrombosis

When a deep vein thrombosis of the pelvis or lower extremity has been diagnosed, total heparinization is the treatment of choice; a loading dose of 7500 to 10,000 units of aqueous heparin solution is administered intravenously, and this is followed by a continuous heparin drip providing 5000 units of heparin every 4 to 6 hours via a heparin-well such that the partial thromboplastin time (PTT) is extended from two to two and one-half times normal. A continuous heparin drip has some advantages: PTT can be obtained at any time; one need not worry about peaks and valleys in anticoagulation. This is usually continued for 6 to 7 days and discontinued after oral anticoagulant therapy has been started. Appropriate medical consulation and follow-up are needed for 3 to 6 months. If embolism occurs despite heparinization, thrombectomy or vena cava ligation should be considered.

## Atelectasis and Pneumonia

Atelectasis and pneumonia occur less frequently after vaginal surgery than after pelvic laparotomy, because the absence of an abdominal incision makes it easier for the patient to breathe deeply and to move about comfortably. This tends to reduce diaphragmatic splinting. Routine deep inspiration should be encouraged after any type of pelvic surgery, beginning the day of operation. Incentive spirometry has proven effective in providing good pulmonary aeration in contrast to intermittent positive pressure breathing devices which, unless the patient forcefully inhales, often do not provide adequate aeration and may, in fact, increase small airway obstruction. It is important to avoid oversedation, for not only does this tend to depress the respiratory center, but, by inhibition of the sensorium, the patient's voluntary efforts are usually noticeably decreased.

Atelectasis results from occlusion of a part of the bronchial tree as a result of hypoventilation, circulatory stasis, and accumulation of intrabronchial secretions that are often associated with a pre-existing acute or chronic bronchitis. Recent or concurrent upper respiratory infections are distinct contraindications to anesthesia and to elective surgery, because bronchial obstruction is followed by absorption of trapped gases with collapse of the distal segment of lung involved. The patient develops fever, tachycardia, and a noticeable increase in respiratory rate. Cyanosis and air hunger are less common unless there is a massive degree of pulmonary collapse. This complication usually occurs early in the postoperative course. Atelectasis represents one of the more common causes of fever during the first 2 or 3 postoperative days. If unresolved by good pulmonary toilet, bronchial pneumonia and consolidation develop rapidly. The chest x-ray is usually of limited value in making an early diagnosis.

There are two principal types of pneumonia: aspiration and bacterial. The former is initiated during the phase of immediate recovery from anesthesia and the latter from inadequate pulmonary ventilation in the later postoperative period, sometimes after unrecognized or untreated atelectasis. There is gradual development of pleural respiratory pain and severe nonproductive cough is present. Treatment for both must be prompt, and for the former includes clearing of the airway of aspirate, correction of hypoxia, administration of steroids such as Solu-Cortef to diminish pulmonary inflammatory reaction, and administration of prophylactic antibiotics. Bacterial pneumonia is best treated by an aminoglycocide together with clindamycin until the specific pathogen has been identified. Failure to effect adequate treatment of either of these types of pneumonia may result in lung abscess, which may or may not be obvious for several weeks. When lung abscess is diagnosed, prompt and intensive antibiotic therapy is indicated. Failure of resolution requires bronchoscopy, and rarely lobectomy.

## Pulmonary Embolism

Pulmonary embolism occurs more frequently in patients with antecedent peripheral venous disease, patients over 50 years of age, those who are obese, and in those with known cardiac or pulmonary disease. The latter include a wide spectrum and may be associated with clinically demonstrable pulmonary infarction, so that a patient displaying pneumonia, atelectasis, or pleurisy with or without effusion should be watched with particular care. Early diagnosis and aggressive treatment by adequate anticoagulation have been responsible for a noticeable reduction in the mortality rate associated with pulmonary embolism.

Dehydration of the patient with hemoconcentration affects heparin activity. Phenobarbital and chloral hydrate have been shown to antagonize anticoagulants. Oral contraceptives are strongly suspect and should, therefore, have been discontinued a month or two before elective surgery.

In summary, prophylaxis begins with preoperative recognition of those patients likely to develop difficulty. Every effort should be made to prevent the development of hypotension by maintenance of an effective circulating blood volume during surgery. Postoperatively, both active and passive motion of the lower extremities should be assured on a regular basis, combined with the use of elastic stockings until the patient is ambulatory. All are of proven prophylactic value. In addition, oversedation is to be avoided, and a positive program encouraging voluntary deep breathing exercises should begin on the 1st postoperative day.

Thrombosis is more likely when swelling of an extremity develops if calf pain and tenderness are localized to the deep venous system than if pain and tenderness are diffuse. When in doubt, x-ray venography, impedance plethysmography, or leg scanning, using human fibrinogen labeled with radioactive iodine, may be considered (8, 12).

Intermittent passive venous compression, as by the Kendall boot, can be initiated with surgery upon the patient at unusual risk. Heparin is, of course, contraindicated in patients with a history of stroke, subarachnoid hemorrhage, peptic ulcer, bleeding diathesis, and hypertension.

Prophylactic heparinization should, moreover, be considered only with great caution in the diabetic patient, because the resultant prolonged elevation of plasma-free fatty acid levels in the diabetic may induce hypercoagulability and cardiac arrythmia, with increased risk of acute myocardial infarction. A massive pulmonary embolism beyond the initial 10th postoperative day (1) may also indicate the use of a thrombolytic enzyme such as streptokinase (250,000 I.U. as a continuous infusion by syringe pump over 1/2 hour, followed by 100,000 units per hour for the remainder of the 24-hour period) as recommended by Hirsh (4), who mentions cardiac arrest or a second major embolism during treatment as an indicator for pulmonary embolectomy. Streptokinase may be contraindicated during the first 10 postoperative days, as its intense lytic activity may interfere with wound healing and initiate bleeding at the site of the operation. Vena cava ligation should be considered if showers of recurrent or of septic emboli have occurred.

Hirsh also recommends ambulation 5 or 6 days after treatment has been instituted. When the patient is pain free, she may be gradually switched to oral anticoagulants, which should be continued for some weeks. Should pulmonary embolism be seriously suspected, even though uncomfirmed, a single intravenous injection of 10,000 units of aqueous heparin may be given followed by 5000 units subcutaneously every 6 hours for 7 to 10 days or until the patient is ambulatory.

Fatal pulmonary embolism now occurs after major gynecologic surgery about once per 1500 major procedures. Prophylactic low-dose anticoagulation, while possibly reducing the risk of fatal pulmonary embolism, increases the otherwise low incidence of significant amount of postoperative bleeding. For this reason alone, anticoagulants are usually employed only if the history or the findings suggest a patient at high risk.

### Differential Diagnosis Between Pelvic Cellulitis and Pelvic Thrombophlebitis

There is little to be found on physical examination that is diagnostic of pelvic thrombophlebitis. Lower quadrant abdominal pain and soreness without cramping are usually present and are aggravated by deep palpation, but when without seemingly related activity in the overlying bowel, are suggestive of the extraperitoneal character of the problem. A sense of fullness may be perceived by the fingers of the examiner, but since some muscle guarding is also present, this is not specific and certainly not pathognomonic. The most characteristic features of the clinical picture are shaking chills accompanying a high spiking fever. A sustained tachycardia does not change even with the abrupt fall in temperature.

In pelvic cellulitis, on the other hand, the pelvic floor is noticeably ligneous and diffusely painful. Chills are usually absent and the temperature elevation is sustained. As the temperature subsides, it does so gradually, and the pulse rate decreases with it.

It is important to make a clinical distinction between infected pelvic thrombophlebitis and pelvic cellulitis, because treatment of the two conditions differs in some respects. Although blood cultures are desirable, they are not always positive and conclusive, but fortunately, broad-spectrum antibiotics are indicated in both situations. The role of anticoagulants in pelvic thrombophlebitis is debatable, and many clinicians use anticoagulants only when embolization has developed or when the patient fails to demonstrate favorable response to intensive antibiotic therapy of several days' duration.

The above distinctions apply only to rather classical thrombophlebitis, in which thrombi are infected and the danger of multiple emboli relate to the vascular dissemination of infected foci. Moreover, areas of thrombosis occurring without infection are equally life threatening and are often totally asymptomatic, until uninfected, large, soft thrombi become dislodged to form massive pulmonary emboli.

The indications for vena cava ligation are often debated, but the certainty of the immediate result keeps the desirability of this procedure from being forgotten. Several observers have noted the frequency with which embolization of massive bland phlebothrombosis occurs a week or so after pelvic surgery when an in-bed patient is having a bowel movement on a bedpan. For this reason, we favor both early ambulation and sufficiently frequent stool softeners, laxatives, or enemas during postoperative convalescence.

### Other Intra-abdominal Complications

The postoperative patient is certainly not immune to an attack of appendicitis, cholecystitis, or diverticulitis, and the characteristic symptoms should never be ignored. Indicated surgery should not be delayed.

## Evisceration

Dehiscence of the apex of the vagina with extrusion of omentum or intestine, or both, often is suggestive of inadequate reconstruction of the supports of the vault or reconstitution of the levator plate at the time of surgery, which have led to a faulty vaginal axis. The rarity of posthysterectomy vaginal evisceration must be noted. This seems independent of whether the vaginal vault is left opened or closed. Perhaps it is the length of the small bowel mesentery that when pathologically long (greater than 15 cm) permits intra-abdominal contents to exert unusual pressure on the surface of the cul-de-sac in the pelvic floor and vaginal vault. Evisceration may occur with sudden massive increases in intra-abdominal pressure, such as violent coughing or postoperative retching. Evisceration may also be seen with extreme overexertions, such as heavy lifting, in which the entire force of increased intra-abdominal pressure is directed to the long axis of the vagina.

Treatment is determined by the viability and integrity of the protruding structure. When loops of intestine protrude, there must be doubt concerning viability. At laparotomy, the loops, after cleansing, may be drawn back into the peritoneal cavity, fully inspected, and the pelvic defect repaired, paying special attention to obliteration of the cul-de-sac and any enterocele that might be present. If intestinal viability or the condition of the base of the mesentery are in question, bowel resection is indicated followed by trimming of any necrotic vaginal tissue and transabdominal closure of the vaginal vault defect during the same operative procedure. If the vaginal portion of the bowel is perforated or necrotic, the specimen may be removed by resection per vaginum and after redraping, the transabdominal anastomosis then accomplished (9, 13).

## Forgotten Foreign Bodies

Instruments are not often left behind or lost during and after vaginal surgery. It is possible, although uncommon, to leave a sponge or pack in the cul-de-sac or in a tissue plane, particularly if there has been noteworthy bleeding during the course of the procedure. A sponge saturated with blood quickly assumes the color of the surrounding tissues when packed into a line of cleavage or beneath a flap or fold of tissue, and it may easily be buried as the tissues are plicated. Periodic sponge counts should be made during the course of a procedure, especially before the peritoneum is closed and again at the conclusion of the operation while the patient is still anesthetized and draped. If a missing sponge is not found in the vagina or in the folds of drapes, an x-ray of the pelvis should be obtained while the patient is still on the operating table. If the patient is obese, it may be necessary to obtain separate films of the lower and upper abdomen. Because only sponges with radiopaque marking should be used in surgery, they will generally be seen on x-ray. Under no circumstances should a sponge be cut in half during the course of an operative procedure, lest a missing but unmarked half be invisible on postoperative x-ray. Because they are so easily lost, small pushers or swabs in the surgical field are never separated from their holding forceps. Although there are reports of foreign bodies having been found incidentally months or years after they have been left behind, the majority will make themselves known by clinical infection within a few days.

Such a patient will usually develop a septic fever, unresponsive to any antibiotic combination, and an abscess may form that will point into the vagina. Probing of this abscess may bring forth a few threads of the offending foreign body. The presence or absence of signs of local peritonitis will indicate whether the foreign body is intraperitoneal; if it is and transvaginal removal cannot be accomplished easily, abdominal laparotomy with drainage and culture of the purulent material may be indicated. When there are signs of extraperitoneal infection, gently opening into the tissue planes of the vagina near the site of the suspected abscess will be necessary. In the presence of the local infection, the sutures of a secondary closure, if any, should be spaced so as not to interfere with drainage from the infected area.

A vaginal examination shortly before discharge from a hospital will permit identification of an unsuspected hematoma, intravaginal adhesions to be broken up, or forgotten intravaginal sponges or packing to be removed. When clinically indicated, this examination is too easily forgotten or omitted. An overlooked intravaginal sponge or packing will invariably give rise to a profuse and offensive vaginal discharge and will cause considerable distress for the patient. Fortunately, there is rarely any damage done by a forgotten sponge or packing in the vagina, and the discharge subsides promptly after removal.

### Cerebral Changes

Hypertensive patients should be watched postoperatively for any signs of cerebral thrombosis which, if significant, may include paralysis and coincident discrepancy in pupillary size. More often, however, minor degrees of cerebral insufficiency may be detected only by careful interpretation of the patient's postoperative course. When the effects of postoperative sedation are superimposed, it is easy to miss a slight slurring of speech, fuzziness of thinking, or memory impairment, but those close to the patient are certain to recognize these changes in the later postoperative weeks. Insidious and unhappy acceleration of the cerebral as well as the vascular aging process may occur more often than we anticipate.

### Coronary Occlusion

Unexplained postoperative tachycardia, especially when combined with dyspnea and substernal pressure, may be indicative of coronary occlusion, especially in a patient with a history of angina or findings of arteriosclerosis. Any patient with preoperative clinical or cardiographic evidence of coronary insufficiency, with or without additional symptoms, should receive a postoperative electrocardiogram and serial enzyme determinations.

### Unexpected Malignancy

The report from the pathology laboratory should be reviewed carefully as soon as available, and preferably before the patient's discharge from the hospital. An unsuspected or more advanced stage of a recognized malignancy occasionally will be demonstrated in the surgical specimen. The patient or a responsible member of her family should be advised promptly of the significance of these findings so that appropriate additional therapy can be instituted when indicated and the advisability and nature of lifetime follow-up studies can be explained. Consultation with an oncologic team is often desirable at this time.

## LATE POSTOPERATIVE COMPLICATIONS

Although genital fistulae may become evident at almost any stage of convalescence, a very small one may not become evident until weeks or even months after surgery. Their treatment is discussed in Chapters 17, 18, and 19. Iatrogenic urinary stress incontinence may also be seen, usually as a result of an overcorrection of a cystocele when inadequate attention has been paid to urethral supports or to preservation of a good posterior urethrovesical angle. When this is socially disturbing, it may necessitate additional surgery. Eversion of the vaginal vault is sometimes seen and is considered in Chapter 16. The significance of the postoperatively shortened vagina and the technical means of avoiding this undesirable result are discussed in Chapter 10 on hysterectomy. Vaginal stricture is discussed in Chapter 20.

The atrophic effects of postoperative estrogen withdrawal some years after a satisfactory repair must be anticipated whenever a colporrhaphy is done upon a premenopausal woman. Atrophy of the vaginal membrane can be detected during a lifetime of periodic pelvic examinations, reversed, slowed, or prevented by the long-term regular instillation of supplemental estrogen cream once a week, particularly in patients who are sexually active.

### Prolapse of the Fallopian Tube

Although prolapse of the tube through the apex of the vagina is a rare complication of vaginal hysterectomy, it does result in a peritoneal fistula. Fallopian tube prolapse is generally a consequence of a hysterectomy technique in which the vault of the vagina is left open at the conclusion of the procedure and the cut ends of the tube have been sutured along a cut edge of the vaginal vault. Since, in the technique herein described, most of the vault is essentially closed in layers, the transected ends of the tubes have been securely buried beneath the wall of the vagina, well away from all vaginal edges. Peritoneal fistulae should be rare, but may be suspected from a watery discharge and by the discovery of a friable soft tissue vaginal vault excrescence that bleeds easily and that, at first, appears to be granulation tissue but fails to heal and disappear after simple cauterization or attempts to curette the suspected granulations away. When local excision fails and discharge persists, salpingectomy may be necessary for cure; otherwise, intermittent hydrorrhea may be reported and a potential route for ascending infection is perpetuated.

A useful transvaginal technique of total salpingectomy for a posthysterectomy fallopian tube prolapse (17) starts with a horizontal incision through the fullthickness of the vagina posterior to the prolapsed tube and the vaginal scar. The peritoneal cavity is incised horizontally and the peritoneal side of the prolapsed tube is inspected carefully. The tube is mobilized and another horizontal vaginal incision is made anterior to the prolapsed tube, and the entire tube and a collar of vagina between the two incisions are removed; the peritoneum and vagina closed separately.

### Colporrhaphy Following Previous Treatment for Cervical or Vaginal Carcinoma

One must be cautious in any recommendation of vaginal repair or reconstruction in patients clinically "cured" by radiation treatment of a cervical or vaginal carcinoma. Cutting through and opening into tissues containing trapped and inactive nests of clinically "dormant" but histologically recognizable cancer cells may seem to reactivate a quiescent malignant neoplasia. Such surgery has been said literally to "open the lid on the casket". Fortunately, this sequence is rather rare, and the fibrosis that follows "cancerocidal" radiation will usually produce sufficient fibrosis, scarring, and shrinkage of the vagina to have arrested the progress of an earlier degree of genital prolapse.

An unexpectedly short and/or narrowed vagina is certain to be a source of dissatisfaction to the patient and to her husband, and consequently, to her surgeon. This result is sometimes achieved deliberately and is of no consequence when it has been an objective with hysterectomy for postmenopausal prolapse when preservation of vaginal function is no longer important. But when this result proves unacceptable, for one reason or another, it must be re-evaluated. This problem is discussed in Chapter 20.

## Depression, Psychiatric and Neurologic Sequelae

A significant degree of depression may develop postoperatively. This result has been discussed in Chapter 6, having to do with the psychological preparation and evaluation of the patient. Peroneal palsy or femoral neuropathy (5) is occasionally seen after vaginal surgery and, while spontaneous recovery is the rule, it is often very slow, extending over a period of 2 to 6 months. In many instances, such injury appears to be idiopathic, although in a few circumstances it may be the result of defective positioning of the patient while on the operating table, with undue flexion of either thighs or knees. With extension of the legs during surgery in the position described in the preceding chapters, there appears to be minimal chance of stretch injury to the sciatic nerve or its peroneal branch; and, furthermore, there is much less tendency for the assistants to lean against the inner aspects of the patient's thigh.

## Anemia

If the patient has experienced hemorrhage, she should have daily, and, if necessary, more frequent postoperative measurements of hemoglobin and hematocrit. In patients in whom there is no history of operative hemorrhage and no visible postoperative bleeding, hemoglobin and hematocrit determinations should be made on the second postoperative day; and if unexpectedly low when compared with the preoperative values, readings should be repeated during the postoperative period until levels have stabilized or begun to improve. Oral iron supplementation may be indicated both during the course of hospitalization and as part of the posthospital postoperative care. If hemoconcentration is present during the first and second postoperative days, a normal or elevated hemoglobin and hematocrit may give a false sense of security. A significantly depressed determination at this time should arouse immediate suspicion and indicate further investigation.

## Arthritis

Acute postoperative monoarticular arthritis strongly suggests exacerbation of unexpected gout and should respond to appropriate treatment.

### References

1. Bell WR: Thrombolytic agents: A better way to treat pulmonary embolism. *Consultant* 16:39–41, 1976.
2. Burchell C: The umbrella pack to control pelvic hemorrhage. *Conn Med* 32:734, 1968.
3. Cruse PJE: Complications. In Beahrs OH, Beart RW (eds): *General Surgery*. Media PA, Harwal, 1984.
4. Hirsh J: Venous thromboembolism: Diagnosis, treatment, prevention. *Hosp Prac* 10:53–62, 1975.
5. Hopper CL: Bilateral femoral neuropathy complicating vaginal hysterectomy. *Obstet Gynecol* 32:543, 1968.
6. Howkins J, Stallworthy J: *Bonney's Gynecologic Surgery*. Baltimore, Williams & Wilkins, 1974.
7. Jacobson HG, Heitzman ER: Pulmonary thromboembolism—update. *JAMA* 243: 2229–2234, 1980.
8. Janisch H, Palmrich AH, Pecherstorfer M: *Selected Urologic Operations in Gynecology*. Berlin, Walter de Gruyter, pp. 21–25, 1979.
9. Kambouris AA, Drukker BH, Barron J: Vaginal evisceration: A case report and brief review of the literature. *Arch Surg* 116:949–951, 1981.
10. Koehler PR, Moss AA: Diagnosis of intraabdominal and pelvic abscesses by computerized tomography. *JAMA* 244:49–52, 1980.
11. Ledger WJ, Campbell C, Taylor D, et al: Adnexal abscess as a late complication of pelvic operations. *Surg Gynecol Obstet* 129:963–978, 1969.
12. Moser KM, Brach BB, Dolan GF: Clinically suspected deep venous thrombosis of the lower extremeties. *JAMA* 237:2195–2201, 1977.
13. Powell JL: Vaginal evisceration following vaginal hysterectomy. *Am J Obstet Gynecol* 115:276–277, 1973.
14. Reich WJ, Nechtow MJ: Ligation of the

internal iliac arteries. *J Int Coll Surg* 36:157–168, 1971.

15. Smith DG, Wyatt JR: Embolization of the hypogastric arteries in the control of massive vaginal hemorrhage. *Obstet Gynecol* 49:317–322, 1977.

16. Thompson JR, Benigno BB: Vaginal repair of ureteral injuries. *Am J Obstet Gynecol* 3:601–610, 1971.

17. Wetchler SJ, Hurt WG: A technique for surgical correction of fallopian tube prolapse. *Obstet Gynecol* 67:747–749, 1986.

# CHAPTER 23

# Horizons and Miscellaneous Conditions

Reconstructive vaginal surgery is a dynamic discipline, constantly being refined. The last word has yet to be said concerning the indications and techniques for reconstructive gynecological surgery. It is essential that the gynecologic surgeon appreciate the phenomenon of individual patient-to-patient anatomic variation, particularly in terms of the branches of the blood vessels, and the relative strengths of muscular and connective tissue components of the individual's pelvic supporting tissues. There are variations related to a relative deficiency or to the adequacy of estrogenic effects in the pelvic tissues of the woman needing a gynecologic repair. While some problems relating to obstetric trauma may come to surgery long before estrogen deficiency is a likely factor, many women develop increased and symptomatic degrees of prolapse during the climacteric and postmenopausal years. To what extent the elastic tissue of the pelvis is dependent upon estrogen and whether its age-related reduction is preventable or reversible by perimenopausal or postmenopausal estrogen supplementation has been suspected but has not been proven.

The appearance of postmenopausal atrophic changes in the vaginal membrane is not a reliable indication of a woman's chronologic age. Changes associated with estrogen deficiency are not to be assumed even several years after a physiologic menopause. Evidence of an estrogenic deficiency effect may be noticeable in the vaginal cytology of less than 50% of women even 5 years after spontaneous cessation of their menstrual periods. Thus, it is evident that individual variations must be taken into consideration. Clinically evident tissue change associated with "atrophic vaginitis" becomes symptomatic in no more than 15% to 20% of postmenopausal women. There appear to be racial differences as well, for atrophic vaginitis appears to be distinctly less common in the black woman than in the white.

There may be many biochemical and biologic differences that have not been recognized but that exist between the black and the white peoples of the world. Such considerations require fundamental biochemical studies as well as clinical observations that might have broad clinical significance, suggesting among other possibilities means by which the individual's endocrines might be manipulated as to prevent the effects of aging. One might suspect that the effects of estrogenic hormone on the tone of the pelvic supporting tissues are insignificant. However, the gynecologic repair, when the vaginal membrane is noticeably atrophic, will be technically easier and healing will be accentuated if the tissues have been primed preoperatively with exogenous estrogen until the vascularity improves. Exogenous estrogen should be resumed throughout the postoperative period, in a dosage adequate to produce a full-blown estrogenic effect and a desirable degree of vascularity and elasticity, at least until healing is complete and the vaginal caliber is re-established.

In our assessment of the tissue of the postmenopausal woman, it is important to recognize that bilateral removal of the ovaries does not deprive many castrates of all estrogenic effects. Interstitial cells in the nonremoved pedicle portion of the ovary, as well as in the adrenal glands, produce androgens that may be converted into significant amounts of estrogens for not less than 40% of castrates. Androstenedione is converted in fat tissue to estrogen in a quantity proportionate to the amount of obesity present, probably due to the ability of fat to aromatize androgens (25). Sex hormone-binding globulin is suppressed in the obese, further increasing free estrogen levels (23). Therefore, symptoms and findings of estrogen deprivation are more likely to be seen in thin women than in the obese. This conversion helps to account for the failure of many women to develop atrophic changes over periods of from 5 to 10 years after oophorectomy. The effectiveness of such continuing estrogenic effects for years after the woman's menopause may be a factor in slowing the individual's aging process, but this effect has yet to be proven.

We do not know the extent to which atrophy and attenuation of elastic tissue might be arrested or reversed by such supplementation or replacement, nor do we know the specific steroid or combination of steroids that are most effective in terms of slowing the more undesirable effects of aging.

There are few data on the suspected long-term effects of the oral progestational agents or "birth control pills" on the ultimate development of the various manifestations of genital prolapse and whether that effect, if any, is related to the intensity of the dose or to the chemical composition of the specific compound. For that matter, we do not know whether the soft tissue components of the pelvis are affected equally or selectively in the attenuating effects of the aging process, just as we cannot accurately predict the individual's tissue response to hormone supplementation or replacement. The degree to which locally applied estrogen equals the efficacy of systemic estrogen replacement certainly must depend upon the effectiveness of the individual's absorption, again emphasizing the importance of the individual's response rather than the magnitude of the dosage given.

Brincat and colleagues (1) have shown that the decline in skin collagen and thickness after the menopause is related to the loss of ovarian estrogens. Comparing skin thickness and collagen content in a group of postmenopausal women treated with sex hormone implants with an untreated group of similar women, they observed

"an inverse relation between skin collagen content and years since the menopause, independent of the actual age of the patient. This suggests that the decline in skin collagen is due to the loss of ovarian estrogens. That effect is lost in the treated group of women indicating treatment with sex hormones prevents or reverses the loss of skin collagen after the menopause."

## POSTMENOPAUSAL ESTROGEN SUPPLEMENTATION AFTER HYSTERECTOMY

Supplemental estrogen appears to lessen the incidence and seriousness of ischemic heart disease if the ovaries have been removed at the time of hysterectomy. This commendable goal appears to be cancelled out by the use of supplemental synthetic progestins, although there is some evidence that it is not removed by the use of natural progesterone. For the most part, therefore, in the absence of the uterus, one might recommend the protective cardiovascular and antiosteoporotic benefits of postoperative supplemental estrogen without progesterone, when there is no contraindication to the use of estrogen.

## PROLAPSE AND DIABETES

There appears to be an increased incidence of prolapse in patients with diabetes. Some observers have suggested that abnormalities in carbohydrate metabolism, as in the diabetic, have an etiologic role in the development of genital prolapse as a result of a characteristic effect on connective tissues. Cohen (2) has discussed the implication of protein glycosylation in the diabetic patient as a possible mechanism of acquired collagen weakness.

"Recent years have witnessed a surge of interest in non-enzymatic glycosylation, which is the attachment of free sugar to certain amino acid residues of proteins . . . Hyperglycemia permits increased non-enzymatic glycosylation not only of circulating proteins such as hemoglobin and albumin . . . but also of tissue proteins, thereby providing insight into pathogenetic mechanisms contributory to chronic complications to diabetes . . . non-enzymatic glycosylation can alter the structure and/or function of involved proteins. Thus, the guilt of glucose can no longer be denied, and has prompted an awareness of the importance of long-term maintenance of euglycemia in diabetic patients in an attempt to prevent the development or arrest the progression of chronic complications. The need for long-term control is further underscored by the recognition that proteins in some of the affected tissues have long biologic half-lives, and hence represent situations in which glycosylation could be relatively permanent since the population of proteins is not quickly replaced . . . Collagen is the main fibrous protein of connective tissues and is a principle constituent of basement membranes. Collagenous proteins are rich in lysine and hydroxylysine, generally have a long biologic half-life, and are continuously exposed to ambient levels of glucose in the vascular compartment and extracellular fluid. Since variables such as the number of free amino groups in and the residence time of a protein determine the extent of glycosylation in vivo, there are a priori reasons to suspect that collagen would be highly subject to excess non-enzymatic glycosylation in vivo. Examination of several collagens has confirmed that this is the case, and a two to three-fold increase has been consistently found when non-enzymatic glycosylation of collagens from tissues of diabetic subjects or animals is compared to that in control samples.

In vitro non-enzymatic glycosylation had been demonstrated with virtually every protein that has been examined to date. It is clear that, at least in vitro, non-enzymatic glycosylation can influence physiochemical properties and packing of collagen fibers. This is further supported by the observation that glucose, in vitro, inhibits the formation of collagen fibrils. This decrease in fibril formation correlates with the loss and the ability of collagen to serve as a substrate for lysyl oxidase (15). (It is possible that) glucoadducts, once formed, would provide a chemical framework for self perpetuating and damaging processes that can continue even if strict diabetic control is instituted. This hypothesis, if correct, provides one of the strongest arguments in favor of early aggressive therapeutic intervention with intensified regimens to establish and maintain normal normoglycemia."

Whether related to a relatively high fat content or to a specific weakening of elastic tissues, the diabetic frequently seems soft rather than "lean and hard." Certainly, the attenuation of elastic tissue strength in the diabetic is not related to a decreased vascularity related to a declining estrogen effect, for studies have clearly shown that the diabetic, like the person suffering from obesity, stores estrogens more efficiently and metabolizes them slowly. As a rule, the diabetic, like the obese individual, tends to continue menstrual-like bleeding at ages beyond that of the average climacteric. Such bleeding is usually anovulatory and related more to the individual's slow metabolism of estrogens rather than to an increased or prolonged production by either the ovary or the adrenal.

The still poorly understood role of lymphangiectasia as an etiologic factor in the markedly hypertrophic changes sometimes seen with genital prolapse needs to be clarified, for it must be related to the metabolic effects of venous stasis and chronic congestion.

When fascial layers are attenuated and barely demonstrable, the usefulness of synthetic subepithelial prostheses, either of permanently placed plastic or of slowly absorbable material, remains to be developed. Evaluation must, of course, be correlated with the predictable connective tissue changes that can be expected as a result of scarring and fibrosis in the later stages of healing.

Much information concerning individual variations in pelvic architecture can be learned from careful and detailed examinations in the morgue. A question that warrants reconsideration from time to time is the extent to which the techniques of surgery can be visualized and developed and improved using postmortem material. In our own experience, certain anatomic questions can best be answered from examination of the fresh postmortem material of many cadavers.

When elongation of the uterus is noted as an apparently dominant feature of genital prolapse, is the cervix actually elongated or is it actually the lower uterine segment? Is such elongation the result of interference with blood or lymphatic circulation, or both, largely because venous and lymphatic channels are compressed as the prolapsed part descends through the genital hiatus and is squeezed between the lateral pelvic soft tissues? Study of the point at which the major branches of the uterine artery enter the cervix should demonstrate whether this elongation is cervical or really represents elongation of the lower uterine segment. Does the site of attachment of the cul-de-sac peritoneum to the surface of the uterus provide a reliable indicator of where the elongation actually begins? A criterion of considerable help to the gynecologic surgeon in making his or her preoperative appraisal would be a reliable means of assuming the actual location of the internal cervical os.

What, if any, are the effects of premature labor, induced labor, or subsequent pregnancy on the integrity of cervical elastic tissue? The clinically incompetent cervix is not always a post-traumatic entity. In instances where conization or cervical amputation has been performed, are the effects on the subsequent pregnancy dependent upon whether the integrity of the internal os was unwillfully damaged?

Although there is documentation of certain positive effects from the voluntary perineal resistive exercises described by Kegel (13), the permanent value of employing galvanic electrical stimulation of the musculature of the pelvic floor and urogenital diaphragm has yet to be established. The stimulation method would seem to provide a more efficient exercise program than the original Kegel-type exercises and may be of greatest value in those patients who seem unable to demonstrate voluntary contraction of the pubococcygeus. Huffman and Sokol (11) suggested that a positive effect from a course of galvanic electrical stimulations was the result of stimulation of both smooth and striated muscle in contrast to the voluntary Kegel perineal resisting exercises, which apparently use only striated voluntary muscles.

## URETHROCOLPOGRAPHY

Although much has been written about the significance of defects of the urethrovesical angle and urinary stress incontinence (5, 8, 24), such factors as a relative deficiency in the support of the levator plate, the course of the pelvic diaphragm, the integrity of the perineal body, and its location may each be of importance in the maintenance of urethral position and tone. By simply applying a thin coating of barium paste within the vagina at the time of bead-chain urethrocystography, one can objectively compare preoperative information with similar postoperative studies concerning deficiencies in each or any combination of these separate systems: the urogenital diaphragm, bladder base-plate, pelvic diaphragm, levator plate, and the perineum (3) (Figs. 23.1 and 23.2). Comparison of preoperative and postoperative films may demonstrate objectively the possible role of a coincident posterior colporrhaphy and a perineorrhaphy in the development of a satisfactory result.

Although there seem few who question the importance of the pubococcygeus portion of the levator ani muscle in the normal voiding process, there remains considerable question as to the role of this muscle and its possible deficiencies in the etiology of urinary stress incontinence.

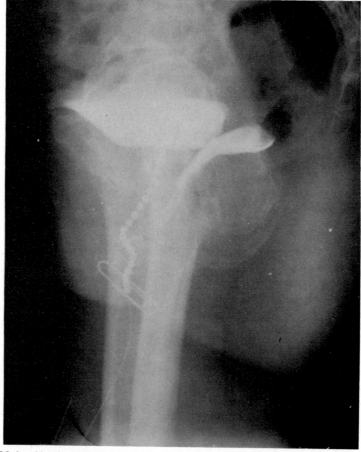

**Figure 23.1.** Urethrocolpography is shown. Radiopaque fluid has been instilled into the bladder, a urethral marking chain inserted, and the vagina lightly coated with barium cream. A lateral standing radiograph of the patient at rest is obtained, and the organ relationships to one another and to the bony pelvis are observed. (Courtesy of the X-ray Department, St. Francis Hospital, Buffalo, NY, Dr. Paul deMarsovszky, radiologist.)

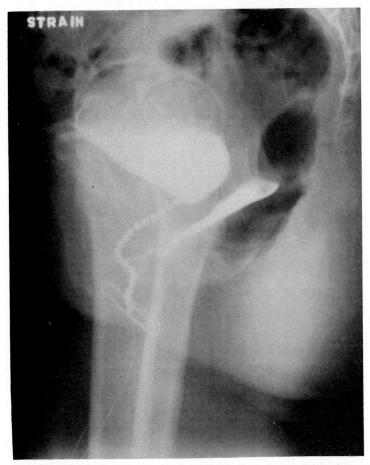

**Figure 23.2.** The patient is asked to strain or bear down as by a Valsalva maneuver and the altered relationships are observed. Note that there is flattening of the posterior urethrovesical angle with some rotational descent of the bladder neck. The vaginal axis is altered, indicating tipping of the levator plate beneath it. (Courtesy of the X-ray Department, St. Francis Hospital, Buffalo, NY.)

## NEUROGENIC DEFECT AND IMBALANCE AS A FACTOR IN GENITAL PROLAPSE

There appears to be considerable variation in the innervation of the voluntary muscles of the pelvis. Although the pudendal is the principal nerve to the levator ani, it is inconstant in its distribution as there is often an independently arising and variously located accessory pudendal nerve that assumes a variable share of total pudendal nerve function. When viscera possess a triple innervation, (i.e., the somatic, sympathetic, and parasympathetic nerve supply of the bladder), the opportunity for physiologic imbalance is very great. This may be influenced not only by congenital defect, but also by trauma or surgery. Sensitive direct electromyography may provide objective information of both muscular and neuromuscular efficiency in a particular situation, and thereby provide a more logical basis for the choice of operation and improvement in the prognosis. Several questions immediately come to mind: Is there a difference between the interpretation of direct and of indirect electromyography? To what extent is genital prolapse caused by secondary damage to the structures or nerves involved (21, 22), and when might it result from a primary or congenital defect in muscle innervation? Can such a possible etiology and pathology of genital prolapse be studied and perhaps effectively measured by electromyography (14)? Is a correlation possible between an abnormal electromyogram and the results of reconstructive surgery?

To be valid, the long-range effectiveness of transvaginal surgical denervation of the bladder (Fig. 23.3) to relieve socially disabling and medically refractive detrusor instability must be established by long-term follow-up of a large number of patients before its place can be determined as a treatment for this condition. To what extent does nerve regeneration reduce the long-term effectiveness of the procedure? The results of such a surgical approach must be compared prospectively to the effectiveness of treatment by drugs and by bladder retraining.

The development of absorbable buried prostheses should also be investigated, both as a reinforcement of the layers of tissue developed during an operative repair as well as a meshwork stimulating the development of fibrous tissue.

## Vesicovaginal Fistula

The selection of surgical treatment technique and its effectiveness may depend partly upon the relationship between the fistula location and the vesicovaginal space. At the very vault of the vagina, there is no vesicovaginal space, as the vagina and bladder capsule are fused to one another at this point. A fistula location more distal in the vagina and through the vesicovaginal space gives the option of separate closure of the wall of the bladder and of the wall of the vagina.

A fistula located near the base of the trigone may very likely be in a nonexpansile layer of the bladder that may influence the time at which the indwelling catheter may be safely removed postoperatively. If in a nonexpansile area, in theory, the catheter may be removed after 48 hours but, in an expansile area, the bladder should be decompressed for 14 to 21 days. If the vesicovaginal fistula transgresses the vesicovaginal space, the postoperative

**Figure 23.3.** Bladder denervation is depicted. An inverted U-shaped incision has been made through the full thickness of the anterior vaginal wall, and by dissection between the bladder pillar and the pelvic diaphragm, the hypogastric plexus has been exposed deep in the wound on the patient's left. The fibers, along with branches of the inferior vesical artery if necessary, are clamped between two forceps, cut, and ligated. A similar procedure can be performed on the patient's right, if necessary, and the vaginal incision closed using interrupted sutures.

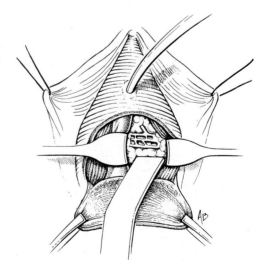

physiology will be closer to normal if the wall of the vagina and of the bladder are closed separately. This is true when the fistula is found distal to the vault of the vagina. A fistula located at the vaginal vault will normally be in an area cranial to the vesicovaginal space. Whether this is closed in one layer or two, it will postoperatively fuse during the course of healing to become a single layer of scar unless an intermediate layer of insulation such as peritoneum, omentum, or a bulbocavernosus muscle fat pad transplant is brought in.

## Suture Placement and Knot Security

Should the placement of sutures and the security of the knots that are tied in such sutures take into account:

1. tissue edema preceding repair;
2. tissue edema at the time of the repair;
3. tissue edema after the repair?

When sutures are placed in edematous tissue, there are two risks to the integrity of the suture line.

1. When the edema has subsided, these stitches will no longer be holding the edges in firm apposition.
2. If one attempts to overcome this by tying the knots tightly or pulling the sutures too tightly, there is a risk of increasing the edema rather than decreasing it yielding "necrosis" at the suture line. Therefore, one would not ordinarily operate on tissues that are edematous if a reduction in edema is likely during the time that healing is taking place.

Because vaginal fistulae represent the development of communication by an epithelialized track between two organs, might this be effectively treated by simple excision of the epithelialized track at a site other than at the vaginal vault and watertight but gentle approximation of the freshly trimmed vaginal edges without tension by some simple device such as the Wachenfeldt clip applied by an applicator suitably modified by a 90-degree bend in its tip (Figs. 23.4 and 23.5)? Any tension developed by the approximation of the vaginal edges could be relieved by suitable relaxing incisions in the lateral vaginal walls. After how many days should such clips be removed? Would this not be the essence of the Sims closure?

## Cervicovaginal Fistula

This may be seen after traumatic dilation and curettage or elective pregnancy terminations in which the forces of induced labor have pushed the products of conception into the vagina through the upper and often posterior wall of an otherwise insufficiently dilated cervix. The endocervix pouts and bulges through the fibromuscular wall of the upper cervical laceration. The fistula should be excised and the cervix closed over a no. 3 Hegar dilator. Because there is considerable tension upon the outermost sutures, they should be of a long-acting synthetic material such as 00 polydiaxanone (PDS) or polyglyconate (Maxon). For patients with no desire for further childbearing, Martius (16) suggests cervical amputation at the level of the fistula, possibly covering the raw wound with a Sturmdorf suture.

The effectiveness, dosage, and patient convenience of newer antibiotics and antibacterials needs adequate assessment, particularly for the patient with demonstrated sensitivity to penicillin. Are intravenous doses or rectal suppositories (12) of metronidazole (Flagyl) an effective substitute?

**Figure 23.4.** The modified Wachenfeldt clip forceps are shown.

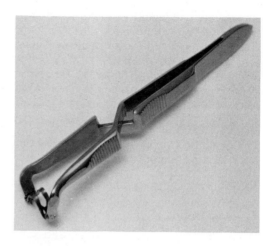

## OBSTETRIC PRACTICE

Current obstetric practices are being subjected to even greater skepticism and modification than is evident in the care of women with gynecologic complaints. Will an increased popularity of home delivery and of spontaneous delivery without episiotomy result in significant increases in soft tissue damage incident to delivery and in a greater need for gynecologic repairs in the future?

The significance of changes in pelvic organ relationships consequent to increased intra-abdominal pressure from unusually heavy work or physical exertion must be considered as a possible etiologic factor in the development of genital prolapse. Equal rights and equal opportunities are certain to bring the

**Figure 23.5.** The patient is in the knee-chest position and a urinary fistula has been excised. The vagina is being closed using the modified Wachenfeldt clip forceps bringing the freshened edges of the cystotomy in contact with one another.

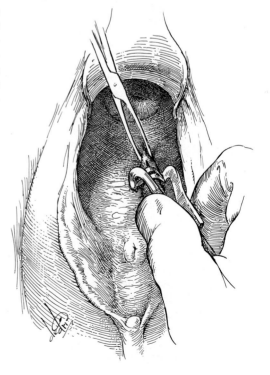

sexes to more equal risks and, more frequently, to similar injuries. More women have become involved in performing the heavy physical types of work previously undertaken only by men. When such strains are superimposed upon (a) pre-existent tissue damage as a result of childbirth; or (b) congenital deficiency; or (c) the secondary attenuations of aging, more realistic guidelines for Worker's Compensation must be established so that all concerned can be treated fairly and equally. There is need to provide a reasonable basis for recommendations concerning work restrictions in an effort to lessen the development of genital prolapse or to decrease the likelihood of genital prolapse or to decrease the likelihood of recurrence after reparative surgery. When such guidelines are established, agreement should also be developed as to the appropriate duration of convalescence after childbirth and the agreement should be reached as to an appropriate time to be allowed for recovery after gynecologic reparative surgery. Hopefully, this will take into consideration not only the nature and the magnitude of the operative procedure but also the particular type of work to which the individual will be returning.

We do not, as yet, know the effects of frequent jogging on the integrity of the urogenital and pelvic diaphragms. There are many women with urinary stress incontinence who are finding the condition aggravated by jogging. We suspect but lack objective evidence that the sport significantly aggravates pre-existing damage to the supports of the vagina, urethra, or to the pelvic diaphragm, while actually strengthening some of the pelvic supports of the patient without pre-existent damage.

The long-term surgical and economic effects on complications and end results of same-day admission and early discharge, as promoted by third party payors, must be studied in detail to determine whether or not this policy is in the public interest. Can society continue to support the activities of the surgeon who has an excessive proportion of postoperative complications and increased length of stay? The surgeons consistently obtaining the best results will become busier at the expense of the less successful. Our individual surgical successes will always improve with continued attention to technical precision and knowledge, learning from the experiences of all, and within an affordable framework of compassion, empathy, and understanding.

What is the place for synchronous combined abdominovaginal hystero-colpectomy for cancer of the cervix (9, 27)? The radical vaginal hysterectomy with extraperitoneal lymphadenectomy (19, 20)?

Observations can be made without the diagnostic use of ionizing radiation through magnetic residence imaging (MRI), which makes visible the soft tissue organs themselves, as seen in Figure 23.6 (10, 17). What effects will these examinations have on anatomic and physiologic studies and clinical diagnosis and relevance?

Is there a place for the paradoxical incision (18) through the external anal sphincter in the reoperation of failed surgery for sphincter restoration of continence?

In the construction of a neovagina using the Abbe-McIndoe technique, the patient is often annoyed by the pain and cosmetic disfigurement at the donor site. It has been suggested that an alternative method of obtaining skin sufficient to cover the obturator introduced at surgery might be the development of large sheets of squamous epithelium, even those of but one cell thickness derived from *preoperative* tissue culture of a skin biopsy taken long before the neovaginal construction. This would require an initial donor site of only a tiny biopsy of skin relieving the patient of pain and discomfort and cosmetic scarring of a large donor site.

We have long been concerned about the effectiveness of low-dose heparin in

**Figure 23.6.**   MRI of sagittal section through the pelvis, showing uterus and vagina and adjacent organs. Note the relatively thin endometrium. (Reproduced with permission of the Radiologic Society of North America from McCarthy S, Tauber C, Gore J: Female pelvic anatomy: MR assessment of variations during the menstrual cycle and with use of oral contraceptives. *Radiology* 160:120, 1986.)

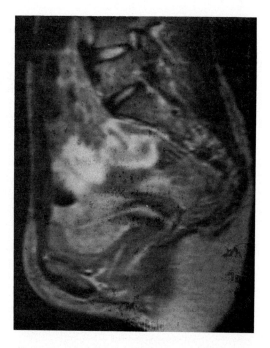

reducing the incidence of postoperative pulmonary embolus, fearing the increased incidence of intraoperative bleeding and postoperative wound hemorrhage. Preliminary reports of the new compound Defibrotide in the prevention of deep thrombosis are most encouraging. It apparently has no association with increased bleeding, has no anticoagulant effect, and no adverse effect upon blood platelets. Its molecular structure resembles heparin, but its mechanism of action is not yet known. The effective dose seems to be in the range of 200 mg four times daily or 400 mg twice daily starting 24 hours before surgery. Because it is not an anticoagulant, no monitoring is necessary.

Autotransfusion using blood retrieved through the Cell-Saver is apparently not suitable for the vaginal surgical patient due to its probable contamination by vaginal bacteria, but autologous transfusion of banked blood is useful, sparing the patient the risk of unexpected innoculation with the virus of hepatitis, non A and non B hepatitis, AIDS, and the risk of transfusion reaction. It probably should not be used in the patient with coronary artery insufficiency or liver or respiratory failure.

## CHRONIC INVERSION OF THE UTERUS

Under certain circumstances, usually postpartum, the uterus can turn inside out. When the condition is acute, there may be accompanying shock, and the uterus can be reverted by intravaginal manipulation. Rarely, when the patient has survived this event and a diagnosis not previously established, the condition may be discovered months later in the course of a pelvic examination to evaluate a chronic bloody discharge. This is so-called "chronic" inversion and requires surgical relief (7). When the patient no longer wishes to retain the uterus, hysterectomy is offered, usually by the vaginal route. If she wants to retain her fertility, the integrity of the uterus must be surgically restored, and this can be done transvaginally using either the Spinelli technique or the lesser known Küstner operation. Both will be described. The surgeon should choose whichever technique seems to fit best the needs of a particular patient. The

Spinelli technique requires dissection of the bladder from the inverted uterus, however, it poses a more complex surgical problem than does the Küstner. In the Küstner technique, the incision through the cervix and myometrium is made in the posterior wall of the uterus, sparing any dissection of the bladder but putting the repair on the posterior uterine wall instead of the anterior uterine wall. Whether the scar on the back of the uterus is equally strong and resistant to future rupture has not been proven.

The Küstner operation as described by Halban (6) is performed as follows: The cul-de-sac of Douglas is opened by posterior colpotomy. The index finger of the operator's left hand is inserted into the peritoneal invagination of the uterus. The posterior uterine wall is incised (Fig. 23.7). The surgeon's thumbs make pressure upon the rear wall of the uterus leading to reversion, restoring it to its normal position within the pelvis. The corpus is flipped through the posterior colpotomy and the incision in the posterior uterine wall is repaired, having trimmed any myometrium if necessary to achieve reapproximation of the serosal surface. The uterus is replaced within the pelvis and the colpotomy is closed.

Technique of the Spinelli operation for treatment of chronic inversion of the uterus (Fig. 23.8) was described by Graves (4):

"A transverse anterior vaginal incision is first made and the bladder separated from the uterus, as described for anterior colpotomy. A median incision is then made through the cervix, dividing completely the constricting ring. This incision should be carried toward the fundus, through the anterior uterine wall, until a point is reached which will allow the reversion of the inverted uterus. It is, as a rule, necessary to continue the incision as far as the fundus.

The uterus is reverted by placing the forefingers at the cervix for counterpressure,

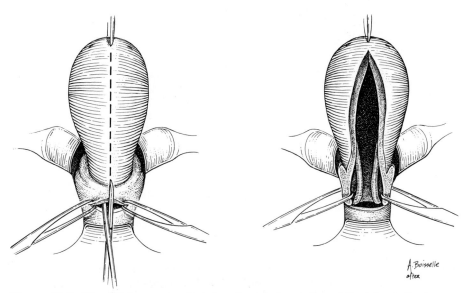

**Figure 23.7.** The Küstner operation for chronic inversion of the uterus is shown. The posterior cul-de-sac has been opened, and the cervix and posterior wall of the uterus should be incised along the path of the *broken line* as shown in the drawing on the *left*. When this has been completed, as shown in the drawing to the *right,* thumb pressure along the sides of the uterus produce reversion, the wounds are closed with interrupted sutures, and the uterus replaced in the pelvic cavity. The colpotomy is then closed.

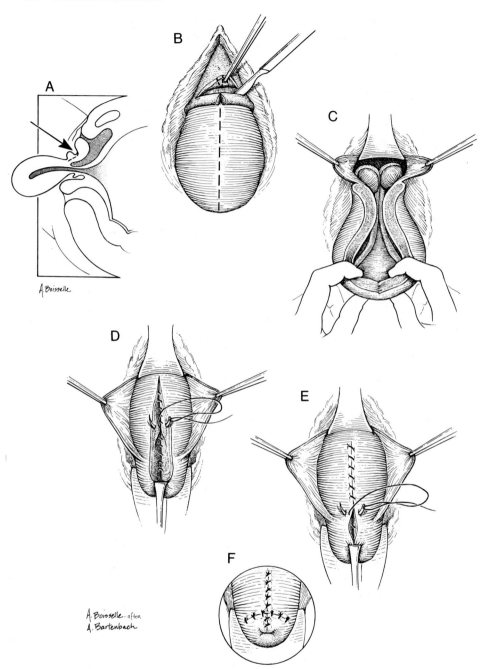

**Figure 23.8.** The Spinelli operation for chronic inversion of the uterus is illustrated. The cervix is split in the midline and carefully separated from the bladder as shown by the *dotted line* in *A*. The anterior wall of the everted uterus is split along the path of the *dotted line* in *B*. By pressure with the operator's index fingers and thumbs, as shown in *C*, the uterus is turned outside-in. The myometrium is reapproximated by two layers of running PGA suture, as shown in *D*, and the serosal surface by a single layer as shown in *E*. The vaginal skin is reapproximated with interrupted sutures, as identified in *F*, as is the full thickness of the cervix.

and forcing the fundus upward by the thumbs in the manner that one would naturally use in turning a tennis ball inside out through a cut in its side.

When the uterus has been restored to its original form the next step is to close the incision in its wall. It will, however, be found that, owing to the shrinking which the peritoneum has undergone in its inverted position, it cannot be approximated, the tissue of the uterine wall pouting out in the manner of an ectropion. The excess of tissue must be trimmed away in the form of longitudinal wedges, when the peritoneal edges may be coaptated without difficulty. The wound of the uterine wall is closed with two rows of continous sutures. The first suture includes and firmly unites the muscular wall; the second is superficial and approximates the peritoneal surfaces. The wound of the cervix is closed with interrupted sutures . . . The vaginal wound is sutured.''

## References

1. Brincat M, Moniz CJ, Studd JWW, et al: Long-term effects of the menopause and sex hormones on skin thickness. *Br J Obstet Gynecol* 92:256–259, 1985.
2. Cohen MP: *Diabetes and Protein Glycosylation*. New York, Springer-Verlag, 1986.
3. DeMarsovszky PJ, Nichols DH, Randall CL: Urethrocolpography. *Arch Gynäkol* 215:351–358, 1973.
4. Graves WP: *Gynecology*, ed 4, Philadelphia, WB Saunders, 1928, pp 841–844.
5. Green TH: Develolpment of a plan for the diagnosis and treatment of urinary stress incontinence. *Am J Obstet Gynecol* 83:632–648, 1962.
6. Halban J: *Gynäkologische Operationslehre*. Wien, Urban and Schwarzenberg, 1932, pp 196–197.
7. Hanton EM, Kempers RD: Puerperal inversion of the uterus. *Postgrad Med* 36:541–545, 1964.
8. Hodgkinson CP: Stress urinary incontinence. *Am J Obstet Gynecol* 108:1141–1168, 1970.
9. Howkins J: Synchronous combined abdomino-vaginal hysterocolpectomy for cancer of the cervix-a report of fifty patients. *J Obstet Gynaecol Br Emp* 66:212–219, 1959.
10. Hricak H: MRI of the female pelvis: A review. *Am J Radiol* 146:1115–1122, 1986.
11. Huffman JW, Sokal JK: The management of stress incontinence. *Geriatrics* 7:225–231, 1952.
12. Ioannides L, Somogyi A, Spicer J, et al: Rectal administration of metronidazole provides therapeutic plasma levels in postoperative patients. *N Engl J Med* 305:1569–1570, 1981.
13. Kegel AH: Progressive resistance exercises in the functional restoration of the perineal muscles. *Am J Obstet Gynecol* 56:238–248, 1948.
14. Kerremans R, Rosselle N: The parameters of the EMG activity of the external anal sphincters and M pubo-rectalis in normal adult and elderly subjects. *Electromyography* 8:89–104, 1968.
15. Lien HY, Stern R, Fu JCC: Inhibition of collagen fibril formation in-vitro and subsequent crosslinking of glucose. *Science* 225:1489–1491, 1984.
16. Martius G: In Friedman EA (ed): *Operative Gynecology*. New York, Thieme-Stratton, p. 165, 1982.
17. McCarthy S, Tauber C, Gore J: Female pelvic anatomy: MR assessment of variations during the menstrual cycle and with use of oral contraceptives. *Radiology* 160:119–123, 1986.
18. Miller NF, Brown W: The surgical treatment of complete perineal tears in the female. *Am J Obstet Gynecol* 34:196–209, 1937.
19. Mitra S: *Mitra Operation for Cancer of the Cervix*. Springfield, IL, Charles C Thomas, 1960.
20. Navratil E: Radical vaginal hysterectomy (Schauta-Amreich Operation). *Clin Obstet Gynecol* 8:676, 1965.
21. Parks AG: Anorectal Incontinence. *Proc Roy Soc Med* 68:681–690, 1975.
22. Percy JP, Neill ME, Swash M, et al: Electrophysiological study of the motor nerve supply of the pelvic floor. *Lancet* 1:16-17, 1981.
23. Plymate SR, Fariss BL, Bassett ML, et al: Obesity and its role in polycystic ovary syndrome. *J Clin Endocrinol Metabol* 52:1246, 1981.
24. Roberts H: Cystourethrography in women. *Br J Urol* 25:253–259, 1952.
25. Speroff L, Glass RH, Kase NG: *Clinical Gynecologic Endocrinology and Infertility*, 3rd ed, Baltimore, Williams & Wilkins, 1983, pp 110–111.
26. Vidakovic S: The vagino-abdominal approach to the extended operation. *Arch Gynäkol* 186:420, 1955.

"Everything should be made as simple as possible,
but not one bit simpler"
Albert Einstein

# Index